T0215437

The Sanctity of Social Life: Physicians' Treatment of Critically Ill Patients

The Sanctity of Social Life: Physicians' Treatment of Critically Ill Patients

Diana Crane

With a new preface by the author

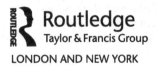

Routledge
Taylor & Francis Group

LONDON AND NEW YORK

First published 1975 by Transaction Publishers

Published 2017 by Routledge
2 Park Square, Milton Park, Abingdon, Oxon OX14 4RN
711 Third Avenue, New York, NY 10017, USA

Routledge is an imprint of the Taylor & Francis Group, an informa business

New material this edition copyright © 1977 Russell Sage Foundation,
112 East 64th Street, New York, New York 10021. Copyright © 1975 Russell
Sage Foundation.

All rights reserved. No part of this book may be reprinted or reproduced or
utilised in any form or by any electronic, mechanical, or other means, now
known or hereafter invented, including photocopying and recording, or in
any information storage or retrieval system, without permission in writing
from the publishers.

Notice:
Product or corporate names may be trademarks or registered trademarks,
and are used only for identification and explanation without intent to
infringe.

This study was originally supported by the Russell Sage Foundation.

The Russell Sage Foundation was established in 1907 by Mrs. Russell Sage
for the improvement of social and living conditions in the United States. In
carrying out its purpose the Foundation conducts research under the direction
of members of the staff or in close collaboration with other institutions, and
supports programs designed to develop and demonstrate productive working
relations between social scientists and other professional groups. As an inte-
gral part of its operation, the Foundation from time to time publishes books
or pamphlets resulting from these activities. Publication under the imprint of
the Foundation does not necessarily imply agreement by the Foundation, its
trustees, or its staff with the interpretations or conclusions of the authors.

Library of Congress Catalog Number: 77-80862

Library of Congress Cataloging-in-Publication Data
Crane, Diana, 1933-
    The sanctity of social life.

    Bibliography: p.
    Includes index.
        1. Terminal care—Social aspects. 2. Critical care medicine—Social
    aspects. 3. Critical care medicine—Decision making. 4. Physicians—
    Psychology. I. Russell Sage Foundation, New York.

[R726.8.C7 1977]   174'.24   77-80862
ISBN 0-87855-648-6 pbk.

ISBN 13: 978-0-87855-648-9 (pbk)

To the memory of my mother, my grandmother, and my aunt.

Contents

Foreword   **xi**

Preface   **xv**

Preface to the Paperback Edition   **xvii**

1. INTRODUCTION   **1**
   Redefinition of Dying and Death: A Source of Controversy, *2*
   Normative Criteria for Medical Decision-Making, *6*
   Origins of Popular Interest in Dying and Death, *8*
   Decisions to Treat Critically Ill Patients: Social vs. Medical
     Considerations, *10*

2. CONTROVERSY AND THE CLINICAL MENTALITY: SOME
   METHODOLOGICAL PROBLEMS AND THEIR EFFECTS
   ON THE RESEARCH DESIGN   **17**
   The Clinical Mentality and Medical Decision-Making, *19*
   Perceptions of Controversy and the Treatment of Critically Ill
     Patients, *21*
   Development of Questionnaires and Scales, *22*
   Design of Samples, *26*

PART I: CRITERIA FOR DECISION-MAKING   **33**

3. DECISIONS TO TREAT CRITICALLY ILL PATIENTS:
   SOCIAL VERSUS MEDICAL CONSIDERATIONS   **35**
   The Case Histories: An Overview of the Patients, *36*
   Prognosis and Type of Damage, *40*
   The Role of the Patient and his Family, *46*
   Social Potential versus Social Value, *51*
   Acute versus Chronic Illness: Emergence of New Norms, *61*

4. THE TERMINAL PATIENT: TREATMENT OF THE DYING
   AND THE DEAD   **67**
   The Terminal Phase, *68*
   Terminal Acts: Euthanasia and Definitions of Death, *71*
   Decisions to Reverse Death: Norms Concerning Resuscitation, *78*
   Conclusion, *83*

5. DECISION-MAKING VIEWED THROUGH
   HOSPITAL RECORDS   85
   Critically Ill Patients in the Hospital Records: Research Design
     and Data Collection, *86*
   Treatment of Critically Ill Patients: Hospital Records versus
     Questionnaires, *88*
   Non-Private Service Patients: Observations of Treatment, *95*
   Mongoloid Children with Heart Defects: Hospital Records, *96*
   Conclusion, *100*

PART II: SOURCES OF VARIATION AMONG PHYSICIANS:
         SOME ORGANIZATIONAL, SOCIAL, AND
         CULTURAL VARIABLES   103

6. CONTEXT FOR DECISION-MAKING: THE HOSPITAL
   SETTING   105
   Type of Hospital Setting and Quality of Patient Care:
     A Review of the Literature, *105*
   Medical School Affiliation and the Care of Critically Ill Patients, *107*
   Effects of Hospital Settings: Some Explanations, *114*
   Physicians versus Residents: Two Medical Cultures? *116*
   Colleague Consensus and Decision-Making in Surgery, *123*
   Departmental Policy and Decision-Making in Internal Medicine, *127*
   Departmental Policy and Decision-Making in Pediatrics, *129*
   Conclusion, *134*

7. THE ACTIVE PHYSICIAN: CULTURAL INFLUENCES
   UPON MEDICAL DECISIONS   137
   Religious Prescriptions toward Dying, Death and the Newborn, *138*
   Religious Affiliation and Religiosity in the Four Medical
     Specialties, *140*
   Religion, Religiosity, and the Adult Patient, *143*
   Religion, Religiosity, and the Infant, *157*
   Cultural and Religious Attitudes Toward the Medical Role, *163*
   A Note on Age, Social Class and Sex Differences, *170*
   The Active Physician, *173*
   Conclusion, *178*

8. DEPARTMENTAL DYNAMICS AND THE DEVELOPMENT
   OF NEW MEDICAL TECHNOLOGY   181
   Ethical Issues in Cancer Chemotherapy Research, *183*
   Social Organization and Ethical Experimentation: Ward I, *184*
   Social Organization and Ethical Experimentation: Ward II, *188*
   Social Organization and Ethical Codes, *190*
   Ethical Treatment of Unsalvageable Patients, *194*
   Conclusion, *197*

9. CONCLUSION 199
Summary of Findings Concerning the Treatment of
Critically Ill Patients, *199*
Social Control over Medical Care for the Critically Ill Patient:
Some Recommendations, *203*
Current Medical Practice on Euthanasia and Its Social
Implications, *206*

Appendix 1: Charts 213
Appendix 2: Questionnaires 219
Glossary of Medical Terms 269
Bibliography 271
Index 279

Foreword

For most of the recorded history of man, death has been accepted as a natural event and frequently as a relief from life's pain and sorrow. "Swing low sweet chariot, comin' for to carry me home," was, even in my youth, a meaningful and heartfelt spiritual. If the world's food supply and population continue to become more and more out of balance, early death will be for many not only an inevitable but also perhaps a desirable possibility. In one country with recent crop failures mothers reportedly were praying for the early death of their children as an escape from the agony of prolonged starvation. So, too, in cases of extreme ill health, death may be the preferred alternative to continued suffering or meaningless living; certainly there was much truth in Sir William Osler's statement that "pneumonia was the old man's friend."

It has been estimated that it was not until about 1912 that a random patient with a random illness consulting a random physician had a better than 50-50 chance of being benefited by the encounter. Indeed, until four or five decades ago, physicians could do little with the exception of performing some surgical procedures and administering a very few effective drugs to restore health and prolong life. Most treatment was ineffective and in many cases harmful. The physician's usual role was to diagnose, reduce suffering, advise, and comfort.

Recently physicians have been faced with an entirely new set of problems. As man has developed more understanding of nature and more ability to control his environment he has been confronted with the discrepancy between his advancing technological competence and the deficits in his wisdom, in his ability to find enduring ethical guidelines. Furthermore, many have come to believe unrealistically that death *should* be a preventable event and to view life as desirable, and see death as not only undesirable but as a shameful defeat. At the same time large numbers of people have lost their belief in some sort of existence after death and to them death no longer represents release to a better fate.

The availability of new therapeutic techniques places today's physician in a moral dilemma; the very techniques that can restore patients to a functional state can, at times, prolong life, and thus, in some patients prolong suffering and illness. Physicians must now decide what techniques are appropriate and ask themselves "Is it in the best interests of the patient and his family to continue to support this life?" It is this question that Diana Crane has put to internists, pediatricians, neurosurgeons, and pediatric heart surgeons. In all, more than 3,000 physicians, both those in training and those already trained, have responded to her simulated cases. Her data and insights should be of great interest and value to the medical profession, for at present there are few guidelines for coping with this highly charged ethical dilemma in which the quality of the patient's life is given significant weight in deciding about appropriate treatment.

Patients, family members, and physicians are bombarded with pressures and even threats as they try to make these most crucial decisions. And while the questions Crane raises may be based on simulated cases, they are neither rare nor hypothetical; almost daily, medical personnel must face similar dilemmas. Physicians who say they do not encounter such ethical issues in their practice may be denying or avoiding them.

In the past few years, physicians and others who have examined the implications of the new medical technology have acquired a new interest in the problems of death. There is now a journal of Thanatology (Thanatos = death in Greek) and there have been a number of symposia on the subject[1]; yet most writings are the expressions of one individual's beliefs. Crane has done us all an invaluable service by sampling a broad section of medical opinion. Thus, whether deciding for prolongation of life at all costs or for euthanasia in one form or another, a physician no longer has to feel completely alone in his existential decisions; he can find that many of his colleagues agree with him whichever point of view he adopts, and he will realize that there is room for honest disagreement in these agonizing confrontations.

But Crane has gone further; she has tried to see if actual behavior in cases requiring heroic lifesaving methods is consistent with the questionnaire results. Within the limits of the methodology, there does seem to be agreement. Furthermore, on two wards set up for research on and treatment of patients with malignancies, she asks whether patients themselves appreciate the extra weeks or months of health—or illness—that medical science can now offer them. Because death is still seen by many physicians as almost an obscene event and as the ultimate professional failure and affront, they have frequently not listened to patients who say "stop." It appears that a dying patient often may not be allowed the right to prepare for and participate in his death and, indeed, during this critical period the

---

[1] Ramsey, P., Morison, R.S., Kass, L.R., Ariès, P., May, W., Cassell, E.J., and Smith, D.H., *Facing Death.* The Hastings Center Studies, Institute of Society, Ethics and the Life Sciences 2 (2):3–80, May, 1974.

patient and family ironically may be abandoned by the doctor.

Crane does not prescribe pat answers or guidelines about the "right" things to do in the cases she presents, but she will make physicians think about these ethical matters and realize that they do not struggle in isolation. Her data show that there are no simple answers, no rules that will fit all situations. The recent newspaper article about the extended dying of a 35-year-old physician, who demanded prolongation of attempts at treatment beyond the limits thought reasonable by his doctors, reminds us that some desperately want, and certainly have the right, to postpone death and demand the use of heroic techniques even in the face of extreme and hopeless illness. Thus, it seems fair to ask: For individual patients, should not the options be made as explicit as they wish and, within reason, should not their choices be honored?

Crane may also make physicians realize that the consumer-public and their elected officials have roles that have not yet been defined in these life and death decisions. Their interests and those of the physicians may not always coincide. She makes it clear that we must return again to the Hippocratic Oath, "Do no harm," and try to decide as best we can, with our limited wisdom, the definition of "harm." Indeed we must redefine life and death and recognize the many gray zones in between. And we must come to terms with death as the most constant part of life. It cannot be escaped. Only its timing may be controlled by modern medical techniques. The use of that control is at once a personal, family, professional, and public issue that must be confronted in order to avoid the consequences of blind actions.

Charles D. Cook, M.D.

Yale University School of Medicine
New Haven, Connecticut

Preface

This book is the result of research which has been in progress for more than five years. At the request of Russell Sage Foundation, I began in 1968 to review the literature concerning the treatment of dying patients. By the end of that year, the problem of doctors' decisions to treat critically ill patients had been defined. During 1969–1970, I conducted more than 125 interviews with physicians and house staffs in a variety of medical specialties in a university hospital and in non-university hospitals. By the fall of 1970, I had prepared questionnaires that were appropriate for several medical specialties. These were mailed during the winter of 1970–1971. Subsequently I obtained materials for two studies of hospital records pertaining to two of the specialties in the university hospital where the interviews were conducted.

These activities would not have been possible without the cooperation of a large number of people. First and foremost, I am enormously grateful to over 3,000 physicians who either returned questionnaires or who were interviewed for the study. I am especially grateful to members of the house staffs at the various hospitals where interviews were conducted who shared with me their day-to-day problems in the treatment of critically ill patients and who permitted me to accompany them on morning rounds. I am also greatly indebted to the physicians who helped me to develop the medical aspects of the questionnaires, particularly Doctors Leigh Thompson, Vincent Gott, and Perry Black, and to Dr. David E. Rogers who signed letters asking physicians to return the questionnaires. I thank Dr. Thompson and Dr. Charles D. Cook for reviewing the manuscript prior to its publication.

Howard E. Freeman of Russell Sage Foundation functioned as the project's chief critic and troubleshooter. I am very grateful for his careful reading of the early versions of research designs and of various versions of the manuscript. Two other colleagues, Sol Levine and Renée Fox, contributed greatly by providing environments in which the research could be effectively pursued. I thank also Edgar F. Borgatta and Jacob J. Feldman for their assistance with technical aspects of the project.

Nancy Karweit provided invaluable assistance with computer analysis of the data. Evelyn Roberts and Tony Winner were of great help with the two studies of hospital records. My students at the University of Pennsylvania were a stimulating and challenging audience for the first draft of the manuscript.

Finally, the many and varied phases of the project could not have been completed without the help of numerous assistants. I thank especially Elsie Bull, Elisabeth Yager, and Jane Rubin for their devoted assistance with many facets of the project. I am also grateful to Melissa Anderson, Susan Daggett, Barbara Florian, Yvonne Flowers, Stephanie Garrett, Stephen D. Goldbloom, Lois Hess, Carla Jensen, David Meister, Joan Moody, and John Weiss for their assistance with particular phases of the project.

Diana Crane

University of Pennsylvania
Philadelphia, Pennsylvania

Preface to the Paperback Edition

I argue in this book that physicians are moving toward a social definition of life—toward defining an individual as being alive if he is capable of performing his social roles, at least to some degree, rather than if he simply meets physical criteria for life. I show, however, that physicians are more willing to apply a social definition of life to some kinds of patients than to others. Even concerning a particular type of patient, there is nothing like the unanimity—regarding the application of the social criteria for life—that has existed in the use of physical criteria.

That the controversy concerning the Karen Quinlan case erupted in public view shortly after the book's publication in September 1975 is perhaps an indication that its thesis is valid. Since the Quinlan case is an excellent example of the social definition of life, I will briefly review the facts of her case. She is a 23-year-old woman who has been in a coma since April 15, 1975. In the fall of 1975, her parents took legal action to obtain the withdrawal of intensive medical procedures—specifically the use of the respirator which was maintaining her breathing. Quinlan's case was complicated by the fact that she does not meet the technical criteria for brain death that had been set by a committee at Harvard in 1968 (Ad Hoc Committee of the Harvard Medical School to Examine Brain Death). All the physicians who examined her agreed that she was in a "chronic vegetative state" and would never recover her ability to function as a human being. They disagreed on what should be done for her.

The Superior Court of the State of New Jersey refused the parents' request stating: "The power of the parents to exercise the constitutional right is found lacking . . . . The right to life and the preservation of it are 'interests of the highest order' and this Court deems it constitutionally correct to deny plaintiff's request." A few months later, the Supreme Court of New Jersey reversed the Lower Court decision provided that attending physicians and the hospital's ethics committee could agree that there was "no reasonable possibility" that she would recover "a cognitive, sapient state." Extraordinary treatments were withdrawn, and, surprisingly, Karen Quinlan continued to live. At this writing, she is still alive in a nursing home in New Jersey.

This case and others like it have led to considerable discussion concerning how doctors should handle such cases. For the most part, such discussion has been based on speculation. For this reason, when I was asked a few years ago by Russell Sage Foundation to undertake some research on problems surrounding dying and death, I thought it would be useful to find out how physicians actually treat such difficult cases—not only cases like Quinlan's but a broad range of difficult medical cases.

Originally, I had planned to examine the relationship between behavior observed in the hospital setting and what doctors say they do in situations where controversial medical decisions are involved. I wrote at that time (Crane 1969, p. 16): "Lack of congruence between the data would suggest strong pressures to deviate from formal norms, failure of social control mechanisms, and the need to reformulate policy so that ideal and actual behavior achieve a greater degree of isomorphism. A high degree of congruence would suggest that the system is functioning adequately at present."

In the fall of 1969 I undertook a number of exploratory interviews in a major teaching hospital, and as a result my thinking about the problem underwent a number of changes. It was clear that physicians saw these problems in very specific terms and disliked to generalize about their experiences. They have what Freidson (1970, Chapter 8) has called the "clinical mentality." They prefer to consider each case as unique. It appeared that the best procedure for examining the problem would be to concentrate upon specific disease entities and to interview doctors who were treating such diseases. I planned to interview entire departments—groups of physicians handling similar problems in the same unit—and to corroborate the interviews using patient records and notes on staff meetings and conferences.

In effect, I was studying medical subcultures with varying norms toward the prolongation of life. I surmised that, while doctors are expected by society to treat patients as long as physical criteria for life are present, this norm is so general that it cannot be followed in many situations. I hypothesized that subcultures develop their own normative systems. The content of the norms would depend upon the social and physical effects of the diseases with which physicians were dealing. Thus doctors working with one type of cancer would develop norms different from those of doctors dealing with another type of cancer. It could be expected that the social organization of medical departments would affect conformity to values of the subculture and types of sanctions imposed.

During the winter of 1969-70, I conducted over 125 interviews with physicians in several teaching hospitals on the East Coast. I gradually came to the conclusion that in order for my findings to be convincing to skeptical members of other disciplines and professions, I would need a large number of cases, many more than I could hope personally to interview. Therefore, a mailed questionnaire seemed desirable. I decided to send questionnaires to physicians in four medical specialties—neurosurgery, pediatric heart surgery, internal medicine, and pediatrics—in order to obtain their attitudes toward the treatment of specific types of critically ill patients. Over 3,000 physicians returned the questionnaire. By shifting to a large questionnaire survey, the study lost the richness of detail it might have had if it had remained a study of medical subcultures. However, it gained in precision and comparability of results.

As one of the very small number of studies of the social and ethical implications of medical technology (for a review of this literature, see Fox 1976), there were a number of problems to be solved in studying a sensitive area of medical practice never examined before. For example, it was not possible to send the same questionnaire to members of four different medical specialties. The questions in each questionnaire had to be suitable for a particular specialty, yet in such a way that the results of the different questionnaires were comparable. In order to tap the effects of the social characteristics of patients, it was necessary to resort to the unusual practice of constructing different versions of the same questionnaire in which the social characteristics were varied.

One of the most difficult problems to solve was that of validating the questionnaire results using hospital records. Although they are often inaccurate and incomplete, these records represent a virtually untapped resource for sociological studies. After much searching and several false starts, I finally located data on all deaths and resuscitations on a nonprivate hospital service during a calendar year and on all cases of mongoloid children who had been catheterized during a five-year period by the pediatric cardiology department of a major teaching hospital.

The study shows that many physicians no longer approach certain types of critically ill patients as if physical life were sacred. Social life has replaced physical life as the criterion for active treatment in such cases. At the same time, there is by no means complete agreement among physicians on the application of social criteria in the evaluation of the patient's potential for treatment. Examination of hospital records showed that physicians tended to overestimate in the questionnaires their likelihood of treating critically ill patients. In other words, there may be more consensus about not treating certain types of patients than the questionnaires suggest.

One of the discouraging aspects of doing a study of this kind is the transience of the results. We seem to be witnessing a gradual shift in the attitudes toward life and death in Western culture. It is not unlikely that replication of the study a decade later will show significant changes. There is a need for further research not only on physicians' perceptions of these problems but on the perceptions of other medical personnel, as well as of patients and their families. Given the lack of consensus on these issues in other social institutions such as the law and religion (as illustrated during the controversies concerning the Quinlan case), studies of the attitudes of judges and theologians toward the prolongation of life would be of considerable interest.

The policy implications of adopting a social definition of life are exceedingly complex and have been the subject of considerable debate among physicians, philosophers, theologians, and others. Unfortunately, discussions of these problems are generally presented from the point of view of a single individual. A physician will present his views based on his personal experiences with patients. A philosopher or a theologian will likewise present his opinions, sometimes on the basis of observations made in one or two hospital settings. This study was undertaken in the hope that information about the practices of large samples of physicians would provide a useful factual basis for ethical, moral, and policy discussions. More than many sociological studies, this one was intended to speak not only to sociologists but also to members of the many other disciplines and professions that concern themselves with these pressing issues.

Paris   Diana Crane
June 1977

References

Ad Hoc Committee of the Harvard Medical School to Examine Brain Death. A definition of irreversible coma. *Journal of the American Medical Association*, 205 (August 5, 1968), 85-88.

Crane, D. *Social Aspects of the Prolongation of Life*. Social Science Frontiers, No. 1. New York: Russell Sage Foundation, 1969.

Fox, R.C. Advanced medical technology: social and ethical implications. *Annual Review of Sociology*, 2 (1976), 231-268.

Freidson, E. *Profession of Medicine*. New York: Dodd, Mead and Company, 1970.

Chapter 1: Introduction

In recent years, the subject of death and dying has become increasingly popular in the mass media. It appears that death is no longer, as it was once described (Lester 1967), a matter of indifference to the average person. Numerous popular articles describe the plight of families facing the dilemmas posed by hospitalization of dying relatives. The number of courses on dying and death offered to college students has multiplied. At the same time, there has been an increase in interest in this subject among physicians and social scientists who have produced a steady stream of articles and books.

What are the reasons for the surge of interest in this topic? One reason is that technology, which has affected virtually every aspect of modern life, has also altered the process of dying. Chronic rather than acute diseases are now the most prevalent causes of death in industrial societies (Lerner 1970). Due in part to the nature of chronic diseases and in part to the availability of increasingly sophisticated technology, the physician's control over the exact timing of death has increased. In some cases, if treatment is not withdrawn, the patient can be kept alive almost indefinitely. Unusually difficult interpersonal problems are thus created for the physician, for the patient, and for his family.

As the physician's capacity to treat illness and control the timing of death has increased, the traditional norms that have guided medical practice have become more difficult to apply. In the past, when the majority of patients suffered from acute illness, aggressive treatment was almost always appro-

1

priate. Gradually it has become apparent that some chronically ill patients do not benefit from such treatment and that they or their families may in fact be adversely affected by such efforts.

Since, to a large extent, it is the physician who makes decisions concerning life and death, it is important to understand the factors which influence his decisions. This book reports the results of an inquiry concerning doctors' attitudes toward the prolongation and termination of life. Under what conditions does the physician do everything possible to save the life of the patient? Under what conditions does he withdraw medical treatment and permit the patient to die? Does the physician, under certain circumstances, actively bring about death — in popular terms, engage in the practice of euthanasia?

Redefinition of Dying and Death: A Source of Controversy

Decisions concerning what types of patients should receive aggressive therapy have been the subject of considerable controversy in recent years. The literature which explores this problem can be divided into two parts: one which upholds the traditional ethic that decisions should be made entirely on the basis of the physiological aspects of illness and another which suggests that social as well as physiological considerations should play a role in deciding whether or not a patient is treatable. In general, three types of patients are described: (1) the conscious terminal patient; (2) the irreversibly comatose patient; (3) the brain-damaged or severely debilitated patient whose chances of long-term survival in his present state are good.

The conscious terminal patient who is suffering a slow and painful demise is the most frequently discussed of the three. How actively should such a person be treated and why? The conservative view is that treatment should be continued as long as it is possible to sustain respiration and heartbeat. Social considerations are irrelevant. Karnofsky (1960) answers the question, "Why prolong the life of a patient with advanced cancer?" in the following manner:

> It is ethically wrong for a doctor to make an arbitrary judgment, at a certain point in his patient's illness, to stop supportive measures. The patient entrusts his life to his doctor, and it is the doctor's duty to sustain it as long as possible. There should be no suggestion that it is possible for a doctor to do otherwise, even if he were to decide that the patient were "better off dead." [p. 9]

Others have argued that, as these lives become less and less satisfying for the patients and their families, social aspects of the case should be taken into consideration in decisions to continue treatment. Morison (1971) expresses this point of view:

... the life of the dying patient becomes steadily less complicated and rich, and, as a result, less worth living or preserving. The pain and suffering involved in maintaining what is left are inexorably mounting, while the benefits enjoyed by the patient himself, or that he can in any way confer on those around him, are just as inexorably declining. [p. 696]

Those who advocate the use of physiological criteria exclusively argue that if we permit other considerations to influence our decisions in these matters, we will move toward a policy of convenience in which little will be done for severely deformed or dying patients who will be shoved out of existence as rapidly as possible. The argument in their favor is the ambiguity in the application of social criteria. The adoption of social rather than physiological criteria to define life creates new problems for the physician. While physiological death occurs at a specific point in time, social death is much more gradual. Except in its most extreme form, brain death, it is very difficult to say at what point the alert individual ceases to interact meaningfully with his social environment.[1] A Swedish writer (Giertz 1966, p. 43) comments: "The central point is whether we can establish the moment when life ceases to have any human value."

The question of social criteria is one on which the euthanasia movement has foundered. In its advocacy of direct measures to end the suffering of dying patients, it has been unable to define precisely at what moment such measures should be used. As a result, critics claim that its recommendations are arbitrary and, because of their vagueness, open the way for more objectionable practices (Kamisar 1969).

The comatose terminal patient is less frequently discussed in the literature although he is no less of a problem to physicians. Fortunately, the cessation of electrical activity in the brain can be measured unambiguously and this has become a criterion for declaring such patients to be dead without waiting for cessation of heartbeat and respiration. This definition of death has been widely accepted although not without considerable controversy.

Probably the most difficult cases are those which are least discussed in the literature on the treatment of the critically ill patient, those of brain-damaged or severely debilitated patients whose chances of survival for a considerable period of time are very good in their present partially functioning state. These patients can be considered to be critically ill, not in the sense that their death is imminent but in the sense that they require considerable medical care and expense in order to maintain their conditions. These prob-

---

[1] Responding to this dilemma, Morison (1971) argues that death is actually "a process not an event." He suggests that the process of dying begins when life begins and does not end until after what has traditionally been defined as death, that is, "when the last cell ceases to convert."

lems are vividly described by Sackett (1969), a physician who turned state legislator:

> On a recent legislative inspection trip, my colleagues and I observed the following situation. A severely retarded male patient, age twenty-five, with marked contractures of all his extremities, had been bedfast during his entire life. He was being fed through a gastrostomy tube, which required major surgery for its insertion. He lay on his side; his eyes were wide open and gazing up at the corner of the ceiling; he responded neither to the calling of his name nor to a sharp tap on his shoulder. [p. 27]

Into this category fall many senile, severely debilitated geriatric patients as well as mentally defective or severely deformed newborns. Here again, opinions differ on whether social considerations should play a role in the decisions to treat these patients. These issues have been discussed more thoroughly in connection with the question of abortion but some writers have discussed the newborn infant. Shils (1968), for example, is willing to accept abortion on the grounds that the fetus is not yet a social being but he has serious doubts about euthanasia of grossly defective newborns. He argues that because the infants are separate from their mothers, their lives are worth saving.

> ... they have a putative capacity for individuality. If we affirm the principle of the sanctity of life, euthanasia in marginal cases of idiocy or monstrosity is reprehensible, and in extreme cases too it is repugnant. [pp. 29–30]

In other words, the infant, no matter how grossly deformed, is a human being because he is part of a network of social relationships while the fetus is not. Tooley (1972), a philosopher, argues alternatively that the fetus and the infant both lack awareness or consciousness of life and therefore are equally without the inherent right to life.

Some physicians writing about grossly deformed infants have used social criteria in evaluating such cases. Discussing the value of neurosurgical techniques for infants with myelomeningocele whose cases are so severe that their lower extremities are paralyzed, that they have no control over bladder or bowel function, and that their intellects are impaired, Bucy (1960) writes:

> ... we are *not* justified in prolonging the lives of these infants to an existence of misery and suffering both for them and for their families. [p. 65]

His argument is essentially a social one, that such a child cannot lead a life which is rewarding either to himself or to his parents. On the other hand, two neurosurgical colleagues, Bluestone and Deaver (1956), argue that these children should be treated no matter how serious their condition. Their argument is also a social one, that these children can in some cases expect to become "useful, independent, and self-supporting members of the community." In each case, the argument is posed in social terms, although the definitions of social welfare differ.

A pediatric surgeon has stated publicly that he feels no obligation to perform complicated cardiac and intestinal surgery upon mongoloid infants, if the parents do not wish their children to be treated. The fact that it is unlikely that such a child will be able to participate in the life of his family in a satisfactory manner is for him the deciding factor (Shaw 1972).

The senile geriatric patient can also be maintained for long periods of time and is not capable of expressing his own views concerning his treatment. This problem is complicated by the fact that, among the seemingly senile, an unknown proportion have simply withdrawn from active social participation without having completely lost the potential for social relationships. With psychiatric intervention, they are sometimes capable of interacting in a meaningful way (Weisman and Kastenbaum 1968).

The question of what should be done for these different types of patients is ambiguous. Ramsey (1970, p. 132) argues that the salvageability of the patient should be the criterion: ". . . in judging whether to try a given treatment one has to estimate whether there is reasonable hope of success in saving the man's life." For those whose lives cannot be saved, their comfort should be the criterion in determining what and how much should be done for them. If aggressive treatment cannot reasonably be expected to prolong an alert terminal patient's life, it should not be used because it would be of no benefit to him. There is, however, one dilemma that Ramsey does not consider. Although a patient's illness may be incurable, it is sometimes possible, using heroic therapy, to give the patient additional months or even a couple of years of comfortable existence. Under what circumstances should such procedures be used? How much additional life justifies the acute discomfort which is often the side effect of such procedures?[2] Many physicians would argue that any amount of additional life makes the use of such procedures worthwhile.

---

[2] The best known example of such a procedure is the heart transplant operation which is extremely onerous for the patient and which, on the average, adds only a few weeks or months to his life, part of which must be spent recuperating from the operation itself. American and Canadian cardiac surgeons who had performed heart transplant operations between 1968 and mid-1969 (N = 28) were asked to indicate the minimum amount of additional life which would justify performing such an operation (Crane and Matthews 1969). They varied widely in their answers. Seven said that the operation would be justifiable if it lengthened the recipient's life by three months, another seven said six months, and six said a year or more. Four refused to answer on the grounds that merely lengthening life was not the justification for the operation. Some of these (as did some of the others who did indicate a time span) stressed that the quality of life rather than the quantity of life was the important factor.

A situation where the amount of additional life does not justify the use of such a procedure has been described by a neurosurgeon (Bucy 1960). He argues that an additional year to eighteen months of life are not sufficient reason to subject the parents of a young child with proven malignant tumor in the cerebellar midline to the ordeal of such an illness on two subsequent occasions:

> If the child is treated successfully . . . he will become so well that the parents will take hope again . . . In a year or eighteen months, he will show signs of local recurrence of metastases . . . The parents will go through all the agonies of the original illness and this time the child will die. Has anything been gained by subjecting these parents to the same dreadful fire twice? Have we been justified in saving this child's life on the first occasion, knowing full well that the tumor will recur and prove fatal? [p. 68]

There is clearly a dilemma regarding the appropriateness of social as compared to physiological criteria in deciding to treat critically ill patients. In the following section, the influence of cultural values upon these types of decisions will be discussed.

Normative Criteria for Medical Decision-Making

American culture contains various norms and values which influence the conduct of both medical personnel and laymen in their decisions regarding dying persons. There is not a single set of normative prescriptions regarding the prolongation of life but a number of inconsistent and contradictory orientations. The first involves the sanctity of life. The norm that medical personnel should attempt to prolong life as long as it is medically possible to do so is based upon the belief in the sanctity of life which is strong in Western culture (Shils 1968). This ideal has its source at least in part in Christian religion and stems from the belief that man's survival is part of God's design.[3]

Those who define life in social terms and those who define it in physiological terms do not disagree about the sanctity of life. They disagree about the definition of life, not about its value. There is some indication that, if this value is to continue to guide human behavior now that its religious bases have been considerably eroded, it must be redefined in social terms. Shils (1968, p. 32) suggests that a belief in the sanctity of individuality will eventually replace the belief in the sanctity of life. For him the problem with such a redefinition is that of assessing accurately the absence or cessation of individuality. The very concept of individuality is difficult to define.

---

[3] Ethical positions which are identified with various religions will be discussed in Chapter 7.

A number of other values influence medical decisions. For example, humanitarian norms prescribe the alleviation and prevention of suffering. It is only recently that this value has begun to conflict with the value that life is sacred since life can now frequently be prolonged even though it entails considerable suffering. It is their commitment to this value that puts the proponents of euthanasia in opposition to those who argue that life defined in physiological terms is sacred.

One of the problems with attempting to redefine the sanctity of life in social terms is that this is often interpreted by those who maintain the traditional definition as a resort to the use of utilitarian values in assessing the need for treatment. There is a strong emphasis in Western culture upon a cost-benefit analysis in the allocation of scarce medical resources. The use of utilitarian norms in assessing the needs of an individual patient is considered unethical. Norms prescribing prolongation because life is sacred and those prescribing humanitarianism are altruistic in the sense that the welfare of the patient is the primary consideration. Utilitarian norms tend to be instrumental since the goals of an organization, institution, or society as a whole are placed ahead of the welfare of the individual patient. Ethical behavior follows altruistic rather than instrumental norms.

One of the objections to defining death in terms of the cessation of electrical activity in the brain has been that the motives of the proponents of the new definition were primarily utilitarian rather than humanitarian since the dying patient's organs could be used to save the lives of others. Jonas, for example, responds positively to Beecher's question, "Can society afford to discard the tissues and organs of the hopelessly unconscious patient so greatly needed for study and experimental trial to help those who can be salvaged?," because he rejects the utilitarian implications of Beecher's question (Beecher 1970, p. 5).

It is, however, absolutely essential to use utilitarian values in assessing medical needs in the aggregate, since resources for medical care are and probably always will be less than what is needed. During wars, when medical resources tend to be critically strained, utilitarian values are usually applied to the selection of individuals for treatment. It is unclear whether medical resources are sufficiently scarce in peacetime to justify withdrawal of treatment from the terminally ill on the grounds that others who could benefit more from it would otherwise be deprived of such care. Morison (1971, p. 696), for example, in discussing the dying patient, comments: "As the costs mount higher and higher and the benefits become smaller and smaller, one may well begin to wonder what the point of it all is." To which Kass (1971, p. 702) in a rejoinder replies: "The hastening of the end should never be undertaken for anyone's benefit but the dying patient's."

Unfortunately the use of social criteria for defining life can easily be confused with utilitarian criteria. The patient who is not participating in social relationships is presumably not contributing anything to society either. If social criteria are to be used ethically, it must be possible to argue that treatment is of no benefit to the patient rather than that its withdrawal would benefit others.

Still another set of norms which plays a role here are legal norms. Euthanasia, defined as measures which in themselves produce the death of a patient, is legally murder in the United States (Rosner 1970). However, there is no case in the Anglo-American tradition in which a doctor has been convicted of murder or manslaughter for having killed to end the suffering of his patient (Fletcher 1968). There is also no case where a physician has been convicted for withdrawing or omitting therapy (Sanders 1969). Juries also tend to be sympathetic toward mercy killings by relatives (Sanders 1969, Rosner 1970). These facts suggest that law, like medicine, is moving toward a social interpretation of life.

Origins of Popular Interest in Dying and Death

Popular concern with dying and death appears to be the result of a series of gradual changes in cultural values and attitudes. The first of these changes is a trend toward humanitarianism in Western civilization. While this trend is too amorphous to document definitively, it appears that, as our personal experience of suffering has declined due to medical advances, our sensitivity to its occurrence in others increases. This can be seen in a growing concern for the quality of life of the poor and of members of minority groups, the treatment of convicted criminals and mental patients, and the rights of human research subjects as well as dying patients.

A second and probably related trend is an increasing desire to exert autonomy in areas where formerly the individual had been content to permit others to make decisions for him. Examples of this attitude can be seen in areas as diverse as religion where traditional forms of organized participation are currently being rejected in favor of individualized religious expression, and the consumer movement, where the hegemony of big corporations is being challenged by a formerly submissive public of buyers. Concomitantly, the average person is more anxious to control not only his own life but his own death and the factors contributing to it. One indication of this is the increasing acceptance of suicide. Suicide is no longer illegal in any state. There is also some indication that the average person prefers suicide to enduring the discomfort of chronic illness. A study which examined all suicides occurring in a town in England during a seven-year period found that only one-third had no organic disease. The remaining two-thirds had either severe hypertension or a wide variety of "painful, disabling, or fear-engendering diseases" (Stewart 1960). An examination of suicides in Seattle yielded similar results (Dorpat and Ripley 1960).

Although the patient has always had the legal right to refuse treatment, the physician has in fact exercised the right to decide when treatment is appropriate on the grounds that the layman lacks the expertise to make such decisions. When disagreements occurred, the physician has occasionally taken the issue to court; until recently, he has generally been granted the right to treat the patient against his wishes or those of his family. The legal right of the patient to control the administration of life-sustaining medical procedures is beginning to be enforced. This right has been recognized in recent legal decisions concerning the refusal of life-saving medical procedures (which will be discussed in greater detail later) as well as in the American Hospital Association's recently issued "Bill of Rights" for patients which states that refusal of medical treatment is one of the rights of patients.

These cultural changes are taking place in the context of many other socioeconomic and technological changes which facilitate these alterations in values and attitudes. Only those which are directly related to the medical area can be discussed here, specifically, technological changes which have affected the character of illness itself. The shift from acute to chronic illness as the leading cause of death has already been mentioned, as well as technological improvements which have given the physician greater control over the process of dying and the timing of death. Less obvious is the way in which improvements in medical technology have produced increasing levels of disability in Western society (Ford 1970). Some of this increase in disability is a side effect of medical progress itself, of the use of new drugs (for example, thalidomide) and of the use of new diagnostic techniques. Another source of increased levels of disability is the survival of more or less severely disabled persons who would formerly have died, such as diabetics and infants with myelomeningocele. Moreover, the presence of increased numbers of older persons in the society — partly a matter of medical advances and partly one of improvement in the quality of life generally — also leads to increased levels of disability. A study of all deaths in Glasgow of those aged 65 or older at the time of death concluded (Isaacs *et al.* 1971):

> It seems that many of those who survive into old age enter a phase of "predeath" in which they outlive the vigor of their bodies and the wisdom of their brains. The century which followed Darwin has yielded a new biological phenomenon: the survival of the unfittest. [p. 1118]

The development of certain kinds of extraordinary medical techniques such as organ transplantation and dialysis for renal disease has also stimulated changes in public attitudes and values. They have attracted popular attention to the negative side effects of the use of medical technology and

led to considerable questioning about the quality of lives which are prolonged in this way, and about the allocation of scarce resources to these
rather than to other social needs. In this area, too, some individuals prefer
to die rather than to adjust to the psychological and physiological stresses
of such treatments (Abram *et al.* 1971).

All of these social and technological changes provide the context for the
emergence of a loosely coordinated, norm-oriented social movement (Smelser 1962, Chapter 9; Fox and Crane, forthcoming) with two principal goals.[4]
The first goal appears to be improvement in the quality of interaction between dying persons and both professionals and non-professionals. This
aspect of the movement is exemplified by the best-selling book by Kübler-
Ross (1969) which describes her detailed studies of individual responses to
the process of dying. A second goal of the movement is the enactment of
legislation to strengthen the patient's right to refuse treatment (Veatch
1972) and to define death (Capron and Kass 1972). The movement, which
has attracted a wide variety of active participants including physicians and
other medical professionals, lawyers, social scientists and theologians, is
based in a number of organizations, most of which are of recent origin, such
as the Institute of Society, Ethics and the Life Sciences and the Foundation
of Thanatology. An older organization, the Euthanasia Society, is in some
ways a forerunner of the present movement. It has adapted its goals to fit
those of the newer organizations. Formerly it was concerned with pressing
for legal changes which would permit direct killing of patients. The new emphasis is upon withdrawal of treatment. It is offering "living wills" which
permit people to request in writing that they not be treated actively in the
last stages of terminal illness. Living wills have been very popular and thou-
sands have been distributed.

Decisions to Treat Critically Ill Patients: Social vs. Medical Considerations

Most discussions of the ethical dilemmas concerning the treatment of
critically ill patients are presented in evaluative terms, in other words, in
terms of what the physician ought to do rather than in terms of what he
actually does. In this book, the criteria which physicians say they use in treating critically ill patients will be examined. Do they evaluate their patients'
potential entirely in physiological terms or do social considerations play
a role? How much consensus about these matters is there among them? Does
analysis of the records of hospital patients confirm or contradict their statements of their attitudes?

---

[4] Smelser (1962, p. 270) defines a norm-oriented movement as "an attempt to
restore, protect, modify, or create norms in the name of a generalized belief. Participants may be trying either to affect norms directly . . . or induce some constituted
authority to do so . . . Any kind of norm — economic, educational, political, religious
— may become the subject of such movements."

The hypothesis being tested here is that physicians evaluate the chronically ill or terminally ill patient not only in terms of the physiological aspects of illness but also in terms of the extent to which he is capable of interacting with others. In other words, the treatable patient is one who, if treated, is capable of resuming his social roles even minimally and temporarily. The untreatable patient is one for whom this possibility must be permanently excluded. For example, the severely brain-damaged patient is completely incapable of performing his social roles while the physically damaged person may be able to resume some of them. For the terminal patient, resumption of social roles is of necessity temporary.

Sociological studies of medicine have been strongly influenced by two models, one which defines the social nature of illness and another which delineates the professional role of the physician. At least in part as a result of Parsons' model of the Sick Role, there is a sizable literature on the factors affecting the patient's decision to seek medical care (Kasl and Cobb 1966). On the other hand, there has been very little research on how the doctor perceives the patient and how he decides to treat the patient. What has been lacking is a model which could predict the conditions under which an individual will be likely to receive treatment, given different categories of debilitating conditions such as acute illness, chronic conditions and terminal illness.

The widely accepted sociological interpretation of illness which derives from the work of Talcott Parsons (1951, 1958) is that illness is a type of deviance. The sick person is considered deviant in the sense that he is incapable of performing his social roles and must be encouraged to seek help in order that he may return to a state of normalcy or health. While this model may be useful in explaining social responses to acute illness, it cannot be used to explain social reactions to chronic or terminal illness. Freidson (1970, p. 238), in an attempt to extend the model to cover such cases, says that the chronically ill patient is granted "unconditional legitimacy" for his illness, which means that he is not required to perform his social roles and may be given additional privileges. Neither of these authors consider the effect of variations in patients' potential capacities to perform their social roles upon physicians' decisions to treat such patients. As a result, the model cannot predict the conditions under which attempts will be made to alleviate the symptoms of chronic illness so as to permit the patient, if only temporarily, to resume his social roles. The model does not explain medical or lay reactions to these very complex cases. In effect, Parsons' model assumes that all patients have the potential capacity to resume their social roles, while Freidson in considering the chronically ill patient appears to rule out this possibility entirely.

Parsons' model of the physician's role does not include the patient's capacity to resume his social roles as an element in the physician's treatment of the patient. It specifies that the physician will make his decisions to treat entirely on medical grounds without considering, for example, the patient's social background and without becoming emotionally involved in his problems.

Both Parsons' sick-role model and his model of the physician's role by-pass the ethical issues surrounding the treatment of critically ill patients. The sick-role model emphasizes that it is normative for the patient to seek treatment while the practitioner model emphasizes that the physician should limit his attention to medical rather than social characteristics of the patient. Consequently these models implicitly accept the traditional medical ethic that life should be preserved as long as it is possible to do so.

Studies of the doctor's role in medical care have come primarily from the symbolic interactionist tradition in sociology rather than from the functionalist tradition. In the symbolic interactionist tradition, a greater emphasis has been placed upon studying the interactions between occupants of different roles. For example, Glaser and Strauss (1965) provide some information about how medical resources are allocated to terminal patients although their interest is primarily in the patient, not in the physician. They are concerned with how the patient's perception of the situation affects his reactions to terminal illness and the reactions of others to him.

Sudnow (1967), who works in a related tradition, ethnomethodology, was directly concerned with the characteristics of the patient which influenced doctors' decisions to treat him. He showed that those whom health professionals perceive as contributing more to society are most likely to be the objects of heroic life-saving efforts. Age is frequently used as a criterion of social value. Concomitantly, those who are perceived as deviant or marginal, such as drug addicts, chronic alcoholics, or prostitutes, are likely not to receive even the minimal attention that could prolong their lives. In other words, Sudnow argues that the individual's social value or social worth is the important factor in determining whether or not he will receive treatment.

However, it can be argued that this model incorporates only one aspect of a larger phenomenon which is the individual's capacity to perform his social roles. Those who are not deviant in the sense that Sudnow has in mind may also lose their capacity for social interaction and be less likely to receive treatment than those who have not lost this capacity.

The individual's capacity to participate in his social milieu may be affected in different ways by his condition. He may be completely unable to perform some roles, for example, occupational roles, but able to continue in a modified form other roles, such as marital and parental roles. The individual who is physically incapacitated may continue to interact in a meaningful way with his family who may in turn be very anxious that he continue to do so even though he may be incapable of resuming a completely normal life. For the terminal patient, resumption of social roles may be possible temporarily. The severely brain-damaged person is no longer capable of performing any social roles and may in fact be rejected by his family on the grounds that the individual is no longer the person they once knew.

Unlike the Parsonian model, the model which is being proposed here can be applied equally well to patients of all ages. For example, it can be used to predict the extent to which attempts will be made to treat critically ill newborns. One would expect that those newborns who have the capacity to develop normal social relationships with their families and others will be actively treated. Those whose relationships are expected to be abnormal due to severe physical disability or brain damage will be less actively treated. The willingness of the parents to attempt to develop normal relationships with such children is also an important consideration.

Similar issues are posed in relation to the unborn fetus. Western society has been gradually moving in recent years toward legalized "abortion on demand." Implicit in this position is an interpretation of life in social rather than in physiological terms. It is not enough for the fetus to be physiologically present in the mother's body; the mother must be willing to accept the social relationship with her child that its birth will impose upon her. If she is unwilling to accept this social relationship, she may no longer be required to bear the child.

The patient's potential capacity to perform his social roles can be determined in a number of ways. First, the physician attempts to decide whether or not the patient is "salvageable." Can the patient be restored to health or can a chronic condition be maintained for an indefinite period of time? Alternatively, is the patient's condition one which will sooner or later be the cause of his death? Cassell (1972) presents a dramatic illustration of how the physician's judgments are affected by the patient's prognosis. The prognosis indicates whether or not the physician can do anything for the patient.

> Case I, the 42-year-old man with acute leukemia is seen by physicians *as dead the moment the diagnosis is made!* It does not matter whether the patient knows or does not, to the physician he is a dying man. On the other hand, the patient with the numerous myocardial infarcts around whom the many physicians and their machines are crowded *is not dying until he is dead!* The response of a surgeon clarifies the point: "A dying patient is someone that I can't help."[5] [p. 532]

In general, as Cassell implies, decisions concerning salvageability are based on the known prognoses of various types of diseases. Obviously, from

---

[5] Italics added by the author.

time to time, the prognoses of certain diseases change but at any particular time there is likely to be a high degree of consensus among physicians concerning the prognoses of most diseases. For example, most physicians would agree that patients with metastatic cancer are unsalvageable. Physicians engaged in research on experimental treatments for this type of disease would undoubtedly be more optimistic concerning the amount of time which a patient could be expected to live but would not disagree that the patient is suffering from what will ultimately be a terminal disease.

A second decision concerns the quality of life which the patient can expect to lead. Is the patient physically damaged or mentally damaged in the sense that he has suffered irreversible physical or intellectual impairment or both? These factors obviously affect the individual's capacity to perform his social roles.

The salvageability of the patient indicates whether it is likely that the individual will resume his social roles; the degree of irreversible damage indicates his capacity for resuming them. If physicians are following the traditional medical norm regarding medical treatment, that is, defining the patient's potential solely in physiological terms, no distinction should be made among cases which differ on these two variables with respect to level of treatment. If the patient's potential is being evaluated in social terms, distinctions will be made depending upon the patient's prognosis and the type of damage which he has sustained. The priorities based on the extent to which the patient is likely to be incapacitated in the performance of his social roles are: (1) salvageable patients with physical damage; (2) salvageable patients with mental damage; (3) unsalvageable patients with physical damage; (4) unsalvageable patients with mental damage.

A third consideration, if the patient is conscious and intellectually aware, is his attitude toward the resumption of his social roles. How do relevant others in his environment view his potential capacities?

Finally, while he may have the potential capacity to resume his social roles, the relative value or social worth of these roles may influence the efforts which the physician is willing to make on his behalf. Some patients occupy roles which, while not normatively deviant, have low social value relative to other social roles, such as the aged and persons in low status occupations. Can one discern an independent effect of the relative social worth or value of the roles the individual would resume as opposed to the effect of his potential capacity to perform social roles regardless of their content?

For reasons which will be discussed in the following chapter, it seemed appropriate to study these decisions using detailed case histories of critically ill patients which were presented on questionnaires to samples of physicians in internal medicine, neurosurgery, pediatrics, and pediatric heart surgery.

These case histories are described in detail at the beginning of Chapter 3. While there is probably no ideal technique for studying these problems, it is clear that there are certain difficulties involved in using case histories to elicit information concerning physicians' attitudes toward these problems. These will also be discussed in Chapter 3.

The data obtained from the surveys can be examined from two points of view: (1) What are the criteria which physicians say they use in deciding to treat critically ill patients? Is it possible to detect the presence of norms concerning treatment that are different from the traditional norm? (2) Given the variation among physicians in the responses to these types of decisions, is it possible to identify the characteristics of those physicians who, by indicating their preference for heroic treatment, appear to support the traditional norm rather than the more permissive norms preferred by some of their colleagues? The first topic will be discussed in Chapters 3 through 5 and the second topic in the remaining chapters.

Chapter 2 discusses the problems that had to be solved in designing a study of doctors' decisions to treat critically ill patients and describes the methodology and sampling procedures which were used.

Chapter 3 presents the findings concerning physicians' decisions to treat critically ill patients and assesses the extent to which social considerations play a role in these decisions.

Chapter 4 describes physicians' decisions to resuscitate (i.e. to reverse cardio-respiratory arrest) patients who have died as well as various types of decisions to withdraw treatment from patients who are about to die.

In Chapter 5, an attempt is made to validate the data from two of the four medical specialties, internal medicine and pediatric heart surgery. A series of decisions to resuscitate patients who had died on the clinical service of a university hospital is examined as well as decisions to operate upon a series of mongoloid children with heart defects who had been catheterized in the same university hospital.

In Chapter 6, the effect of different types of hospital settings upon doctors' decisions to treat critically ill patients is examined. In this chapter, also, the effects of the attitudes of a physician's colleagues, and of the policy of the department in which he practices, upon his decisions are considered.

In Chapter 7, the effects of personal characteristics of the physician such as his religious affiliation, age and social class are examined.

Chapter 8 analyzes the problems which medical experimentation poses for the treatment of terminally ill patients using data obtained from two case studies of cancer chemotherapy wards.

The final chapter includes some policy recommendations for dealing with the dilemmas which critically ill patients pose for physicians.

Chapter 2: Controversy and the Clinical Mentality: Some Methodological Problems and Their Effects on the Research Design

Few physicians write about the ethics of medical practice. Those who do are probably not representative of their colleagues. They are usually committed to a relatively extreme view and either defend the traditional belief in the preservation of life or advocate a position close to that of the euthanasia movement. In order to develop a framework in which to study decisions to treat critically ill patients, it was essential to discuss the issues with physicians who fell at different points along the continuum between these two categories. Critically ill patients were defined as patients (1) who probably would die if not treated during the course of a hospital admission for an acute illness superimposed upon a chronic condition or for aggravation of a chronic condition or (2) who suffered from a debilitating chronic condition which seriously impaired their quality of life. How do the problems of these patients appear in the context of medical practice? Initially, interviews were conducted in a large university hospital. The first physicians were selected from specialties that have frequent contacts with terminal patients, such as oncology and intensive coronary care units. Gradually it became evident that problems concerning the treatment of critically ill patients occur in almost every specialty and with almost every type of patient. Eventually interviews were conducted with pediatricians, internists, oncologists, neurosurgeons, pediatric heart surgeons, pediatric cardiologists and urologists.

In the beginning, interviewees were selected on the basis of recommendations of previous informants but quite soon after the interviewing began, it became apparent that it would be desirable to interview intensively in particular settings. It was evident that the interviews would benefit from increasing knowledge of the setting. An attempt was made to interview all physicians, residents, and interns in certain departments and some auxiliary personnel, such as nurses, social workers, and psychiatrists. In the smaller departments, such as pediatric cardiology and pediatric heart surgery, and in two oncology divisions (one at another hospital), most members of the medical staff were interviewed. Almost all residents and interns rotating through the nursery for premature babies during the academic year 1970–71, as well as some attending physicians in the setting were interviewed. Approximately one-third of the interns and residents in internal medicine were interviewed as well as a few private physicians and full-time staff physicians. Several interns and residents in internal medicine at a community hospital in the same city were interviewed. A few physicians and residents in neurosurgery, neurology, and urology were also included. In addition, the investigator observed ward rounds in pediatrics, internal medicine, and oncology, and sat in on staff meetings in the surgical specialties in order to see how the problems of critically ill patients were discussed outside the interview context.

At first it was difficult to find a way to discuss these problems with physicians. Although they would allow themselves to be interviewed, useful information was often not obtained. Either they would talk in vague generalities or they would refuse to generalize in any way. It became apparent to the investigator that the way to approach the subject was by encouraging them to discuss particular cases.

The reason for this type of behavior on the part of these physicians is explained by what Freidson (1970) has called "the clinical mentality." In making judgments concerning patients, physicians prefer to consider each case as unique. They dislike making generalizations about the ways in which they treat patients. In part, this is a reaction to the fact that the situations which they face are exceedingly complex and varied. Even when questions were phrased in quite specific terms, some physicians demanded even more information and it was clear that, without describing an actual patient in all his complexity, their demand for details could never be completely satisfied.

For this reason, it was useful to begin the interviews with a general question: "I'm interested in factors affecting doctors' decisions to prolong the lives of (or treat) patients with potentially fatal diseases or severely debilitating diseases. Is there ever any controversy in your department surrounding decisions of this kind?" This permitted the respondent to define the problem in his own terms and to describe patients whom he perceived as belonging to these categories.

These interviews as well as the comments which were written by many respondents on questionnaires which were sent to samples of physicians (see below) will be used to illustrate points in the text. Many such quotations will be used since it seems desirable to allow physicians to speak for themselves as much as possible.[1]

The Clinical Mentality and Medical Decision-Making

In the course of the interviewing it became obvious that the process of making decisions about critically ill patients is not entirely rational or scientific. A great many variables enter into a particular decision and these variables can be combined in many different ways; the physician often finds it difficult to see patterns in his own decisions. Many physicians, both informants and respondents, described these decisions as highly individualized. Each case appears to be different; it is impossible to apply general rules. The following comments give an indication of some physicians' perspectives on patient care:

Medicine is an art not a science. [Internist.]

No patient resembles any other patient really. [Neurosurgical resident.]

Each case has to be analyzed individually. You can't make a general statement. You have to look at the individual merits of the case. [Pediatric surgical resident.]

I personally have no set rules as to the vigor of patient care but try to consider each patient as an entity. [Medical resident.]

Physicians cope with the complexities of the clinical situation in various ways. Some are convinced that the decision is not entirely rational, that it is at least in part intuitive. Such physicians spoke of the intangibles which influenced their decisions while others emphasized the inconsistencies in their own behavior.

This sort of thing is very difficult to get at. People come to these decisions without verbalizing them and without really thinking about them very clearly. [Pediatric heart surgeon.]

It is very hard to define how you make decisions. It is not rational or scientific and they are very difficult decisions to make. [Neurologist.]

When asked why he had vigorously treated a woman with terminal renal

---

[1] In this and in subsequent chapters, interviewees will be described as informants and physicians who filled out questionnaires as respondents. Physicians practicing internal medicine will be described as internists, and residents in this specialty as medical residents. Physicians practicing pediatrics will be described as pediatricians, and residents in this specialty as pediatric residents.

disease whose kidneys had ceased to function and who was essentially a vegetable, a medical intern said in an interview:

> There was no specific reason. It just happened. After I thought about it, I wasn't so vigorous. It was sort of a reflex.

Others stressed the inconsistencies in their own behavior:

> Each patient is so different that the consideration I give to any factor is usually different with each patient. [Medical resident.]

> Answers to questions like these are as contradictory and confused as my actual behavior. I believe and espouse one concept and find I am actually practicing another. [Internist.]

Such inconsistencies in their behavior were enhanced by the emotional aspects of the situation, both their own emotional reactions and those of others:

> Very few physicians have spent enough time studying philosophy to have philosophies of their own. I have opinions and rationalizations only ... I am sure my decisions have been uncontrollably influenced by my emotional responses to the infants and families. [Pediatrician.]

> It is not possible to make decisions, 1, 2, 3, etc. in an atmosphere which is usually emotionally loaded and in situations which may make us use varying responses depending upon the reactions of the family, nurse, house staff, etc. These answers could easily change with the same disorder in different families. [Pediatrician.]

Still others were influenced by their recollection of exceptional cases which had colored their subsequent attitudes toward similar cases. While the physician who actually makes a decision may feel that it is not altogether a rational one, some, perhaps especially younger physicians, find themselves incapable of making decisions in difficult cases so that in the end the decision is made for them by events or changes in the patient's condition.[2]

A pediatric resident said:

> I never had to make the decision regarding prolongation. The decisions were made for me by the conditions of the infants themselves.

A neurosurgeon said:

> Many of these questions you ask are not resolved by confrontation by the physician. He waits and waits and the question is answered.

---

[2] Simmons *et al.* (1972) in a study of decisions by family members to donate kidneys to relatives in need of transplants found that some family members postponed making a decision until they were "locked into" donation or non-donation through a series of smaller decisions to take or not to take preliminary tests and work-up procedures.

Rather than make a difficult decision each time it arises, some physicians fall back upon what they describe as "standard practice":

Some of the answers reflect what I do — not what I think — i.e. usual and standard practice. [Neurosurgeon.]

When I check what I would do, this is not always what I would do of my own volition. My check mark is often a concession to hospital demands and to legal concerns. [Internist.]

The way in which these various pressures can interact to influence the physician in a particular situation was summarized very well by a pediatrician respondent:

Your approach here may seem a bit naive to those who make this sort of decision in close, small community, private practice settings.

1. The individual physician may not make the decisions at all . . . they may be forced by the availability of information to the entire community, by previously agreed upon staff policies, by the desire of the patient's parents to bring the infant to a known activist center, by the commitments undertaken during the diagnostic evaluation of the infant's status in looking for a correctible lesion, by the arrival of the anesthesiologist with his damn machine before your own arrival, etc.

2. Or the decision-making process may be so interwoven with the process of education of the parents and dealing with the parents' confused sense of responsibility for decision-making and underlying guilt that it is very unclear exactly when and by whom the decisions were made, even though the physician then announces them as being his own.

Regardless of whether his decisions are inconsistent, nonexistent or dependent upon standard practice, one other mode of dealing with these cases is available to the physician, that of differentiating between the type or level of treatment which he selects. Most physicians appeared to have a concept of degrees of treatment ranging from minimal supportive therapy to aggressive, sometimes called "heroic" therapy. Definitions of what would be considered heroic or supportive therapy varied considerably, but the concept of degrees of treatment was widely understood except by those who felt that everything should be done for a patient under all circumstances.

Perceptions of Controversy and the Treatment of Critically Ill Patients

How much controversy about decisions to treat critically ill patients did these physicians perceive? This question was not asked on the questionnaire since the amount of consensus in these areas can be inferred from the distribution of responses. Most interviewees were aware of some controversy with respect to critically ill patients. How much controversy they perceived seemed to depend upon the number of such cases which they handled from day to day. Controversy appeared to be most intense in the premature nursery where difficult cases were practically routine. Controversy seemed to be least intense among the pediatric heart surgeons partly because decisions to operate are shared by them with pediatric cardiologists who do much of the preliminary work of assessing patients' potential for surgery.

In internal medicine and pediatrics, controversy is likely to arise due simply to the nature of the decision-making process itself. Few residents and interns make their decisions entirely alone and without any consultation whatsoever. Even senior physicians frequently consult other physicians and many will be influenced to some extent by the patient's or his family's views. This type of situation inevitably engenders disagreements which can be quite intense at times.[3]

Those who perceived little or no controversy either felt that the decision was entirely their own or had worked out very clear guidelines for treating difficult cases which they had found from experience to be satisfactory. For example, a medical intern said in an interview:

> No, I haven't seen any controversy. The intern is the patient's doctor. He makes the decisions and the others go along with it.

A pediatrician said:

> There is no controversy but there is discussion ... I have a strong personal philosophy ... The house staff welcome the opportunity to talk about these kinds of cases ... I tell them what I would do.

Development of Questionnaires and Scales

The exploratory interviews indicated clearly that there were controversies surrounding the treatment of critically ill patients and that physicians could only respond meaningfully to questions about their decisions to allocate or withdraw treatment in terms of specific cases. Since it was not practical to attempt to interview enough physicians to obtain systematic information about these decisions, the only alternative was to develop a questionnaire. It was clear that the questionnaire had to consist of specific medical cases described in some detail.

With the assistance of physicians who had previously been interviewed, questionnaires were developed for each specialty using the following format: (1) several case histories followed by precise descriptions of possible medical treatments; (2) attitude questions; and (3) social and professional back-

---

[3] See Chapter 6 for a discussion of mutual influences upon these decisions.

ground questions. The questionnaire for physicians in pediatrics is concerned with the treatment of infants born with congenital anomalies and severe birth defects. The questionnaire for physicians in internal medicine examines the treatment of progressive chronic disease. The questionnaires for neurosurgeons and for pediatric heart surgeons are concerned with the types of cases which occur in the practice of those specialties.[4]

One justification for the use of case histories to assess physicians' attitudes toward these issues is that the technique resembles to some extent the tests which physicians take in order to become board-certified. These examinations also present typical cases and ask the physician to indicate what treatments he would use.

The chronic conditions which are used in the questionnaire were those which the interviews suggested create the most difficult problems for physicians in these specialties. Some of these conditions occur very frequently. For example, cancer which figures in the internal medicine questionnaire is the second of the ten leading causes of death in the United States (Lerner 1970). Other conditions such as anencephaly which appears in the pediatric questionnaire are relatively rare. Such a relatively rare condition is included because it poses with particular acuity the type of ethical problem which is being studied here.

The patients described in the case histories vary in terms of brain damage, physical damage, physical pain, patient attitude, family attitude, social class and age. In the neurosurgery and pediatric heart surgery questionnaires, physicians were asked to indicate whether they would usually, sometimes, or rarely perform such an operation. The questionnaires for internists and pediatricians provided lists of appropriate treatments for each case. The treatments ranged from supportive therapies such as intravenous fluids to aggressive diagnostic and therapeutic procedures such as gastroscopy and tracheostomy to "heroic" procedures such as resuscitation.

Since the interviews suggested that physicians often deny the influence of social variables such as social class and family attitude toward the patient, an attempt was made in the internal medicine and pediatric questionnaires to present these variables relatively unobtrusively. Three versions of the internal medicine questionnaire and two versions of the pediatric questionnaire were developed. The same cases were presented in each version but the social variables were changed. The different versions of the questionnaire were assigned randomly to hospitals in the samples (see following section). They were assigned to hospitals rather than to individuals to avoid the possibility that individuals would see different versions of the questionnaires since this would have spoiled the effectiveness of this device. Not a single

---

[4] Copies of the questionnaires are included in Appendix 2.

comment on any of the questionnaires suggested that respondents did see alternative versions of the questionnaires or that they even suspected that different versions existed. In the neurosurgery and pediatric heart surgery questionnaires, different versions of the same question with the social variables varied were presented in a single questionnaire. Summaries of the research designs for the four specialities appear in Charts A.1–A.4 (see Appendix 1).

The questionnaires were pretested informally upon physicians, some of whom had been informants in the earlier phase of the study. The internal medicine and pediatric questionnaires were formally pretested during the summer of 1970. Subsequently a number of changes were made in the format of the questionnaires.[5] The pretest indicated that physicians would respond to questions of this sort on a questionnaire.

In general, reactions to the questionnaires by physicians were favorable. Aside from the response rates which will be presented in the following section, an indication of this is to be found in the comments which respondents wrote on the questionnaire. Respondents were specifically requested to write such comments. Twenty-one percent wrote a comment of some sort. Extremely favorable and extremely negative comments occurred in about the same proportions and relatively rarely. The majority of comments described the respondent's philosophy of medical practice or made specific comments upon some aspect of the questionnaire. Two case histories in the internal medicine questionnaire in which the diagnosis was deliberately left ambiguous in order to test hypotheses concerning the effects of uncertain prognosis upon medical decisions particularly troubled internal medicine respondents. Others objected to certain questions in the remainder of the questionnaire. Questions in which respondents were asked to rank diseases in terms of how actively they would treat them and to rate the effect of professional or social factors upon their treatment of patients elicited many negative comments. A few physicians also objected to the request for information about religious affiliation and social class origin on the grounds that this information was entirely irrelevant.

---

[5] Nevertheless a few errors still remained in the questionnaires in the final printing. In one version of one of the case histories in the internal medicine questionnaire, the description provided conflicting information concerning the attitude of the family. In another case history, the patient was described as having damaged kidneys and then being a candidate for kidney donation. The data based on these materials were omitted from the analysis. Finally, in the first mailing of one of the versions of the pediatric questionnaire, a set of boxes indicating responses was omitted next to one of the items on one case history. The non-respondents for this case (Blb) are omitted in calculations involving this case for pediatric residents since the percentage of non-respondents on this scale among the pediatric residents was substantially higher (35 percent) than for the other scales.

The non-response rates to specific questions varied depending upon the type of question. In general, response rates were highest for the case histories and for background questions, and lowest for questions which required the respondent to rank items or to estimate numbers of patients in various categories which he treated.[6] The questions where response rates were poorest were used very little in the analysis.

A number of respondents doubted whether the case histories defined in sufficient detail the complexities of the clinical situation which physicians actually face. On the other hand, there was an upper limit to the amount of information which could be presented in a questionnaire due to the fact that respondents were unlikely to be willing to devote a great deal of time to complete it.

Others were concerned that they would not respond to the questionnaire in the same way if it were administered on two different occasions. In technical terms, they were concerned about "test-retest reliability." While data were not obtained concerning responses to the questionnaire when it was presented at two or more points in time, it can be argued that this problem is not detrimental to the study for the following reason. The decisions which are being studied are central to the physician's daily activity and they are decisions which he takes very seriously; his answers are unlikely to be superficial or ill-considered.

Others felt that no hypothetical situation could accurately reflect actual practice. In other words, confronted with an actual situation, the respondent might react very differently from the way he had indicated in the questionnaire. This is the problem of the validity of the responses: Do responses of this sort reflect actual medical practice? Information about actual medical practice in these areas can be obtained from hospital records which are frequently incomplete. An attempt to validate the questionnaire findings through studies of hospital records in internal medicine and in pediatric heart surgery will be discussed in Chapter 5.

For the pediatric and internal medicine questionnaires, scales were constructed in the following manner. All items representing hypothetical treatments for the entire set of cases were factor-analyzed as a single group.[7] The

---

[6] The percentage of non-responses for specific items in the case histories ranged from 0 to 1 percent in the surgical samples and from 1 to 3 percent for most items in the medical and pediatric samples. On the scales which include several items from each case history the percentage of non-responses ranged from 0 to 6 percent. On some of the questions involving rankings or estimates of numbers of patients in certain categories treated by the physicians, the proportion of non-responses rose as high as 16 percent. On the standard questions concerning the respondent's professional and social history, the percentage of non-responses ranged from 0 to 6 percent.

[7] A varimax rotation was used.

factor analysis indicated that each of these cases represented separate dimensions of behavior although not all items under a single case were included in that dimension. A scale was developed for each question which included only those items which were highly correlated with one another as shown by the factor analysis.[8] Each pediatric scale includes between four and seven items. The tables show the proportions of respondents who would perform all of the items in a particular scale for the patients described (i.e., a "yes" response). Each internal medicine scale includes six to seven items. The tables show the proportions of respondents who would perform all or all but one of the items in a particular scale (i.e., a "yes" response).

Scales were also constructed with items from different questions in order to obtain a measure of a tendency to be consistently active regardless of the nature of the case. Three such scales were constructed for internal medicine, using three different types of behavior: initiation of resuscitation, performance of heroic operations, and utilization of heroic treatments. Each scale measures a consistent tendency to perform or not to perform these types of procedures on different types of patients. A similar scale representing a tendency to initiate resuscitation procedures was constructed for pediatrics. These scales are discussed further at the end of Chapter 7.

Design of Samples

Since the numbers of physicians practicing the specialties of neurosurgery and pediatric heart surgery are small, lists of members of these specialties were sampled. The World Directory of Neurological Surgeons provides a complete list of neurosurgeons in the United States. A 50 percent sample was drawn from this list. All members of the American Association for Thoracic Surgery were polled.

Pediatrics and internal medicine are large medical specialties, comprising physicians who practice in a wide variety of medical settings. The exploratory interviews and other studies of physicians (Kendall 1963, Mumford 1970) suggested that hospital environment is an important influence upon the behavior of physicians. Staffs of hospitals which are closely connected

---

[8] The items which were used in the scales are the following: *Internal Medicine: Question 1:* 12, 13, 15, 16, 17, 18; *Question 2:* 21, 22, 23, 24, 25, 26, 27; *Question 3:* 30, 31, 32, 33, 34, 35, 37; *Question 4:* 40, 41, 42, 43, 44, 45, 47; *Question 5:* 50, 51, 52, 54, 55, 56, 57; *Question 6:* 60, 61, 62, 63, 64, 65, 68; *Question 7:* 71, 72, 74, 75, 76, 77, 78. *Pediatrics: Questionnaire A, Question 1 (a):* 10, 11, 12, 13, 14; *Question 1 (b):* 17, 18, 19, 20, 21; *Questionnaire B, Question 1 (a):* 10, 11, 13, 14; *Question 1 (b):* 17, 18, 20, 21; *Questionnaires A and B: Question 2:* 25, 26, 28, 29; *Question 3:* 31, 32, 33, 34; *Question 4:* 38, 39, 40, 41; *Question 5:* 45, 46, 47, 48, 49, 50, 51.

with medical schools are more likely to be interested in the scientific aspects of disease while physicians in community hospitals are more likely to be personally acquainted with the patients they treat. These factors related to the organizational setting could affect decisions to treat critically ill patients. There is also some evidence that standards for treatment are higher in medical school settings which might also mean that doctors in these settings would be more active in their treatment of patients (Goss 1970, Kendall 1963). For these reasons, it was decided to select pediatricians and internists practicing in hospitals which represent different types of hospital environments. Since residents also participate in these decisions, and since the exploratory interviews suggested that they may be more active in their treatment of patients than older physicians, they were also included.

The sampling procedures were modeled upon those used by Kendall (1963) in her study of the learning environments of hospitals. A sample of hospitals was drawn from the American Medical Association's *Directory of Approved Internships and Residencies*.[9] The Directory classifies hospitals into four categories: (1) those which are *major* units in a medical school's teaching program; (2) those which have *limited* roles in such a program; (3) those which are used for *graduate* training only; (4) those which have *no affiliation* with a medical school. Since the number of residencies in pediatrics is not large, all hospitals with more than 300 beds which offered residencies in 1970–71 were selected for the study.[10] The number of residencies in internal medicine is considerably larger so that it was necessary to draw a random sample of hospitals stratified in terms of the four categories described above. A sample of 14 percent of the hospitals which are major units in medical school teaching programs was drawn, since these hospitals have larger numbers of residents. A sample of approximately 40 percent of the hospitals was drawn from the remaining three categories. Hospitals were asked to provide lists of their residents in pediatrics and internal medicine and of physicians who had admitting privileges in these specialties. Ten percent of the pediatric hospitals and 15 percent of the internal medicine hospitals refused to participate in the study.

---

[9] Hospitals with less than 300 beds were excluded from the sample since preliminary interviews suggested that such hospitals did not ordinarily treat many of the types of cases with which the study is concerned. Federal hospitals were also excluded in order to reduce the number of independent variables since it was inferred that medical practice in such hospitals would be different from medical practice in non-federal hospitals.

[10] Information about sampling procedures for both pediatrics and internal medicine is summarized in Chart 2.1 (p. 28).

CHART 2.1
SAMPLING DESIGN: HOSPITAL AND PHYSICIAN SAMPLES

A: INTERNAL MEDICINE

MEDICAL SCHOOL AFFILIATION	NUMBER OF HOSPITALS WITH APPROVED RESIDENCIES AND 300 OR MORE BEDS[a]	NUMBER OF HOSPITALS EXCLUDING THOSE NOT OFFERING RESIDENCIES, 1970–71	SAMPLE SIZE	REFUSALS AND NO ANSWERS	DELETIONS[b]	REMAINING HOSPITALS
Major	168	148	30	6	4	20
Limited	76	50	27	3	4	20
Graduate training only	60	39	21	2	4	15
None	170	105	57	9	9	39
Total	474	342	135	20	21	94

PERCENT OF TOTAL HOSPITAL SAMPLE (I.E. COLUMN 2)	TOTAL NUMBER OF RESIDENTS (ESTIMATE)	SAMPLING RATE	TOTAL NUMBER IN SAMPLE (ESTIMATE)[c]	TOTAL NUMBER OF PHYSICIANS (ESTIMATE)	SAMPLING RATE	TOTAL NUMBER IN SAMPLE (ESTIMATE)[d]
14	609	2/3	406	2,373	20%	403
40	210	100%	210	1,134	20%	193
38	128	100%	128	976	20%	166
37	308	100%	308	2,244	20%	382
27	1,255	—	1,052	6,727		1,165

[a] Includes only short-term general hospitals; if a hospital has more than one affiliation, it is classified with the most prestigious type.

[b] Deleted if it had not obtained any residents for 1970–71 or if it was used in pretest.

[c] The actual number in the sample was 1,065.

[d] The actual number in the sample was 1,165.

Samples of residents and physicians were drawn from the lists provided by the hospitals. The sampling rates were as follows: (1) pediatric sample: 25 percent of the pediatric residents and 10 percent of the pediatricians in the top category of hospitals; 100 percent of the pediatric residents and 30 percent of the pediatricians at hospitals in the remaining categories; (2) sample of internists: 67 percent of the medical residents in the top category of hospitals and 100 percent of the residents in the remaining categories; 20 percent of the internists in all four types of hospitals.

B: PEDIATRICS

MEDICAL SCHOOL AFFILIATION	NUMBER OF HOSPITALS WITH APPROVED RESIDENCIES AND 300 OR MORE BEDS[a]	REFUSALS OR NO ANSWERS	DELETIONS[b]	REMAINING HOSPITALS
Major	124	12	26	86
Limited	28	3	11	14
Graduate training only	17	1	6	10
None	52	6	12	34
Total	221	22	55	144

TOTAL NUMBER OF RESIDENTS (ESTIMATE)	SAMPLING RATE	TOTAL NUMBER IN SAMPLE (ESTIMATE)[c]	TOTAL NUMBER OF PHYSICIANS (ESTIMATE)	SAMPLING RATE	TOTAL NUMBER IN SAMPLE (ESTIMATE)[d]
1,485	25%	371	4,700	10%	470
90	100%	90	630	30%	126
77	100%	77	220	30%	44
190	100%	190	1,053	30%	210
1,842	—	728	6,603	—	850

[a] Includes all short-term general hospitals and all Children's Hospitals (N = 6) with more than 300 beds which offered a pediatric residency in 1970–71. If a hospital has more than one affiliation, it is classified with the most prestigious type.

[b] Deleted if it had not obtained any residents for 1970–71, if it shared a residency with another hospital in the sample, or if it was used in pretest.

[c] The actual number in the sample was 651.

[d] The actual number in the sample was 763.

There were a number of problems involved in sampling from these lists, since the lists often included names of individuals who were not relevant to the sample. This was particularly the case with the samples of internists and pediatricians. The lists included names of physicians who were retired or dead, who were not specializing in either pediatrics or internal medicine, or who said they were not practicing at the hospital despite being listed by the hospital. The lists of residents in these specialties were more accurate.

Questionnaires were mailed to members of all four samples during the winter of 1970–71. The questionnaire was anonymous but respondents were asked to return a postcard indicating that they had sent back the questionnaire under separate cover. Since many physicians practice in more than one hospital, respondents in the samples of pediatricians and internists were asked to respond in terms of their practice in the sample hospital which was named in the covering letter. The neurosurgeons and pediatric heart surgeons received up to three mailings of the questionnaires. The pediatricians and internists received up to three mailings of the questionnaires plus two letters from a prominent physician introducing the study. All pediatric heart surgeons who had not replied after three mailings of the questionnaire were contacted by telephone and urged to reply. Since the other samples were larger, it was not practical to contact all non-respondents. An attempt which was not always successful was made to contact 50 percent of the physicians and neurosurgeons and 100 percent of the residents. Since the questionnaires were too complex to be administered by telephone, the effect of these calls on the response rate was slight.

The response rates were as follows: neurosurgery, 71 percent; medical residents, 71 percent; internists, 57 percent; pediatric residents, 73 percent; pediatricians, 59 percent. As discussed above, drawing a sample from lists of hospital staff and from specialty directories meant that a number of physicians were included who were not appropriate for the sample. Excluding from the sample those in the following categories: (1) address and phone number unknown; (2) retired, dead, ill, medical school graduate before 1930; (3) not qualified to answer because not specializing in that type of practice; (4) not practicing at hospital listed in covering letter (internal medicine and pediatrics only), the response rates were higher: neurosurgery, 78 percent; medical residents, 80 percent; internists, 76 percent; pediatric residents, 78 percent; pediatricians, 79 percent. In the case of pediatric heart surgery only a small proportion of the members of the American Association for Thoracic Surgery were actually performing pediatric heart surgery at the time the study was conducted. Based on questionnaires returned and telephone contacts with virtually the entire non-respondent sample, it was estimated that the population of active surgeons was 287 of which 72 percent responded to the questionnaire. Excluded from the population were 44 pediatric heart surgeons who were part of a pre-test sample.

Comparisons between the non-respondents (excluding those in the categories described in the preceding paragraph) and the respondents were made on several variables:[11] type of hospital affiliation for the internal medicine and physician samples, citizenship for the two samples of residents, and board certification and professional age (year of M.D.) for the physician and surgical samples. This analysis showed that board-certified physicians were represented in greater proportions in the sample than among the nonrespondents in neurosurgery and pediatrics. There were no differences between

---

[11] Here and in the analyses presented in the next paragraph, the chi square test was used to assess the differences between the various samples and subsamples.

internists and neurosurgeons in the samples and the nonrespondents on professional age (year of M.D.). Pediatricians and pediatric heart surgeons in the samples were younger than the nonrespondents.

Since part of the analysis involved comparisons between subgroups in the samples of internists and pediatricians who received different versions of the questionnaire, these subgroups were also compared on a number of variables. There were no differences between the subgroups of residents and physicians which received the two types of pediatric questionnaires on the following variables: number of births per year in the hospital with which they were affiliated, professional age of physician, social class origin, importance of religion, and, among physicians only, board certification (few residents were board-certified). The pediatric subsamples differed on prestige[12] and type of hospital affiliation, type of hospital control (government, private, religious), and religious affiliation. Among residents, there were no differences with respect to citizenship (94 percent of the physicians were U.S. citizens). The subgroups in the sample of internists did not differ on these variables except for type of hospital control and size of hospital (number of hospital beds). The subgroups in the sample of medical residents differed on type of hospital affiliation, prestige of hospital affiliation, type of hospital control and size of hospital.

In stratified samples of the type used in the samples of internists and pediatricians, it is necessary to weight responses when generalizations are being made to the population as a whole (i.e. without controlling for the variable on which the sample is stratified). In the tables which appear in subsequent chapters, responses for physicians and residents who were affiliated with hospitals in the first category in the samples of pediatricians and internists are weighted so that they have the same weight in the tables as they do in the population from which the sample is drawn.[13] However, the totals which are shown in the tables represent the sizes of the unweighted samples and subsamples. The tables in Chapter 6 are unweighted since one of the variables being examined is the variable on which the sample is stratified.

In order to assess the significance of the findings, a number of statistical tests were used. The first was a test which compares two distributions to determine whether there are meaningful differences between two groups (see McNemar 1962, pp. 79–83). The groups compared may be two different groups or the same group tested twice in different ways. In the first case, a test for the difference between independent means is used, and in the second case, a test for the difference between correlated means. This test produces

---

[12] For the definition of this variable, see Chapter 6, pp. 107–108.

[13] The weights are as follows: medical residents, 5; internists, 3; pediatric residents, 4; pediatricians, 3.

a z score which if sufficiently large is statistically significant, meaning that there is a high probability that the difference found in the sample exists in the population from which the sample was drawn. These z scores are shown in the tables where this test was used. A variation of this test is a test for the difference between proportions which has been used to compare the proportions of very active physicians or the proportions of physicians who would resuscitate particular types of patients in two groups of physicians (Blalock 1960, pp. 176–178). This test also yields a z score which is reported in the tables where this test is used.

The chi-square test which compares the observed frequencies with the expected frequencies of responses in various categories was used to test for differences among three or more sub-groups (Blalock 1960, pp. 212–221). This test also produces a score with a known level of significance and this is reported in the tables where this test was used.

In some cases, we are interested in the extent to which a change in one variable is associated with a change in another variable. Two measures are appropriate here. One is Goodman and Kruskal's gamma which is used to measure the degree of association between two variables whose components can be ranked but which do not constitute a continuous or interval scale (Freeman 1965, pp. 84–87). Probability levels shown next to the gamma coefficients in the tables represent the levels of significance of chi squares computed for the same data. The other measure is Pearson's r correlation coefficient which is generally used to measure the association between two variables which can be measured continuously or scored in such a way that a continuous variable is simulated (see Chapter 7 where this type of analysis is used).

Tests of statistical significance are appropriate only for random samples. Therefore in this study they are not used in samples which are not random, i.e., the pediatric heart surgery sample and the hospital records samples (see Chapter 5). Measures of association are appropriate for use on such samples, however, and therefore Goodman and Kruskal's gamma was used in assessing the association between variables in these samples.

Finally, in order to increase the credibility of the study for physicians and others in health-related professions, the actual medical terms have been used in discussing the cases used in the questionnaires. Difficult terms are explained in the Glossary (p. 269).

Part I: Criteria for Decision-Making

Chapter 3: Decisions to Treat Critically Ill Patients: Social Versus Medical Considerations*

In the first chapter, a model was proposed which predicts the conditions under which an individual will be likely to receive treatment, given different categories of debilitating conditions ranging from acute illness, chronic conditions, and terminal illnesses or conditions. According to this model, the patient's potential capacity to perform his social roles is the decisive factor determining how actively he will be treated.

If the traditional norm governing medical practice were being followed consistently, social considerations would have no weight in these decisions. All the hypothetical cases which were presented to specialists on the questionnaires would be treated actively. This point of view was well expressed by a neurosurgeon who responded to the questionnaire:

> If one resolves in advance to do *everything* possible for *every* patient, one is spared many of the "difficult decisions" you ask about. Our training is to preserve life and function wherever possible — not only where it is desirable and convenient, but where it is possible. We are not trained (and should not be!) to decide who is "better off dead."

Alternatively, the patient's potential capacity to perform his social roles may influence the physician's decision to treat him and thereby to attempt

---

* Portions of material in this chapter appeared in the article: Diana Crane, "Decisions to treat critically ill patients: a comparison of social versus medical considerations," *The Milbank Memorial Fund Quarterly/Health and Society*, Winter 1975.

to restore his social capacities, temporarily or permanently. We will also examine the relative effect of the social value or worth of the roles which the patient could be expected to perform as compared to the effect of his capacity to perform social roles *per se*.

The Case Histories: An Overview of the Patients

The patients were selected to represent various combinations of salvageability and physical damage. A few of the cases will be described in detail here. All the cases for each of the four specialties are summarized in Charts A.1 through A.4 (see Appendix 1). The questionnaires are printed in Appendix 2.

In *neurosurgery* (Questionnaire 1), two of the salvageable cases were based on a patient who was described by a neurosurgeon in an interview with the author. The patient had developed a large hematoma (a swelling filled with extravasated blood) in his brain. The location of the hematoma in the brain was such that his mental faculties were affected before and after its surgical removal. After recovering from the operation, the patient had an IQ of 90, he could no longer practice his profession, and his right arm was paralyzed. If the operation had not been performed, the patient would have died. As a result of the operation, he can be expected to live a normal life span. The informant, a neurosurgeon, said that he sometimes wondered whether or not he had done the man a favor by operating upon him. This case is described in Operation 1 (a). Since this condition can affect the physical capacities of the patient rather than the mental faculties, depending upon the location of the hematoma in the brain, a parallel case, Operation 1 (b), was constructed in which the patient had suffered visual impairment and some paralysis on the left side of his body but no intellectual or speech impairment.

The neurosurgical unsalvageable cases involved a patient with a solitary metastatic brain tumor. The presence of metastases indicates the transfer of cancer cells from one part of the body to another and is considered to be a sign that the disease is irreversible and terminal. Again, depending upon the location of the tumor in the brain, the patient's physical or mental capacities are affected. Both possibilities were presented to the neurosurgical respondents in Operation 3 (a) (i) and (ii) and they were asked to indicate whether or not they would remove such a tumor in a 40-year-old man. The same pair of cases was repeated in Operations 3 (b) (i) and (ii) with the subject being a 65-year-old man. Another unsalvageable case, that involving a metastatic tumor in the spine which had produced paraplegia in the patient, was also included (Operation 4) since it could be corrected by a fairly simple surgical procedure and therefore was more likely to be performed.

In *internal medicine* (Questionnaire 2, Versions A, B and C), the salvageable patient with physical damage was suffering from chronic pulmonary fibrosis, a severe respiratory disease. The case (Question 6) is described as follows in version A of the questionnaire:

> A 35-year-old man is brought to the hospital by his wife. He has a history of severe chronic pulmonary fibrosis and for three years has been unable to climb stairs or walk more than 10 feet due to shortness of breath. He is found to have pneumococcal pneumonia, but during his first hospital day he becomes cyanotic and semi-comatose. If a tracheostomy is performed, he will probably survive without further impairment of lung function. His wife is reluctant to authorize this procedure. Which of the following would you be likely to perform? (Check yes, maybe, or no for each of the following.)
>
> 60. Would you attempt to persuade his wife to authorize tracheostomy?
> 61. Intravenous feeding for dehydration.
> 62. Antibiotics.
> 63. Arterial puncture for blood gas analysis.
> 64. Urine culture for pyuria.
> 65. Urethral catheter for urinary obstruction.
> 66. Appendectomy for incidental suspected appendicitis.
> 67. Small bowel resection for suspected infarcted bowel.
> 68. If cardiac arrest occurred, would you begin resuscitation?
> 69. If resuscitation was unsuccessful after 15 minutes, would you continue?

The items which are included in the scale of activism for this case are 60, 61, 62, 63, 64, 65, and 68. Although the patient is severely debilitated, he is considered salvageable since patients with this chronic condition can be maintained over considerable periods of time. The age of the patient is varied on the three versions of the questionnaire and in one version the patient is presented as a drug addict to test the role of deviant statuses in the decision to treat.

The salvageable internal medicine patient with moderate mental damage (Question 2, versions A and C) is described as follows in version A:

> A 65-year-old woman had a severe stroke one year ago. As a result, she cannot walk, eats with difficulty, and has mild difficulty expressing herself. She is admitted to the ward service dehydrated and septic. Her family is unwilling to care for her at home if discharged from the hospital following treatment. Which of the following would you be likely to perform? (Check yes, maybe, or no for each of the following.)
>
> 20. Intravenous feeding for dehydration.
> 21. Lumbar puncture for stiff neck and fever.
> 22. Urine culture for pyuria.
> 23. Six blood cultures for fever and murmur.
> 24. Appendectomy for incidental suspected appendicitis.

25. Small bowel resection for suspected infarcted bowel.
26. If respiratory insufficiency due to pneumonia became severe, would you use endotrachial tube and respirator?
27. If respiratory distress lasted 2 days, would you perform tracheostomy?
28. If cardiac arrest occurred, would you begin resuscitation?
29. If resuscitation was unsuccessful after 15 minutes, would you continue?

The items which are included in the scale of activism for this case are 21, 22, 23, 24, 25, 26, and 27. In versions A and C, the willingness of the family to care for the patient was presented negatively and positively, respectively. In version B of the case, a similar patient with more severe brain damage was presented as "a 65-year-old woman with severe cerebral atrophy (who) cannot walk, feed herself, or communicate meaningfully with others."

Two cases of unsalvageable physical damage were presented to the internists (Questions 1 and 5). The first case (Question 1) involved a particularly painful form of cancer, cancer of the esophagus (part of the passage through which food is transmitted from the mouth to the stomach). In the three versions of the question, the patient's social class and financial need were varied.

A second unsalvageable case with physical damage (Question 5: versions A and C) presented a man with "melanoma (a type of cancer) of the leg that has metastasized to the spinal cord" causing paraplegia. This case was presented in two versions which varied in terms of the patient's desire to be treated. Question 5, version B, presented another unsalvageable disease involving physical damage, multiple sclerosis (which causes severe muscular weakness and lack of physical coordination), in order to compare physicians' reactions to a terminal disease which does not have such negative connotations as cancer.

In addition, two other cases, Questions 4 and 7, were presented in which the diagnosis was deliberately left ambiguous in a situation where it was necessary for the physician to take some action immediately. This was done in order to study the effects of uncertainty of diagnosis upon the physician's willingness to treat these patients.

In *pediatrics* (Questionnaire 3, Versions A and B), the salvageable patient with physical damage (Question 2) was an infant who had been born with myelomeningocele, a hernial protrusion of the spinal cord through the vertebral column, usually containing a watery fluid. The infant is described as having "no nerve function in his legs and no bladder or rectal sphincter control." If an operation to close the defect is performed soon after birth, the child's condition can be maintained for many years, although the associated paraplegia and absence of bladder and bowel control remain. If the operation is not performed, the infant may eventually die a slow and painful death. Children with myelomeningocele are often but not necessarily mentally retarded but this variable was not introduced in Question 2. The two versions of this case (A and B) were varied in terms of the social class of the parents. A similar case of myelomeningocele was presented to the neurosurgeons.

Two cases of salvageable infants with mental damage were presented to the pediatric respondents. One was an infant with mongolism (Down's syndrome). The other was a case in which, due to difficulties during delivery, the infant had been deprived of oxygen. A similar case had been the subject of considerable controversy in the premature nursery where field observations were made in connection with the study (see Chapter 6: Departmental Policy and Decision-Making in Pediatrics). An electroencephalogram indicated brain damage. Associated muscular problems developed. The case is described as follows in version A of the questionnaire (Question 4):

> As a result of premature separation of the placenta, an infant was without oxygen in the uterus for an indeterminate period. He weighs 1500 grams. Seizures develop within two or three hours of birth and persist in spite of therapy. Marked spasticity and hypertonia develop. An electroencephalogram is highly abnormal. This is the first birth for a professional woman who has had several miscarriages. She wants the child very much. Which of the following would you be likely to perform? (Check yes, maybe, or no for each item.)
>
> 38. Intravenous fluids for maintenance.
> 39. Monitor blood pH and correct as needed.
> 40. Antibiotics for infection.
> 41. If he develops pneumothorax, would you aspirate the chest?
> 42. If he stops breathing for more than two minutes, would you bag-breathe him for two to three hours?
> 43. Would you place him on a respirator if he continues to have apneic spells?
> 44. If he then has a cardiac arrest, would you resuscitate him?

The items used in the scale of activism for this case are: 38, 39, 40, and 41. The different versions of these two cases (Questions 3 and 4) were varied in terms of the social class of the parents and the mother's desire to have the child.

The two unsalvageable pediatric cases were (a) the statistically rare but philosophically interesting case of the anencephalic child, who, because it is born without portions of the brain that control conscious and voluntary processes and coordinate muscular movements, can be considered to be sub-human; (b) the case of a rare and incurable heart defect, hypoplastic left ventricle, which is difficult to diagnose without performing a catheterization, which in turn may be fatal to the patient if he has the condition. The condition, like that of anencephaly, leads rapidly to the demise of the patient.

The cases which were presented in *pediatric heart surgery* (Questionnaire 4) were all cases of salvageable patients with physical or mental damage associated with cardiac defects, since unsalvageable cases are uncommon in their practice. Two cases of children with mongolism (Operations 1 and 2) were described as having associated heart defects of varying degrees of severity (tetralogy of Fallot is less severe than atrio-ventricular canal). These cases were varied in terms of parental interest in and concern for the child. The same types of cardiac defects were presented in Operations 4 and 5 in association with a physical defect, a "severe but treatable urogenital anomaly." In these cases, parental concern and financial resources were varied. Finally, a case (Operation 6) of a relatively minor cardiac defect, patent ductus arteriosus, combined with rubella syndrome (congenital effects upon the infant of German measles contracted during pregnancy by the mother) was presented in two parts: with and without associated developmental retardation.

Obviously case histories of this sort can only partially simulate the actual medical situation which the physician faces. On the one hand, cases were chosen which were mentioned in the interviews as creating difficulties for physicians in these specialties. The details of the cases and the treatments suggested were realistic. However, there is an element of artificiality in the use of such case histories in that the physician generally interacts with a patient over a period of time, during which his assessment of the case gradually changes. In the case of an adult, the physician is likely to be most active during the first phase of his encounter with a patient on the grounds that the patient could perhaps be saved. Later when the exact nature of the patient's condition has been determined, a decision may be made to withdraw treatment. In the newborn infant, the effects may be reversed. The longer the seriously damaged infant lives, the greater may be the efforts to save him on the grounds that he has become a member of a family which has developed certain expectations for him. In the case histories, these phases are combined in the sense that the physician is presented at once with all the information on which he can base his decision.

However, regardless of the difficulties involved in using this technique, it is superior to the very general questions on euthanasia which have been used in previous studies (Williams 1969, Brown *et al.* 1970). Field data on these types of decisions are very difficult to collect (see Chapter 5) and would be virtually impossible (because of constraints of cost and time) to collect on a scale sufficient to adequately test the hypotheses being examined here.

Prognosis and Type of Damage

Among the neurosurgeons and the internists, salvageable patients with physical damage were more likely to be actively treated than any of the other types of patients (see Tables 3.1 and 3.2). For example, a salvageable patient with physical damage was more likely to be actively treated than a salvageable patient with mental damage. Of those sampled, 55 percent indicated that they would usually operate upon cases of intracerebral hematoma when

Table 3.1
Percent of Neurosurgeons Who Would "Usually Operate"
By Patient's Prognosis and Type of Damage[a]
(N = 650)

PERCENT OF NEURO-SURGEONS "USUALLY OPERATING":	PATIENT'S PROGNOSIS: SALVAGEABLE		PATIENT'S PROGNOSIS: UNSALVAGEABLE		
	PATIENT HAS PHYSICAL DAMAGE	PATIENT HAS MENTAL DAMAGE	PATIENT HAS PHYSICAL DAMAGE CASE (1)	CASE (2)	PATIENT HAS MENTAL DAMAGE
	89	55	76	50	22

Salvageable-physical vs. *Salvageable-mental* Cell 1 vs. Cell 2: z[b] $= 14.66$, p $<$ .01	*Unsalvageable-physical vs.* *Unsalvageable-mental:* Cell 3 vs. Cell 5: $z = 22.31$, p $<$ .01 Cell 4 vs. Cell 5: $z = 11.44$, p $<$ .01
Salvageable-physical vs. *Unsalvageable-physical:* Cell 1 vs. Cell 3: $z = 6.45$, p $<$ .01 Cell 1 vs. Cell 4: $z = 16.33$, p $<$ .01	*Salvageable-mental vs.* *Unsalvageable-mental:* Cell 2 vs. Cell 5: $z = 13.37$, p $<$ .01

[a] Cell 1: Salvageable Prognosis-Physical Damage: cerebral hematoma affecting physical capacities.

Cell 2: Salvageable Prognosis-Mental Damage: cerebral hematoma affecting mental capacities.

Cell 3: Unsalvageable Prognosis-Physical Damage (Case 1): tumor metastatic from kidney to thoracic epidural space producing paraplegia.

Cell 4: Unsalvageable Prognosis-Physical Damage (Case 2): solitary metastatic brain tumor affecting physical capacities.

Cell 5: Unsalvageable Prognosis-Mental Damage: solitary metastatic brain tumor affecting mental capacities.

[b] In this and in subsequent tables, the z statistic measures the difference between correlated means and independent means, depending upon which samples or subsamples are being compared. The probabilities shown are for one-tailed tests of significance.

the patient would be brain-damaged while 89 percent said that they would usually operate upon a similar salvageable case when the damage would be physical only (see Table 3.1). Among unsalvageable patients, a similar distinction was made between those who were physically or mentally damaged (see Table 3.1).

Internists were also influenced by the nature of the damage sustained by the patient in deciding to treat salvageable patients (see Table 3.2).

Respondents indicated that they would treat less actively a brain-damaged patient than one whose symptoms affected his physiological but not his mental functioning. In addition, the more severely brain-damaged patient was perceived as requiring less active treatment than the less severely brain-damaged patient. A resident commented in an interview:

> A female patient who has had a stroke is paralyzed and can't speak. She has been here a month. She spiked a fever for two days and we are not going to give her antibiotics. There is no hope of getting her back to normal functioning.

Table 3.2

Percent of Internists[a] Who Would Treat Very Actively
By Patient's Prognosis and Type of Damage[b]

PERCENT OF INTERN-ISTS WHO WOULD TREAT VERY ACTIVELY:	PATIENT'S PROGNOSIS: SALVAGEABLE			PATIENT'S PROGNOSIS: UNSALVAGEABLE		
	PATIENT HAS MODERATE PHYSICAL DAMAGE	PATIENT HAS MODERATE MENTAL DAMAGE	PATIENT HAS SEVERE MENTAL DAMAGE	PATIENT HAS MODERATE PHYSICAL DAMAGE CASE (1)	CASE (2)	PATIENT HAS SEVERE PHYSICAL DAMAGE
	67 (1,410)	30 (909)	16 (501)	36 (909)	28 (501)	3 (1,410)

Salvageable-physical vs. Salvageable-mental:	*Salvageable-physical vs. Unsalvageable-physical:*
Cell 1 vs. Cell 2: $z = 28.68$, $p < .01$	Cell 1 vs. Cell 4: $z = 24.70$, $p < .01$
Cell 1 vs. Cell 3: $z = 33.13$, $p < .01$	Cell 1 vs. Cell 5: $z = 20.95$, $p < .01$
Cell 2 vs. Cell 3: $z = 18.15$, $p < .01$	Cell 1 vs. Cell 6: $z = 72.30$, $p < .01$

Salvageable-mental vs. Unsalvageable-physical:
Cell 2 vs. Cell 4: $z = 3.57$, $p < .01$
Cell 2 vs. Cell 5: $z = 2.78$, $p < .01$
Cell 3 vs. Cell 6: $z = 3.82$, $p < .01$

[a] Physicians and residents combined.

[b] Cell 1: Salvageable Prognosis-Moderate Physical Damage: chronic pulmonary fibrosis.

Cell 2: Salvageable Prognosis-Moderate Mental Damage: stroke with moderate brain damage.

Cell 3: Salvageable Prognosis-Severe Mental Damage: severe cerebral atrophy.

Cell 4: Unsalvageable Prognosis-Moderate Physical Damage (Case 1): melanoma of the leg metastasized to the spinal cord.

Cell 5: Unsalvageable Prognosis-Moderate Physical Damage (Case 2): multiple sclerosis.

Cell 6: Unsalvageable Prognosis-Severe Physical Damage: cancer of the esophagus.

There are no cases of unsalvageable prognosis with mental damage in this questionnaire.

Not all physicians would withdraw treatment for infection in such a case. Another resident reported more active treatment for such a patient:

> We have an old lady on the floor who is a vegetable. She's been a vegetable for a year and she was half a vegetable before then. She came in dehydrated and septic. We treated her and hoped that she would perk up. Then we decided that she had reached her baseline and was not getting any better. We continue to treat her infection but we have decided that we won't resuscitate her or do any tests on her.

However, these physicians were less likely to distinguish between salvageable patients with mental damage and unsalvageable patients with physical damage. A salvageable patient who had suffered severe mental damage (cerebral atrophy) was less likely to be actively treated than a terminal cancer patient with moderate physical damage only (see Table 3.2). This suggests that the mentally damaged, salvageable patient is seen as being less capable of resuming his social roles than the terminally ill, physically damaged patient.

Both of these types of cases are more actively treated by neurosurgeons than the terminally ill, mentally damaged patient (see Table 3.1). Fifty-five percent of the neurosurgeons said that they would be likely to operate upon a salvageable patient with a neurosurgical problem which had affected his intellectual functioning, while only 22 percent said that they would be likely to operate upon an intellectually damaged patient whose case was definitely terminal. A neurosurgeon commented during an interview:

> If the patient is unsalvageable, you just have to accept it . . . . A lot of our patients are severely ill and incapacitated. Frequently death is the better way out.

Among the pediatric cases, a very clear distinction was made between salvageable and unsalvageable patients (see Table 3.3). In this specialty, the physically damaged, salvageable patient was not more likely to be actively treated than the mongoloid, salvageable patient. The explanation may lie in the choice of the physically damaged, salvageable case. The physically damaged, salvageable pediatric patient had a myelomeningocele and was described as having no nerve function in his legs and no bladder or rectal sphincter control. He was thus unlikely to have a more meaningful social existence than the mongoloid infant with whom this patient was compared. However, the expected priorities do appear in the comparison between the infant with a myelomeningocele and an infant whose brain had been damaged at birth as well as in the comparisons between the former and the other two infants in the decision to resuscitate. Twenty-nine percent of these physicians said that they would resuscitate the patient with a myelomeningocele

Table 3.3
*Percent of Pediatricians[a] Who Would Treat Very Actively
By Patient's Prognosis and Type of Damage[b]*

	PATIENT'S PROGNOSIS: SALVAGEABLE			PATIENT'S PROGNOSIS: UNSALVAGEABLE	
PERCENT OF PEDIATRICIANS WHO WOULD	PATIENT HAS PHYSICAL DAMAGE	PATIENT HAS MENTAL DAMAGE		PATIENT HAS PHYSICAL DAMAGE	PATIENT HAS MENTAL DAMAGE
		CASE (1)	CASE (2)		
TREAT VERY ACTIVELY:	55 (922)	52 (922)	47 (922)	25 (376)[c]	4 (458)

Salvageable-physical vs. salvageable-mental:
Cell 1 vs. Cell 2: n.s.
Cell 1 vs. Cell 3: $z = 4.64$, $p < .01$.

Unsalvageable-physical vs. unsalvageable-mental:
Cell 4 vs. Cell 5: $z = 47.91$, $p < .01$.

Salvageable-physical vs. unsalvageable-physical:
Cell 1 vs. Cell 4: $z = 3.27$, $p < .01$.

Salvageable-mental vs. unsalvageable-mental:
Cell 2 vs. Cell 5: $z = 47.85$, $p < .01$.
Cell 3 vs. Cell 5: $z = 63.66$, $p < .01$.

[a] Physicians and residents combined.

[b] Cell 1: Salvageable Prognosis-Physical Damage: myelomeningocele.

Cell 2: Salvageable Prognosis-Mental Damage (Case 1): mongoloid with severe respiratory disease.

Cell 3: Salvageable Prognosis-Mental Damage (Case 2): seizures with spasticity and hypertonia.

Cell 4: Unsalvageable Prognosis-Physical Damage: hypoplastic left ventricle.

Cell 5: Unsalvageable Prognosis-Mental Damage: anencephaly.

[c] Non-respondents excluded among the residents (see Chapter 2, p. 24).

compared to 16 percent who would resuscitate the mongoloid infant and the brain-damaged infant.

Neither the anencephalic nor the infant with incurable heart disease (hypoplastic left ventricle) will live more than a few days on the average unless extraordinary efforts are taken on their behalf. Even so, the infant with physical damage receives more attention than the one with mental damage (see Table 3.3), although this is possibly due to uncertainties surrounding the diagnosis of the former condition.[1]

---

[1] Some physicians said that clinical diagnosis was not entirely accurate but the most accurate diagnostic technique (cardiac catheterization) may kill the patient. Just over two-thirds of the pediatricians indicated that they would recommend that procedure in this case.

Some of the difficulties involved in making these kinds of decisions were described by a pediatric resident in an interview:

There are some instances where I would let them all die, for instance, if the child had severe congenital anomalies. But it's hard to draw a line between saving them and not saving them. It's hard to set goals in advance and then follow them. You can't say in the actual situation: "This is one of the kids that I decided to let die."

The pediatric heart surgeons were presented with case histories of salvageable patients only. They were much less likely to say that they would perform cardiac surgery upon children with an accompanying brain anomaly, mongolism, than upon children with an accompanying severe, but treatable physical anomaly (see Table 3.4).[2] The brain-damaged children clearly

Table 3.4

Percent of Pediatric Heart Surgeons Who Would "Usually Operate"
Upon Salvageable Patients by Type of Damage in Patient and
Severity of Patient's Cardiac Anomaly[a]
(N = 207)

SEVERITY OF PATIENT'S CARDIAC ANOMALY	PATIENT'S TYPE OF DAMAGE	
	PHYSICAL	MENTAL
Mild	93	56
Moderate	90	59
Severe	82	50

[a] Row 1: patent ductus arteriosus combined with rubella syndrome and (a) no developmental retardation; (b) developmental retardation.

Row 2: tetralogy of Fallot combined with (a) urogenital anomaly; (b) mongolism.

Row 3: atrio-ventricular canal combined with (a) urogenital anomaly; (b) mongolism.

Parental Attitude: Row 1: unspecified; Rows 2 and 3: favorable toward treatment of patient.

Statistical tests are not shown because the sample is not random (see Chapter 2).

---

[2] About 35 percent of mongols have different types of congenital heart disease (Lilienfeld 1969, p. 111). The questions concerning tetralogy of Fallot and atrioventricular canal combined with mongolism were presented in two parts: one in which the child was described as living with his parents who were anxious to have the operation performed; the other in which the child was described as living in an institution for mentally retarded children. The question combining these two conditions with a severe but untreatable urogenital anomaly was also presented in two parts: one in which the parents were described as being financially comfortable and asking the physician to spare no expense in the treatment of their child; the other in which the parents were described as having three other healthy children and having limited financial resources. In Table 3.4, the case of the mongoloid child whose parents are anxious to have the operation performed is compared with the physically damaged child whose parents want no expense spared in his treatment.

have a lower potential for performing social roles than the physically damaged children. The interviews suggested that the medical standards which are applied to mentally retarded children are different from those which are applied to normal children. A pediatric cardiologist said:

> Heart problems are usually fixed in normal children but they are not usually fixed in the mentally retarded. For the mentally retarded they are only fixed if the patient is in gross discomfort. Such discomfort is rare.

While many physicians appeared to be using social considerations in making their decisions to treat critically ill patients, others upheld the traditional medical ethic of not making such decisions. A pediatric cardiologist gave the following rationale for utilizing the traditional approach:

> You can't act as God. Someone once said that you treat everybody or nobody...I know some cardiac surgeons who won't operate on mentally retarded children. I think it's easier for a physician to operate on everyone.

To sum up, the priorities in terms of treatment appear to be the following: (1) salvageable patients with physical damage; (2) salvageable patients with mental damage and unsalvageable patients with physical damage; and (3) unsalvageable patients with mental damage.

The Role of the Patient and his Family

If a physician is basing his decision concerning treatment in part upon the patient's social situation and not entirely upon his physiological status, the attitude of the patient toward himself and of his family members toward him would be expected to influence the physician's decision. In fact the effects of these variables are very specific.

Patient Attitude. Among adult patients, the patient's attitude appeared to influence the physician's decision primarily when the patient was suffering from a terminal illness. For example, in one of the versions of the questionnaire for internists, a terminal cancer patient requests to be treated vigorously. In another version of the questionnaire, he asks that he not be treated actively. Fifty-one percent of the physicians who received the first version of the questionnaire indicated that they would treat this patient very actively. Twenty-two percent of the physicians who received the second version were willing to treat the patient very actively (see Table 3.5). However, although it was not tested in the survey, it seems likely that the effect of this variable would have been smaller with respect to salvageable patients. A resident in internal medicine expressed this point of view in an interview:

> I had a patient with rheumatoid arthritis who was very uncomfortable and

septic. She kept saying, "Let me die," and meant it very much. But I would not let her die because I felt that something could be done to make her more comfortable. But if it was somebody who had metastatic cancer, I would be more sympathetic toward letting him die.

The effect of the patient's favorable as compared to unfavorable attitude toward treatment was much less noticeable in a case where the prognosis was deliberately left ambiguous (see Table 3.5).[3] While internists indicate that the terminal patient's attitude is an important influence upon their decisions regarding treatment, other studies show that many patients have difficulty communicating their attitudes to their physicians (Kübler-Ross 1969, Quint 1964, Glaser and Strauss 1965).

Table 3.5

Influence of Patient Attitude Upon the Treatment of Adult
Patients with Physical Damage by Internists
(percent of internists who would treat very actively)

PATIENT'S PROGNOSIS[a]	PATIENT ATTITUDE TOWARD TREATMENT	
	FAVORABLE	UNFAVORABLE
Unsalvageable	51	22
	(430)	(479)
Uncertain	47	33
	(479)	(430)

[a] Row 1: melanoma of the leg metastasized to the spinal cord; $z = 16.71$, $p < .01$. Row 2: myocardial infarction combined with jaundice and history of lung cancer; $z = 5.98$, $p < .01$.

In spite of his legal right to refuse treatment, there is no guarantee that the patient's wishes will be regarded by the physician who is treating him. In the hospital setting, patients are often cared for by interns and residents who have had little or no previous contact with the patient. The nature of the doctor-patient relationship which ensues was well described by an intern in an interview:

What happens in practice is that we know very little about our patients before they come into the hospital. On the day of admission we usually cannot find a physician who has known the family of the patient and has a long-term perspective on him. We are presented with a patient whom we don't know and who is very ill. Our initial approach is to make every effort

---

[3] In the case of the terminal illness, patient attitude was varied in terms of requests by the patient to be treated or not to be treated actively. In the case of the illness with uncertain diagnosis, the patient was described in one case as talking about his plans for the future and in the other as talking fatalistically about dying.

on their behalf. A week or two later when we have a kind of cross-sectional history and have interviewed the family and dug up old charts, then everyone settles down to some point of view on the patient . . . Conservative therapy suggests that you should support the patient and that any therapy on his behalf is worthwhile if it will help him to maintain the status quo that he had reached in the past. In other words, you try to get him back to the point which he was at before he came into the hospital.

These problems are accentuated when the house staff is dealing with lower-class patients, as is usually the case on non-private wards. In these situations, communication problems between the doctor and the patient are accentuated. These patients who are relatively unsophisticated and inarticulate are not well equipped to engage in the delicate kind of negotiations which are required. Their families are in no better position. Some physicians simply infer from the fact that the patient has come to the hospital for treatment that he desires active treatment. An intern commented in an interview:

If he was sick at home and came to the hospital, then I think you have to treat him. By coming here, it means that he expects me to do something . . . If he says he wants to die, then he's probably delirious. In a rational moment he made a choice to seek aid. They've had a chance to kill themselves at home.

Although the extent of patient influence upon physicians' decisions among those on private wards was not studied systematically, comments by informants suggest that the patient's wishes concerning treatment carried considerably more weight on the private service than on the non-private service, as the following comments by residents illustrate:

There's a tremendous difference between the private and the non-private services. On the private service, a number of patients come in to die for whom nothing can be done. They are allowed to die. On the non-private service, patients are not allowed to die no matter what. The patients' wishes are disregarded. A private-service patient can tell you, "I've been suffering; I don't want to suffer anymore." That influences me. I don't think that this is true on the non-private service. The patients are less articulate.

Patients on the private service are more dependent upon you emotionally and you can talk to them. On the non-private service, more rigorous medicine is practiced. If you have a patient who is salvageable, any procedure is done, even if it causes discomfort to the patient. But on the private service some procedures of potential benefit are foregone for the patient's comfort.

Evidently, while many physicians may be favorably predisposed toward the patient's right to refuse treatment, a number of situational factors influence whether or not the physician is aware of the patient's desires in any particular case and whether or not he follows them.

Family Attitude. The influence of the family's attitude upon the treatment of the adult patient appears to be indirect. The interviews suggested that the internist is often ambivalent toward his patients' families. If they urge him to treat their relatives actively, he suspects them of being motivated by guilt. If they request him to withdraw therapy, he wonders if they have ulterior motives. Such ambivalence is most common when the physician does not know his patient well, for example, among interns and residents who have had little contact with their patients prior to hospital admission. The family physician who has cared for the patient and his family for years is better able to evaluate the attitudes of family members.

The family's attitude appeared not to influence physicians' decisions to treat salvageable patients.[4] For example, internists' decisions to treat actively were not influenced by the family's willingness to care for a moderately brain-damaged stroke patient upon her discharge from the hospital. In the case of the physically damaged salvageable patient which was presented to the internists, the family was described as being opposed to aggressive treatment in all three versions of the questionnaire but this case was more actively treated by physicians than any of the others. However, the family's attitude may have an indirect influence upon the treatment of unsalvageable patients, as is suggested in the following description which an internist gave in an interview of the kinds of reasoning that affected some of his decisions:

> If the patient has a chronic incurable illness and has been maintained over a period of years with some kind of meaningful life, there often comes a point when he simply falls apart at the seams. He begins to grumble that his funds are running out and it is difficult for the family. You know that there is little that you can do about this. So when the fellow comes to the hospital with an acute illness superimposed upon the chronic illness, you know that if you get him over it, he will have to go to a chronic disease hospital. You tend to let him go. After all, he has probably had five great years.

If a family does not define a brain-damaged child as socially dead, will the physician's judgment of the case be affected? Table 3.6 shows that in three medical specialties, pediatrics, pediatric heart surgery, and neurosurgery, the family's concern for a brain-damaged infant or child has a considerable influence upon the physician's decision to treat him.

On the pediatric questionnaire, favorable family attitude was defined in terms of a "precious pregnancy," which means that the mother had tried unsuccessfully in the past to have children and was therefore very anxious for the current pregnancy to be successful. It appeared that this variable influ-

---

[4] Several physicians commented on the questionnaire that the patient's role was more important to them in decision-making than that of the family. Some felt that the questionnaire overstressed the role of the family.

Table 3.6
Influence of Family Attitude Upon the Treatment of
Salvageable Patients with Mental Damage[a]

MEDICAL SPECIALTY		FAMILY ATTITUDE TOWARD TREATMENT	
		FAVORABLE	UNFAVORABLE
Pediatrics[b]	(i)	59	44
		(464)	(458)
	(ii)	58	33
		(458)	(464)
Neurosurgery		47	32
		(650)	(650)
Pediatric heart			
surgery	(i)	59	18
		(207)	(207)
	(ii)	50	12
		(207)	(207)

[a] Treatment is defined as: percent who would treat very actively (see Chapter 2) among pediatricians; percent who would "usually operate" among neurosurgeons and pediatric heart surgeons.

Row 1: mongoloid with severe respiratory distress (newborn); $z = 10.57$, $p < .01$.
Row 2: seizures with spasticity and hypertonia (newborn); $z = 12.24$, $p < .01$.
Row 3: hydrocephaly combined with mongolism (newborn); $z = 8.06$, $p < .01$.
Row 4: tetralogy of Fallot combined with mongolism (child aged 8).
Row 5: atrio-ventricular canal combined with mongolism (child aged 8).
Statistical tests are not shown for Rows 4 and 5 because the sample is not random (see Chapter 2).

[b] Physicians and residents combined.

enced decisions to treat mongoloid and brain-damaged infants actively. A pediatric resident described the following case in an interview:

> For example, take a woman who is 25 and who has been trying for six years to have a child and finally gets through to her 35th week. She develops an infection and they try to induce the child. They damage the uterus which has to be removed and she gives birth to a septic baby weighing 800 grams. This woman can't have more children. I had such a case when I was an intern and I was very vigorous with the child. He went home. *Do you think he will be normal?* He appeared to be. Even if he was spastic, I think that he would be wanted. But with an unmarried mother, you would be less vigorous.

The influence of parental attitude is greatest in the pediatric heart surgery cases, where the family's rejection of the children was strongest. Their rejection of the children was indicated by the fact that the children were described as having been institutionalized. The importance of the family's attitude is indicated by the following comments by a surgeon and a cardiologist:

Would you decide to operate upon a child with severe mental retardation?
I don't own the child . . . If the parents really wanted an operation I would
do it. The patients belong to the parents.

If the child is institutionalized and the parent is not involved, then there is
no need to investigate the heart.

Table 3.6 suggests that physicians who treat children are aware of the
stressful consequences for a family of having a mentally retarded child.
While a few physicians who were interviewed commented upon the happi-
ness which mongoloid children can bring to their parents, others appeared
to be sensitive to the difficulties which such children can create. A considerable literature which is reviewed by Farber (1968) illustrates the effects
upon families of the presence of mentally retarded children. While the level
of parental adjustment undoubtedly varies considerably, these studies indicate that initially there is almost always an emotional shock followed by considerable restructuring of family relationships in order to facilitate the care
of the child, unless the child is institutionalized soon after birth.

However, the effects of parental attitude were once again very specific.
For example, these effects are noticeable in cases involving brain-damaged
children but much less noticeable in cases which were presented to the
pediatric heart surgeons involving physically damaged children with cardiac
defects (see Table 3.7). It seems plausible that the parents' attitude toward
a brain-damaged child would be more important than their attitude toward
a physically damaged child since a greater effort would be required to establish social relationships with the former.

Table 3.7
Influence of Family Attitude Upon the Treatment of Patients with
Physical Damage: Pediatric Heart Surgery[a]

SEVERITY OF PATIENT'S CARDIAC ANOMALY[b]	FAMILY ATTITUDE TOWARD TREATMENT	
	FAVORABLE	UNFAVORABLE
Moderate	90	83
	(207)	(207)
Severe	82	70
	(207)	(207)

[a] Treatment is defined as percent who would usually operate. Both patients are
salvageable.

[b] Row 1: tetralogy of Fallot combined with urogenital anomaly.
Row 2: atrio-ventricular canal combined with urogenital anomaly.

Some of the neurosurgical informants described having performed operations of which they disapproved because the families pressured them to do

so. An operation was included in the questionnaire in order to test the extent to which neurosurgeons would yield to this type of pressure. It described the case of an adolescent with a broken neck which had caused quadriplegia. The operation (cervical fusion) is useless because the case is hopeless whether or not the operation is performed. The likelihood that the operation could improve the patient's condition is estimated to be one in five thousand. The question concerning this operation was presented in two parts, one in which the family was "anxious that everything possible be done for their son" and the other in which the family was "applying no pressure . . . for action." In the first case, 9 percent of the neurosurgeons said that they would usually operate; in the second case, the figure was 7 percent.

Social Potential versus Social Value

In all human societies, members are ranked according to certain characteristics. Certain classes of individuals are considered more important or valuable than others. Those whom physicians perceive as contributing more to society may be more likely to be the objects of heroic life-saving efforts. A few years ago, Sudnow (1967) concluded on the basis of participant-observation in the emergency room of a large county hospital in California that the individual's social worth or value had a noticeable effect upon the amount of effort which was made to save his life. According to his observations, older persons were much less likely to be resuscitated than young persons. Persons who were deviant in some respect were also the object of less vigorous life-saving efforts. The alcoholic was the prime example of this category which included "the suicide victim, the dope addict, the known prostitute, the assailant in a crime of violence, the vagrant, the known wife-beater, and, generally, those persons whose moral characters were considered reproachable."

In this section, we will examine three measures of social value: (1) socioeconomic status in terms of occupation and financial resources; (2) deviance in terms of drug addiction and alcoholism; and (3) chronological age.

Socioeconomic status. In the treatment of a patient with an uncertain diagnosis (myocardial infarction combined with jaundice and history of lung cancer), internists did differentiate to some extent between a patient with a high status occupation (a banker) and one who was described as an unemployed laborer (see Table 3.8). However, in the treatment of an unsalvageable patient (cancer of the esophagus), they did not distinguish between a lawyer whose illness was described as "exhausting the family's resources" and a truck driver in the same situation. Both of these cases were treated less actively than that of a lawyer with the same illness whose family had asked the physician "to spare no expense in treating him" (see Table 3.8). This suggests that physicians are responsive to the financial burden of an illness to the family, presumably because of its effects on family relationships. However, when asked to rank the relative influence of social characteristics upon their decisions to treat chronically ill patients, they ranked this factor sixth out of seven (see Table 3.9).[5]

Several physicians suggested in interviews that the family's financial resources would influence decisions involving children with devastating and permanent damage, such as hydrocephaly and myelomeningocele. The patient with a myelomeningocele, especially, requires enormous amounts of medical care, since he is very likely to have serious neurological, renal, and bowel problems in addition to paraplegia and mental retardation. Responses to the neurosurgical questionnaire did not suggest that financial factors influenced neurosurgical decisions involving infants with such an anomaly. The case was presented to respondents in two parts, the first one involving "20-year-old parents neither of whom have completed high school" and

Table 3.8
*Effects of Patient's Socioeconomic Status and Prognosis
Upon Internists' Decisions to Treat
(percent who would treat very actively)*

PATIENT'S PROGNOSIS[a]	SOCIOECONOMIC STATUS OF PATIENT		
	HIGH OCCUP.; NO FINANCIAL PROBLEMS	HIGH OCCUP.; FINANCIAL PROBLEMS	LOW OCCUP.; FINANCIAL PROBLEMS
Unsalvageable: Physical damage[b]	29 (479)	18 (501)	19 (430)
	HIGH OCCUP.	LOW OCCUP.	
Uncertain: Physical damage	47 (479)	37 (501)	

[a] Row 1: cancer of the esophagus; cell 1 vs. cell 2: $z = 10.99$, $p < .01$; cell 1 vs. cell 3: $z = 12.66$, $p < .01$.

Row 2: myocardial infarction combined with jaundice and history of lung cancer: $z = 4.03$, $p < .01$.

[b] Since the proportions treating very actively are so small for this case, the percentages used for this and subsequent comparisons represent those respondents whose scores fell into the lowest third of possible scores (low scores represent high activism).

[5] The characteristics are listed in Table 3.9. The rankings for each characteristic were coded separately. Some physicians did not rank consecutively but instead assigned the same rank to two or more factors.

Table 3.9

Rankings of Social Characteristics of Patients in Terms of Their Influence Upon Decisions to Treat Patients: Neurosurgery and Internal Medicine (percentage ranking 1st, 2nd, or 3rd)

SPECIALTY	PHYSIO-LOGICAL AGE	PATIENT'S POTENTIAL USEFULNESS	CHRONO-LOGICAL AGE	FAMILY CONCERN	DESIRE TO DIE	FINANCIAL BURDEN TO FAMILY	FINANCIAL BURDEN TO SOCIETY	NUMBER OF RESPONDENTS
Neuro-surgery	77	70	46	40	34	21	7	650
Internal medicine	83	66	50	43	39	19	5	1,410

When you are uncertain about how actively to treat such a patient, how much do the following *characteristics of the patient* influence your decision? Please place a 1 next to the factor which influences you most, a 7 next to the factor which influences you least, and a 2, 3, 4, 5, and 6 next to the factors which have intermediate degrees of influence upon your decision.

_____ a. The patient's chronological age.
_____ b. The patient's physiological age.
_____ c. The patient's desire to die.
_____ d. The family's concern for the patient.
_____ e. The financial burden of his illness to his family.
_____ f. The financial burden to society (i.e. insurance and welfare).
_____ g. The patient's potential usefulness to society or family if he recovers.

Table 3.10
Rankings of Social Characteristics of Patients in Terms of Their Influence
Upon Decisions to Treat Patients: Pediatrics and Pediatric Heart Surgery
(percentage ranking 1st, 2nd, or 3rd)

SPECIALTY	IMPACT OF CHILD ON FAMILY[a] Def.	B.D.	CHILD'S POTENTIAL USEFULNESS	PRECIOUS PREGNANCY	MOTHER'S ATTITUDE TOW. DEF.	MOTHER'S ATTITUDE TOW. MONG.	FINANCIAL BURDEN TO FAMILY	FINANCIAL BURDEN TO SOCIETY	NUMBER OF RESPONDENTS
Pediatric heart surgery	59	59	63	—	36	48	24	14	207
Pediatrics	80		66	62	49	42	38	14	922

When you are uncertain about how actively to treat such an infant, how much do the following *characteristics of the infant* influence your decision? Please place a 1 next to the factor which influences you most, a 7 next to the factor which influences you least, and a 2, 3, 4, 5, and 6 next to the factors which have intermediate degrees of influence upon your decision.

_____ a. The anticipated impact of the severely deformed or brain-damaged infant upon the family with whom he will live.
_____ b. The infant's potential usefulness to society or family.
_____ c. The mother's attitude toward a mongoloid infant.
_____ d. The mother's attitude toward a severely deformed infant.
_____ e. The mother's desire to have a baby combined with the fact that she has been unable to complete previous pregnancies successfully.
_____ f. The financial burden of the infant's condition to his family.
_____ g. The financial burden of the infant's condition to the state (i.e. insurance and welfare).

[a] This item was presented in two parts to the pediatric heart surgeons. In one version the child was deformed, in the other brain-damaged.

the second part involving parents who were "well-educated and financially comfortable." The difference in the proportions usually performing this operation in these two cases was only 2 percent. However, a similar comparison among the pediatricians yielded a percentage difference of 20 percent (see Table 3.11).

Table 3.11

Influence of Family's Socioeconomic Status Upon Decisions to Treat Physically Damaged Newborns: Neurosurgery and Pediatrics[a]
(percent of neurosurgeons who would usually operate; percent of pediatricians who would treat very actively)

| MEDICAL SPECIALTY | SOCIOECONOMIC STATUS OF PATIENT'S FAMILY | |
	HIGH	LOW
Neurosurgery	50	48
	(650)	(650)
Pediatrics	65	45
	(458)	(464)

[a] In both specialties the patient was described as an infant born with high lumbar myelomeningocele, having no nerve function in his legs and no bladder or rectal sphincter control. In one variation, the parents were described as "well-educated and financially comfortable," in the other, they were described as being twenty years old and not having completed high school. These two variations were presented on the same questionnaire to neurosurgeons and on different questionnaires to different subsamples of pediatricians. Row 1: $z = 1.66$, $p < .05$; row 2: $z = 10.60$, $p < .01$.

The explanation for the difference between the two specialties may lie in the relative importance which members of the two specialties place upon the financial burden of an illness to the family. Thirty-eight percent of the pediatricians ranked this factor among the top three on a list of social characteristics of the patient influencing their decisions to treat patients, compared to 21 percent of the neurosurgeons (see Tables 3.9 and 3.10). It seems that the financial burden of an illness to the family is a more important consideration to the pediatrician and this is reflected in their responses to the two versions of the question concerning the treatment of myelomeningocele.[6]

However, when social status measured in terms of financial resources was varied together with family attitude on the pediatric questionnaire, the latter appeared to be the more important factor. The comparison involved two cases which were quite similar: a mongoloid with severe respiratory distress and an infant with seizures combined with spasticity and hypertonia.

---

[6] In all three samples, however, the relationship between attitude toward the financial burden of the illness to the family and decisions to treat these cases was slight.

Brain damage is a very probable result of the latter condition. Table 3.12 shows that when the family's attitude is favorable, the children are actively treated, regardless of the socioeconomic status of their families. When the family's attitude is negative, socioeconomic status of the family is related to treatment.

Table 3.12

Influence of Family's Attitude and Socioeconomic Status Upon Pediatricians'
Decisions to Treat Mentally Damaged Newborns[a]
(percent of pediatricians who would treat very actively)

FAMILY ATTITUDE	SOCIOECONOMIC STATUS OF PATIENT'S FAMILY	
	HIGH	LOW
Favorable	58	59
	(458)	(464)
Unfavorable	44	33
	(458)	(464)

[a] Socioeconomic status is defined in terms of occupation and financial resources; family attitude is defined in terms of a "precious pregnancy" and maternal rejection of the child.
Row 1: seizures with spasticity and hypertonia; mongoloid with severe respiratory distress; not significant.
Row 2: mongoloid with severe respiratory distress; seizures with spasticity and hypertonia; $z = 2.73$, $p < .01$.

These findings are consistent with the pediatricians' rankings of social values. "Precious pregnancy," which was the way in which favorable family attitude was defined on these questionnaires, was ranked third in importance by the pediatricians (see Table 3.10). The anticipated impact of the severely deformed or brain-damaged infant upon his family was ranked first by the pediatricians, which may explain why infants belonging to lower-class families are treated less actively when the family's attitude toward the child is negative than infants belonging to middle-class families. The impact of such a child might be expected to be less favorable in a lower-class family than in a middle-class one.[7]

Deviance. Although Sudnow's (1967) observations in an emergency ward showed that deviants such as alcoholics, drug addicts, and prostitutes are less

---

[7] Farber (1968) suggests that the reactions to a severely mentally retarded child are different in middle- and lower-class families. The middle-class mother is more likely to define the situation as tragic in the sense that her aims and aspirations are frustrated, while the lower-class mother is more inclined to suffer a crisis of role-organization since caring for the mentally retarded child disrupts her relationships with other members of her family.

likely to be actively treated than non-deviants, that did not appear to be the case in this study. In a comparison between two patients with the same salvageable illness (chronic pulmonary disease), physicians indicated on the questionnaires that they would treat a 35-year-old drug addict who had been brought to the hospital by the police as actively as a 35-year-old patient who was described as being brought to the hospital by his wife.

In addition to the questionnaires, information concerning the treatment of 286 critically ill adult patients was obtained by examining the hospital charts for all patients who had died (some of whom had been the subjects of unsuccessful attempts at resuscitation), and all those who had been successfully resuscitated during a calendar year (1969) on the non-private service of a university hospital.[8] These patient histories frequently mentioned chronic alcoholism or history of chronic alcoholism. Occasionally drug addiction and psychiatric problems were mentioned. Twenty-three percent of the sample were chronic alcoholics or were described as having a history of chronic alcoholism. Thirty-one percent were "deviant" in the sense that they were or had been alcoholics or drug users, or had psychiatric problems including suicide attempts. There was no relationship between these sorts of deviance and the use of either resuscitation or major treatment or diagnostic procedures. Since it might be argued that the physician's awareness of these characteristics of his patient might increase the longer he stays in the hospital, this relationship was examined among patients who died or were resuscitated after the second hospital day. There was still no relationship.

Age. Parsons and Lidz (1967) have pointed out that attitudes toward the dying in our society differ depending upon whether death occurs at the end of the life cycle or as a break in the life cycle. The first type of event is considered normal; the second is the object of vigorous intervention. Sudnow found that in the emergency room of a large county hospital in California the aged were less likely to be resuscitated than young persons.

The frequency with which physicians indicated that they would treat older patients actively was somewhat lower than for younger patients in two out of three internal medicine cases and in two neurosurgical cases. In these cases, patients in their thirties and forties were compared with patients in their sixties. The largest percentage difference appeared in the internal medicine questionnaire when a 75-year-old patient was compared with a 45-year-old patient (see Table 3.13A, Row 3).

---

[8] This study is described in greater detail in Chapter 5. Throughout, the term "resuscitation" refers to *attempts* to resuscitate the patient which may or may not have been successful.

Table 3.13
Influence of Social Variables upon the Treatment of Adult Patients

A. *Effect of Age and Prognosis upon the Treatment of*
Internal Medicine Patients
(percent of internists who would treat very actively)

PATIENT'S PROGNOSIS[a]		PATIENT'S AGE	
		LESS THAN 50	65 OR OVER
Salvageable:			
Physical damage	(i)	69	66
		(479)	(430)
	(ii)	61	52
		(430)	(479)
Salvageability uncertain:			
Physical damage		39	23
		(479)	(501)

[a] Row 1: chronic pulmonary fibrosis; $z = 1.44$, $p < .07$.
Row 2: cardiac arrest due to physician error; $z = 5.61$; $p < .01$.
Row 3: dyspnea and hypotension combined with possibility of lung cancer; $z = 3.41$, $p < .01$.

B. *Effect of Age and Type of Damage upon the Treatment of*
Neurosurgical Patients
(percent of neurosurgeons who would "usually operate")

TYPE OF DAMAGE TO PATIENT[a]	PATIENT'S AGE	
	40 YEARS	65 YEARS
Unsalvageable:		
Mild physical impairment	50	40
	(650)	(650)
Unsalvageable:		
Severe mental impairment	22	15
	(650)	(650)

[a] Row 1: solitary metastatic brain tumor affecting physical capacities; $z = 4.20$, $p < .01$.
Row 2: solitary metastatic brain tumor affecting mental capacities; $z = 4.15$, $p < .01$.

When the hospital records sample was examined, it appeared that the age variations which had been used in the questionnaires were not wide enough. Physicians apparently distinguished between three age groups: under 40, 40 to 79, and over 79. As Table 3.14 shows, those under 40 were most likely to have been resuscitated in this hospital. Patients between the ages of 40 and 79 were somewhat less likely to have been resuscitated with no distinction by decade within this group. Those over 79 were much less likely to have been resuscitated. The use of major diagnostic and treatment procedures was also related to age in exactly the same manner.

It might be argued that the relationship between age and resuscitation is due to differences in the types of diseases from which persons in these age groups suffer. However, in this sample it appeared that older people were more likely to suffer from the types of diseases which are considered most amenable to treatment (i.e. the degenerative diseases).[9] There was no relationship between age and brain damage.

It is not clear what these three categories of age represent. Do they represent different social values assigned to the various age groups or differential capacities for resuming social roles? Since Western societies place a high value on youth, it could be argued that, with the exception of exceedingly eminent persons, the aged have low social value. In the interviews, physicians frequently distinguished between physiological and chronological age, arguing that two patients with the same chronological age might have very different physiological potentialities for recovering from illness. When asked to rank the relative influence of social characteristics upon their decisions to treat chronically ill patients, 50 percent of the internists and 46 percent of the neurosurgeons placed the patient's chronological age among the top three out of seven characteristics. The patient's physiological age was rated among the top three by 83 percent of the internists and 77 percent of the neurosurgeons (see Table 3.9). An emphasis upon chronological age as the criterion for resuscitation would suggest that these age groups have different social values while an emphasis upon physiological criteria would suggest that the important factor is the capacity to perform social roles.

If physiological rather than chronological age was affecting their decisions to resuscitate, one would expect that the relationship between age and resus-

Table 3.14
Percent of Patients Resuscitated by Age in a Sample of Deaths and Resuscitations on the Non-Private Service of a University Hospital

	AGE OF PATIENT[a]				
	10-39	40-59	60-79	OVER 79	TOTAL
Percent resuscitated	73 (37)	51 (97)	47 (125)	33 (27)	50 (286)

[a] $G = -.29$ (Goodman and Kruskal's gamma).

---

[9] See footnote 7, Chapter 5, for a definition of "degenerative diseases."

citation would be lower among patients who died or were resuscitated after their second hospital day since it takes time to evaluate the physiological age of an individual. The relationship between age and resuscitation was less strong among patients who were resuscitated after the first two hospital days.[10]

Physicians who were interviewed resisted the idea of setting arbitrary age limits for the withdrawal of treatment. Considerable protest was elicited some years ago by a statement from a British hospital superintendent that persons over 65 in his hospital were not to be resuscitated (Lasagna 1970, pp. 87–88).

Summary. Although the evidence is by no means clearcut, the physician appears to be influenced more by the individual's capacity to perform his social roles than by the social value or rank of these roles. Sudnow did not perceive any relationship between resuscitation efforts and either race or sex, and the same is true in the study of hospital records. Marital status and whether or not the patient lived alone or with relatives also had no effect. Both attitudinal and behavioral data showed that deviants were not less actively treated than non-deviants. In comparisons of attitudes toward treatment, occupants of high status roles were more actively treated than occupants of low status roles. However, when disruption of family relationships was examined concomitantly with social value, it appeared that the effect of the sick person on family relationships was the more important factor. Finally, the aged were less actively treated than younger patients. It appeared that advanced age represented to the physician a decline in social capacity rather than a loss of social value. Further studies of the relationship between social potential and social value are needed.

Acute versus Chronic Illness: Emergence of New Norms

Evidence from the present study suggests that physicians respond to the chronically ill or terminally ill patient not simply in terms of physiological definitions of illness but also in terms of the extent to which he is capable of interacting with others. The treatable patient is one who can interact or who has the potential to interact in a meaningful way with others in his environment.

If some physicians are not reluctant to withdraw treatment and thereby hasten the death of a chronically ill patient, what implications does this be-

---

[10] Gamma coefficients relating age of patient to use of resuscitation procedures were the following: (1) age by resuscitation: $-.29$; (2) age by resuscitation during first two hospital days: $-.43$; (3) age by resuscitation after first two hospital days: $-.12$.

Table 3.15

Ranking of Types of Diseases in Terms of
How Actively They Should Be Treated:
Percent of Internists Selecting Each Ranking Pattern[a]

	RANKING PATTERNS					
SPECIALTY	ACUTE > CHRONIC PHYSICAL > CHRONIC MENTAL	ACUTE + CHRONIC PHYSICAL > CHRONIC MENTAL	ACUTE > CHRONIC PHYSICAL + CHRONIC MENTAL	ALL HIGH OR ALL LOW	OTHER	NO ANSWER
Internists	48	6	29	3	13	2
Medical residents	62	10	17	3	8	1
Total	55 (725)	8 (112)	22 (312)	3 (41)	10 (145)	1 (17)

[a] The question read as follows: "Assuming that the patient is a 45-year-old man with a concerned family, please rank the following illnesses in terms of how actively you would treat them. Place a 1 next to the illness which you would treat *most* actively, an 8 next to the illness you would treat *least* actively, and 2, 3, 4, 5, 6, and 7 next to the illnesses to which you would give intermediate degrees of attention."

Chronic physical	a)	Chronic pulmonary disease
Chronic physical	b)	Chronic uremia
Acute	c)	Meningitis
Chronic mental	d)	Metastatic carcinoma to the brain
Chronic mental	e)	Metastatic carcinoma to the spine
Chronic mental	f)	Multiple strokes
Acute	g)	Myocardial infarction
Acute	h)	Pneumonia

The diseases were not labeled as "chronic physical," "chronic mental," etc., on the questionnaire.

havior have for the treatment of acute illness? The traditional norm regarding medical care — that treatment should be continued as long as it is possible to do so — is most appropriate for acute illness.

Internists were asked to rank eight illnesses — three of which were acute and five chronic — according to how actively they would treat them in a 45-year-old male patient with a "concerned" family.[11] Forty-eight percent of the physicians and 62 percent of the residents ranked these illnesses in the following manner: acute illness highest, chronic illness with physical effects only (uremia and chronic pulmonary disease) next, and chronic illness which involves brain damage last (see Table 3.15). An additional 35 percent of the physicians and 27 percent of the residents ranked the acute illnesses highest but either ranked the physical chronic illnesses equally high or did not distinguish between physical and mental chronic illness in the subsequent rankings. Only 16 percent of the physicians and 11 percent of the residents did not distinguish between these different types of illnesses in any way.

Among the pediatricians, the percentage who said that they would treat an acute condition (primary apnea) actively was much higher than the percentage who would treat a chronic physical condition actively.[12] Perhaps because of the nature of the conditions selected, noticeable differences in the rankings given to conditions affecting physical as compared to mental faculties did not appear among the physicians or residents.

The ratings of disease types suggest that physicians distinguish between acute and chronic illnesses as well as between physical and mental effects of chronic illness and that different levels of treatment are seen as appropriate for each type. There is, however, a substantial number of physicians in internal medicine who do not appear to make some or all of these differentiations. In the absence of data for different time periods, it is difficult to say whether the size of this group is increasing or decreasing. There is, however, some evidence which suggests that acceptance of the norms differentiating between different types of conditions is greater among younger physicians. Residents were most likely to rank acute illnesses ahead of chronic physical conditions and, in turn, the latter ahead of chronic conditions involving mental damage. Younger physicians were also more likely to make this distinction than older physicians.[13] These data suggest that as the proportion of chronic illness increases in the patient population, the younger physicians who are closest to the daily care of these patients are

---

[11] Comparable information was not obtained from the neurosurgeons.

[12] Eighty-four percent for primary apnea as compared to 61 percent for myelomeningocele. Comparable data were not requested from the pediatric heart surgeons.

[13] Goodman and Kruskal's gamma coefficient relating age to acceptance of the pattern was $-.23$, $p < .01$.

most likely to be aware of the necessity of distinguishing between chronic and acute illnesses in the treatment process.

Further indication of the kinds of distinctions which physicians make can also be seen in cases where it is unclear whether the patients are salvageable or unsalvageable. Two cases on the questionnaire were designed to test the hypothesis that a physician will treat very actively when he is uncertain about the diagnosis. The following comment by a resident expresses this point of view:

> In a few of the situations, Cases 4 and 7, one is unsure of the *exact* diagnosis and *extent* of the disease. My belief that all supportive and investigative measures are indicated until these are obtained may have biased my conclusions.

As was discussed in Chapter 2, the cases in which the diagnoses were left somewhat ambiguous disturbed the respondents. It seems likely, however, that such ambiguity is "realistic" in the sense that it must be a fairly common experience for a physician in his daily practice. However, attempts to test hypotheses concerning uncertainty produced somewhat inconsistent results.

In one of the cases where the salvageability of the patient was deliberately made to appear ambiguous, the internists indicated that they would treat the patient less actively than a salvageable patient of comparable age. The case involving the salvageable patient (chronic pulmonary fibrosis) was presented in two versions, one in which the patient was 35 years old and another in which he was 65 (see Row 1 of Table 3.13A). In one of the "uncertain" cases, a patient with dyspnea and hypotension combined with the possibility of lung cancer was presented as 45 in one version and 75 in another version (see Row 3 of Table 3.13A). The 45-year-old with uncertain diagnosis was much less likely to be treated actively than the 35-year-old salvageable patient (but was more likely to be resuscitated — see Table 3.16) while the 75-year-old with uncertain diagnosis was much less likely to be treated actively than the salvageable patient of 65 years (see Table 3.13A) and somewhat less likely to be resuscitated (51 percent compared to 61 percent).

The internists indicated that they would treat the 45-year-old and a 47-year-old man with uncertain diagnosis (myocardial infarction combined with jaundice and history of lung cancer) only slightly more actively than a 30-year-old man with metastatic cancer (see Table 3.16). However, the element of uncertainty was not discounted altogether in these cases since the physicians were much more likely to indicate that they would attempt to resuscitate these patients than the terminal cancer patient (see Table 3.16).

Table 3.16
Treatment and Resuscitation of Adult Patients with Physical Damage
by Certainty of Diagnosis: Internal Medicine (all patients under 50)

PHYSICIAN BEHAVIOR	CERTAINTY OF DIAGNOSIS[a]			
	CERTAIN (SALVAGEABLE)	UNCERTAIN (POSSIBILITY OF LUNG CANCER)	UNCERTAIN (HISTORY OF LUNG CANCER)	CERTAIN (UNSALVAGEABLE)
Percent who would treat actively	69	39	40	36
Percent who would resuscitate	66	72	61	43
Number of cases	(980)	(479)	(1,410)	(909)

[a] Column 1: chronic pulmonary fibrosis.
Column 2: dyspnea and hypotension combined with possibility of lung cancer.
Column 3: myocardial infarction combined with jaundice and history of lung cancer.
Column 4: melanoma of the leg metastasized to the spinal cord.
Row 1: Column 1 vs. Column 2: $z = 3.07$, $p < .01$.
Row 2: Column 1 vs. Column 2: $z = 3.16$, $p < .01$.
Row 1: Column 3 vs. Column 4: $z = 4.30$, $p < .01$.
Row 2: Column 3 vs. Column 4: $z = 13.98$, $p < .01$.

Chapter 4: The Terminal Patient: Treatment of the Dying and the Dead

Modern medical technology combined with the nature of many types of chronic diseases has given the physician considerable control over the process of dying. There are many decisions to be made, most of which are still controversial in one way or another. For example, the physician can choose to accelerate the dying process either by withdrawing treatment or by directly bringing about the death of the patient. It is not clear whether there is a meaningful difference between omission of treatment which is needed to maintain the patient's life (for example, antibiotics in the case of a terminal patient who contracts pneumonia) and the use of measures which are deliberately designed to end his life such as those which the proponents of euthanasia advocate. Omission of therapy has sometimes been called indirect or negative euthanasia. The issue becomes even more obscure when one considers the administration of large doses of painkilling drugs to terminal patients who are suffering from severe pain. Since large doses of such drugs may have the indirect effect of hastening death, their administration can be considered to be a form of euthanasia although the physician's motive may be that of relieving pain, and not of killing the patient.

As we discussed in Chapter 1, cessation of heartbeat was formerly required as an indication that death had occurred. A new definition of death which has been proposed substitutes brain death for cessation of heartbeat as the criterion. As a result, a patient who is still alive in terms of the strictly physiological criterion of heartbeat can be declared dead if it can be shown that he has lost irrevocably any possibility of recovering the capacity for social interaction.

Finally, death itself has ceased to be an irreversible event. For many years, it has been possible to reverse cardio-respiratory arrest by resuscitation techniques. The patient's cardiac and respiratory function can be revived and, in some cases, he returns to a normal life. At what point the physician chooses to declare the state of death irreversible often depends as much upon his judgment as upon the physical state of the patient. While most physicians will automatically resuscitate a patient whose medical history they do not know (providing that they can initiate such a procedure almost immediately), those who are aware of the total life situation of the patient may be influenced by the kind of life that the resuscitated patient could expect to lead.

We will consider in turn: (1) the terminal phase, the period when the patient is actually dying; (2) terminal acts, behavior which defines the patient as dead in social rather than purely physiological terms; and (3) decisions to reverse deaths which have already occurred, in other words, to resuscitate the patient.

The Terminal Phase

In the previous chapter, we found that certain types of patients are less likely to be actively treated than others. Specifically, terminal patients are less likely to be actively treated than salvageable patients. Brain-damaged patients, particularly severely brain-damaged patients, are less likely to be actively treated than physically damaged patients.

This does not mean, however, that treatment is withdrawn entirely in such cases. Only in the case of severely damaged patients (a brain-damaged patient who was described as being unable to walk, feed herself, or communicate meaningfully with others and an unsalvageable patient with cancer of the esophagus) did sizable proportions (32 and 34 percent) of the internists indicate that they would do virtually nothing for the patient.[1] Only

---

[1] These figures represent the proportions of physicians who had the highest scores on the scales. A high score indicates unwillingness to treat. In the first case, and in cases 1, 2, and 3 in the rest of the paragraph, the possible scores ranged from 7 to 21. The percentages shown here represent the proportions of physicians with scores of 17 to 21. In the case of the patient with esophageal cancer, the possible scores ranged from 6 to 18 and the percentage given represents the proportion of physicians with scores of 15 to 18.

A similar procedure was used for pediatric cases discussed below. The possible scores ranged from 4 to 12 and the figures shown represent the proportions of physicians with scores of 10 to 12 except in the case of the anencephalic infant where scores ranged from 5 to 15 and the figure shown represents the proportion of physicians with scores of 12 to 15. Forty percent of the physicians and 31 percent of the residents had scores of 15 for this case (i.e. complete withdrawal of treatment).

21 and 31 percent of the residents respectively were in this category. No more than 6 percent of the physicians and residents in internal medicine were willing to withdraw virtually all treatment from three other cases: (1) a salvageable patient with a severe chronic lung ailment; (2) a moderately brain-damaged salvageable patient who was described as being unable to walk, eating with difficulty, and having mild difficulty expressing herself; and (3) an unsalvageable patient suffering from cancer of the leg which had metastasized to the spinal cord. The patient who is incapable of all but the most rudimentary social interaction is evidently the one from whom treatment is most likely to be withdrawn in spite of the patient's salvageability. Treatment is also very likely to be withdrawn from the unsalvageable patient with cancer of the esophagus. Here the quality of the patient's life probably adds an additional dimension since this condition is one of the most painful types of cancer.

As Table 4.1A shows, internists distinguish between different levels of treatment. Willingness to withdraw these different levels of treatment is also

Table 4.1

A: Withdrawal of Treatment by Internists: Percent of Physicians Saying That They Would Not Perform Specific Types of Treatments

TYPE OF PATIENT	TYPE OF TREATMENT[a]			
	COMFORT THERAPY	DIAGNOSTIC PROCEDURES	EMERGENCY SURGERY	RESUSCI- TATION
1. *Salvageable:* Severe lung ailment	2	9	10	29
2. *Salvageable:* Moderate brain damage	3	8	28	41
3. *Salvageable:* Severe brain damage	11	27	57	77
4. *Unsalvageable:* Cancer of the leg metastasized to the spinal cord	2	20	27	45
5. *Unsalvageable:* Cancer of the esophagus	1	16	36	74

[a] *Comfort therapy:* intravenous feeding; *Diagnostic measures:* lumbar puncture, arterial puncture or pericardiocentesis; *Emergency surgery:* tracheostomy or appendectomy.

Table 4.1 Cont'd
B: *Withdrawal of Treatment by Pediatricians: Percent of Physicians Saying
That They Would Not Perform Specific Types of Treatments*

TYPE OF PATIENT	TYPE OF TREATMENT[a]			
	COMFORT THERAPY	DIAGNOSTIC OR MINOR TREATMENT	"HEROIC" TREATMENT OR SURGERY	RESUSCI- TATION
1. *Salvageable:* Severe physical damage	9	—	18	52
2. *Salvageable:* Brain damage (mongolism)	16	17	66	73
3. *Unsalvageable:* Severe cardiac anomaly	26	13	47	65
4. *Unsalvageable:* Severe brain damage (anencephaly)	64	68	84	92

[a] *Comfort therapy:* Case 1 only: manage urinary infection; Cases 2, 3 and 4: antibiotics for infection; *Diagnostic or minor treatment measures:* Case 2: appropriate cultures (blood CSF); Case 3: medical management of congestive heart failure; Case 4: correct blood sugar for hypoglycemia and hypocalcemia; *"Heroic" treatment or surgery:* Case 1: shunt for hydrocephalus; Case 2: bag-breathing; Case 3: bag-breathing; Case 4: blood transfusion.

related to patient salvageability and type of damage. Residents were less likely to withdraw these various types of treatments but their priorities were similar. A continuum ranging from comfort therapy to diagnostic procedures to emergency surgery to resuscitation can be discerned, with physicians being least likely to withdraw the first and most likely to refuse to perform the last.

The patient's capacity for social interaction is a significant factor in these decisions. The patient from whom treatment is least likely to be withdrawn is the salvageable patient with physical damage. He is presumably seen as having the greatest potential for social interaction upon recovery. The salvageable moderately brain-damaged patient and the unsalvageable physically damaged patient are seen as having approximately the same potential although presumably for different reasons. The relative willingness to withdraw comfort therapy from the severely brain-damaged patient is probably due to the fact that it would be useless for such a patient while it would make a difference to the well-being of the other patients.

Pediatricians were somewhat more likely to say that they would withdraw virtually all treatment from their newborn patients. Again they were most likely to say that they would do so with respect to a case of severe brain damage (an anencephalic infant). Seventy-one percent of the pediatric physicians said that they would withdraw virtually all treatment from such an infant. Eighteen percent said they would withdraw virtually all treatment from an infant with an incurable heart ailment; 13 percent from a mongoloid infant with severe respiratory distress; and 12 percent from an infant with a severe physical defect (myelomeningocele). In each of these cases and particularly that of the anencephalic infant, residents were less likely than physicians to be willing to withdraw virtually all treatment. As Table 4.1B shows, pediatricians also distinguish between different levels of treatment, being more ready to withdraw the "heroic" forms, depending upon the salvageability and type of damage of the patient. These findings also show that a social rather than a purely physiological definition of life is being used by these physicians in deciding whether or not to treat and how much treatment to give.

Similar distinctions were made by surgeons. Among neurosurgeons, the percentage saying that they would rarely operate ranged from 2 percent for a salvageable patient with physical damage, 20 percent for a salvageable patient with brain damage, 23 percent for an unsalvageable patient with physical damage, to 49 percent for an unsalvageable patient with brain damage.

Among pediatric heart surgeons, the percent saying that they would rarely operate ranged from 1 percent in the case of a child with an accompanying physical anomaly whose family situation was favorable, to 5 percent in a similar case where the family situation was unfavorable; and 14 percent in the case of a child with accompanying brain damage (mongolism) where the family situation was favorable, to 51 percent in a similar case where the family situation was unfavorable.[2]

Terminal Acts: Euthanasia and Definitions of Death

We have seen that physicians are reluctant to withdraw all therapy from the dying patient and that they reduce the level of treatment to a minimum only for certain types of patients. Are there situations in which physicians attempt to hasten or to bring about terminal events? Responses to a question in the pediatric questionnaire concerning direct killing of an anen-

---

[2] In both cases a favorable family situation was defined in terms of the family's desire to have the operation performed. An unfavorable situation was defined as the absence of financial resources in the case of the physical anomaly and as institutionalization of the child in the case of the mental anomaly.

cephalic infant were overwhelmingly negative. Among the respondents (both residents and physicians), only 1 percent said they would be likely to give an "intravenous injection of a lethal dose of potassium chloride or a sedative drug" to an anencephalic infant; 3 percent said that they might do so.[3]

Internists were asked to indicate whether or not they would increase the dosage of narcotics for a patient in the last stages of terminal cancer to the point where it might risk or would probably lead to respiratory arrest. Eighty-one percent of the physicians and 68 percent of the residents were willing to take "some" risk or "high" risk of inducing respiratory arrest in the patient by increasing his dosage of narcotics (see Table 4.2). While the same proportions of both groups were willing to incur "some" risk of respiratory arrest (38 percent and 39 percent respectively), the physicians were much more willing to incur "high" risk of respiratory arrest (43 percent) than were the residents (29 percent).

Specific questions to test their perceptions of the act were not included in the questionnaire, but presumably their willingness to prescribe heavy doses of narcotics in this situation is related to the fact that the patient's capacity for social interaction is limited because of his pain and, since his illness is terminal, it will not be renewed. Comments in the interviews suggested that some physicians defined this treatment as euthanasia while others argued that this procedure is not a true example of euthanasia since the physician's *intention* is to suppress pain and not to cause death. The following comment by a physician is an example of the latter:

> *How actively would you treat a patient with disseminated cancer which was accompanied by severe pain?* If it was the kind that couldn't be treated, I would give them as much pain medication as they want and nothing else. *Do you think that giving a lot of pain medication sometimes hastens death?* Yes, but I don't worry about it . . . If you give them a lot of morphine, this could be defined as unintentional hastening.

A resident, on the other hand, clearly perceived this type of behavior as euthanasia:

> If the person has terminal pain and has no chance of survival, then I favor negative euthanasia, that is allowing a disease to follow its downhill course without becoming heroic. Positive euthanasia would be overloading the person with drugs. *Would you do that?* No, I wouldn't.

It is possible, although there are no data to show this conclusively, that the older physician is more likely to make this distinction between intent and ac-

---

[3] These low figures are not due to the fact that the case involves an infant which might be expected to have special significance for physicians since 76 percent of the pediatricians indicated that they would turn off the respirator after brain death had occurred in an infant.

Table 4.2
Willingness to Risk Respiratory Arrest in the Prescription of Narcotics for a Terminally Ill Patient: Physicians and Residents in Internal Medicine

A. *Narcotics Decision: Physicians vs. Residents*[a]
(in percentages)

SPECIALTY: INTERNAL MEDICINE	No INCREASE IN DOSAGE	INCREASE WITHOUT DANGER OF RESPIRATORY ARREST	INCREASE WITH SOME RISK OF RESPIRATORY ARREST	INCREASE WITH HIGH RISK OF RESPIRATORY ARREST	No ANSWER	NUMBER OF RE- SPONDENTS
Physicians	—	18	38	43	—	660
Residents	1	31	39	29	—	750

[a] $\chi^2 = 85.3$, df $= 2$, p $< .01$.

B. *Respirator and Narcotics Decisions: Physicians vs. Residents*
(in percentages)

SPECIALTY: INTERNAL MEDICINE	PERCENT TURNING OFF RESPIRATOR[a]	PERCENT WILLING TO INCUR HIGH RISK TO LIFE OF PATIENT	NUMBER OF RESPONDENTS
Physicians	65	43	660
Residents	72	29	750

[a] See Table 4.3.

tion than the younger physician. In other words, for the older physicians, the important aspect of the use of narcotics with terminally ill patients is that it suppresses pain. The younger physician whose actions are closely supervised by others perceives both functions equally and is afraid that his action will be interpreted in terms of "hastening" death rather than in terms of pain-suppression.

Physicians in all four specialties were asked whether they would consider cessation of brain function, apart from cessation of respiratory and cardiac function, as a terminal event under certain precisely defined conditions. The conditions have been defined by an interdisciplinary committee at Harvard (Ad Hoc Committee of the Harvard Medical School to Examine the Definition of Brain Death, 1968).[4] In the four specialties, respondents were presented with cases appropriate for their specialties which were described as having the criteria of brain death, as defined by the Harvard Committee. The respondents were given several choices: leaving the respirator running until

---

[4] A review of 1,665 cases by a committee of the American Electroencephalographic Society found that in none of the cases which met the criteria described by the Harvard Committee, did brain function reappear (Silverman *et al.* 1969).

spontaneous cardiac activity ceased or turning off the respirator either without consultation with other persons or after consulting either colleagues or the patient's family or both. Most physicians accept irreversible cessation of brain function as a criterion for death permitting them to cease maintaining the patient's respiratory functions (see Table 4.3). In other words, for these physicians irreversible loss of the capacity for social interaction is a more important consideration than the continuation of the physiological indicator of life, heartbeat.

However, among those who accepted the criteria, no more than 18 percent in any of the samples were willing to turn off the respirator without any consultation whatsoever. This suggests that there is some ambivalence toward them since the agreement of either colleagues or family or preferably both is required by most of these physicians.

Why should these criteria be rejected by a quarter or more of the specialists in each of the samples (see Table 4.3)? This question cannot be answered directly from the data but the answer can be inferred from comments by respondents and informants. Turning off the respirator is viewed by some physicians as an act which directly involves the doctor in ending the patient's life. If brain death is not accepted as a definition of death, then turning off the respirator is euthanasia in the sense of "direct killing."

Some physicians feel that such a drastic step is unnecessary. The same result can be accomplished in other ways, for example, by not putting such a patient on a respirator with the result that respiratory arrest is soon followed by cardio-respiratory arrest. A pediatric informant commented:

> Certainly there are some children nobody would put on the respirator. In other words, if you have a severely malformed and damaged child that goes into respiratory arrest, usually you say, that's it, he's died.

An alternative strategy is to fail to maintain the respirator, as described in the following comment by a neurosurgical resident:

> If they have severe brain damage and no reflexes I will try not to put them on the respirator. If they are already on the respirator when they come to me, then I don't support the blood pressure or the heart function. I've never given vasopressor agents. I don't turn off the respirator but I omit therapy which then has the effect of hastening death.

Those who are willing to shut off the machine are also concerned about legal aspects. Consultation with the family is used in part as a method of insuring that they will accept the decision and not take legal action against the physician later. It is not considered appropriate for the family to make the final decision, however, as comments indicated. A pediatrician commented:

> The family should not be given the full responsibility for deciding on the child's life or death as they may subsequently experience considerable guilt.

Table 4.3
Decision to Continue or Discontinue Respirator in Case of
Brain Death by Specialty
(in percentages)

SPECIALTY	LEAVE RESPIRATOR RUNNING	TURN OFF AFTER CONSULTATION				TURN OFF WITHOUT CONSULTATION	NO ANSWER	NUMBER OF RESPONDENTS
		WITH COLLEAGUES ONLY	WITH FAMILY ONLY	WITH BOTH	(SUBTOTAL)			
Neuro-surgery	29	9	21	28	(58)	13	—	650
Pediatric heart surgery	30	14	8	43	(65)	6	—	207
Internal medicine	28	19	9	40	(68)	2	2	1,410
Pediatrics	24	26	8	32	(66)	6	4	922

The amount of recent experience with this type of decision varied widely among physicians in the various specialties. Respondents were asked to indicate how many patients in whom there was a question of brain death they had treated on respirators within the previous year. About 50 percent of the internists and pediatricians reported no cases of this sort within the past year (see Table 4.4). Thirty-nine percent of the pediatric surgeons had had no such cases. Medical and pediatric residents were much less likely to have had no recent experiences with these types of cases (12 percent and 19 percent respectively). Not surprisingly, only 6 percent of the neurosurgeons had had no such cases during the previous year. There did not appear, however, to be any relationship between willingness to turn off the respirator and recent experience with such cases.

The ambivalence which still exists in this area can be seen by comparing the attitudes expressed by pediatricians toward an infant defined as having the criteria of brain death and toward an anencephalic infant whose brain is nonexistent. Both infants lack functioning brains but pediatricians are much more willing to define as dead the infant whose brain has ceased to function than to withhold treatment entirely from an infant who was born without a brain.

While no more than 2 percent of the pediatricians said that they would resuscitate an anencephalic infant,[5] only 40 percent of the *physicians* and 31 percent of the *residents* indicated that they would not use any other forms of treatment. These percentages are substantially lower than the percentages who indicated that they would turn off the respirator when an infant's condition met the criteria for brain death (67 and 80 percent respectively).[6] It appears that the recent controversy over donation of hearts for transplants has made withdrawal of treatment in cases of brain death acceptable while absence of public discussion of an analogous type of decision, that of the anencephalic infant, has meant that it remains unacceptable.

During the interviews, respondents were asked how much treatment they would give to an anencephalic infant. Those who indicated that they would treat such infants were asked to explain why. Few of them could offer an explicit rationale. In general, it appeared that those who would treat such a child did so because the idea of completely withdrawing therapy was simply unthinkable.

Very few doctors seemed to have given such matters enough consideration to have worked out a philosophical position toward them. Only one out of

---

[5] Five percent said that they *might* resuscitate an anencephalic infant. Ninety-two percent said that they would *not* do so (see also Table 4.1B).

[6] This set of percentages includes only respondents who received the question about anencephaly in order to be strictly comparable to the percentages reported concerning anencephaly.

Table 4.4
Percentage of Physicians Who Did Not Treat Any Patients on
Respirators in Whom There Was A Question of Brain Death
Within Previous Year by Specialty[a]

SPECIALTY	PERCENTAGE OF PHYSICIANS WITH NO CASES OF PATIENTS ON RESPIRATORS WHO MET CRITERIA OF BRAIN DEATH	NUMBER OF RESPONDENTS
Neurosurgeons	6	650
Medical residents	12	750
Pediatric residents	19	475
Pediatric heart surgeons	39	207
Pediatricians	50	447
Internists	52	660

[a] This table is based on responses to the following question: In the past year, how many patients (infants, children) have you treated on the respirator in whom there was a question of brain death?

eighteen interns and residents who were interviewed argued that he would treat such an infant on the basis of an innate respect for life:

> I think you probably end up getting religious. Everybody, insofar as these are children who are alive, tends to respect that life. Life has a value in itself . . . I don't think that you can place a value on existence in terms of retardation. Insofar as they are people, they have an absolute value.

Another resident who had recently been involved in the care of such an infant took the opposite point of view:

> I don't think that there is any sense in artificially prolonging the life of an anencephalic child. These are not beings that have a soul. I have an equivalent amount of reverence for all of life and I assume that man is of more worth than other animals. I don't enjoy killing but I could kill an anencephalic child. The residents in the premature nursery said that the decision should have been made in the delivery room. Once it was in the premature nursery, we were obligated to feed and care for it . . . They held a meeting and decided that the child should be fed and allowed to die of its own accord. I think that it's silly to attach worth to something at that point . . . If we were going to let it die, why should we feed it? It's incapable of suffering.

Decisions to Reverse Death: Norms Concerning Resuscitation

Decisions to resuscitate terminally ill patients and infants with congenital anomalies or severe birth defects evoked considerable controversy among physicians and nurses in the settings where interviews were conducted for this study.

Controversial cases tended to be those in which a patient with a terminal illness or severe brain damage had been resuscitated. In some of these cases, the physician had been unaware of the diagnosis at the time of the resuscitation. In cases where they were unfamiliar with the patient's medical history, the house staff believed that it was necessary to resuscitate a patient on the assumption that he might be salvageable. An example of such a case was described by a nurse on the non-private service:

> A lot of people were disgusted about that resuscitation because the patient had no brain function and it shouldn't have been done. The charge nurse and the intern did it. They didn't know the patient had no brain function.

Use of resuscitative procedures upon newborns was also controversial. An argument against resuscitating newborns with congenital anomalies was provided by a pediatric resident who responded to the questionnaire:

> Babies with congenital anomalies who arrest are generally not resuscitated if their prognosis is poor. My own feeling is that we do not often enough consider the financial burden to the hospital, state, and family, the work burden to the nursing staff (detracting from the adequate care of less sick normal infants), and the emotional burden assumed by staff and family as they become more and more involved in and optimistic about an infant whose chances of survival are very low, and of a normal, non-institutional existence zero.

In general, the surveys showed that the same criteria which are used in decisions to allocate treatment to patients are used in decisions to resuscitate. Salvageable patients with physical damage were more likely to be resuscitated than salvageable patients with brain damage or unsalvageable patients with physical damage. Severely brain-damaged salvageable patients were not as frequently resuscitated as moderately brain-damaged salvageable patients and the same distinction was made between severely and moderately physically damaged patients. However, in the cases of moderately mentally damaged salvageable patients and unsalvageable physically damaged patients, the proportions of internists who said that they would resuscitate these patients were higher than the proportions who said that they would treat them actively (see Table 4.5).

Although this technique is not recommended for those who are terminally ill (Charlebois 1968), it is interesting to note that over one third of the internists said that they would be likely to begin resuscitation upon patients with terminal disease (cancer, multiple sclerosis). However, only 14 percent indicated that they would be likely to begin resuscitation upon a patient who was described as being in an advanced stage of a very painful form of cancer, cancer of the esophagus (see Table 4.5).

Unlike the internists, the proportions of pediatricians who said that they would resuscitate salvageable patients were lower than the proportions who said that they would treat such patients actively (see Table 4.6). This is surprising since the technique is much more dramatic when practiced upon adults than upon children.

While it was clear from the interviews and the surveys that norms concerning brain damage and salvageability were perceived as applying to decisions to resuscitate, young physicians sometimes had difficulty using these criteria and resuscitated patients whom others felt should not have been resuscitated. At times the young physician may be upset by the consequences of his own vigorous efforts. A pediatric intern described such a case during an interview:

> We brought a baby back after 45 minutes and now it's in an institution [for mentally retarded children]. I know an intern who feels remorse every night about this. The baby has been readmitted to the hospital twice for feeding problems. The family has been wrecked by the child. The parents were

Table 4.5
Treatment vs. Resuscitation of Adult Patients by Internists

PHYSICIAN BEHAVIOR	PATIENT'S PROGNOSIS[a]				
	SALVAGEABLE		UNSALVAGEABLE		
	MODERATE BRAIN DAMAGE	SEVERE BRAIN DAMAGE	MODERATE PHYSICAL DAMAGE CASE (1)	CASE (2)	SEVERE PHYSICAL DAMAGE
Percent who would treat actively	30	16	36	28	3
Percent who would resuscitate	48	17	43	36	14
Number of cases	(909)	(501)	(909)	(501)	(1,410)

[a] Column 1: stroke with moderate brain damage; $z = 113.4$, $p < .01$.
Column 2: severe cerebral atrophy; n.s.
Column 3: melanoma of the leg metastasized to the spinal cord; $z = 108.1$, $p < .01$.
Column 4: multiple sclerosis; $z = 83.1$, $p < .01$.
Column 5: cancer of the esophagus; $z = 184.6$, $p < .01$.

Table 4.6
Treatment vs. Resuscitation of Salvageable Infants by Pediatricians
(N = 922)

PHYSICIAN BEHAVIOR	PATIENT'S TYPE OF DAMAGE[a]		
	PHYSICAL	MENTAL	
		CASE (1)	CASE (2)
Percent who would treat actively	55	52	47
Percent who would resuscitate	29	16	16

[a] Column 1: myelomeningocele; $z = 62.1$, $p < .01$.
Column 2: mongoloid with severe respiratory distress; $z = 54.7$, $p < .01$.
Column 3: seizures with spasticity and hypertonia; $z = 58.1$, $p < .01$.

very young and very immature. We feel a lot of guilt about it. There's tremendous expense to the state and the federal government involved.

A number of factors contributed to such decisions: the young physician's lack of expertise in determining at what point treatment should be withdrawn in a terminal patient, social pressures to resuscitate, and the desire to improve skill with the technique itself. These factors undoubtedly reinforce each other and contribute at times to unnecessary resuscitations such as the following one described by a nurse:

We had a 46-year-old male who arrested. He had been dialyzed and then arrested. He was resuscitated and lived for one hour. [A senior physician] said: "It was a sin to make this man breathe again." *Why did he say that?* Because the patient would die anyway. He only had one kidney and that kidney was damaged.

The same nurse described the social pressures which can influence the young physician to resuscitate unnecessarily:

You tend to feel helpless if you don't do something. The emergency cart is right there and everyone expects you to do something, so I understand why the intern does it.

Some nurses who were interviewed were highly critical of what they considered to be unnecessary resuscitations. They were more aware than the house staff of the undesirable consequences of such resuscitations—their negative effects on total patient care on the hospital service. A nurse described these problems in an interview:

When we resuscitate a patient, frequently an RN has to spend hours and hours with that patient. A good percentage of the personnel on the floor will be devoted to a particular resuscitation. This means that the rest of the patients are not getting as good care as they otherwise would.

Members of the pediatric house staff said that sometimes they were unable to reach a decision in advance as to whether or not a child with severe problems should be resuscitated if he had a cardio-respiratory arrest. A pediatric resident said:

We discussed whether or not to resuscitate. Each time we discussed it, we were unable to make a decision so that when the child stopped breathing we did resuscitate because we hadn't decided not to.

The technique of resuscitation is one which requires considerable practice before the requisite skill is achieved. A resident commented on the questionnaire:

As a university teaching service we tend to attempt resuscitation in all patients, particularly at the beginning of the academic year.

In the pediatric nursery, this was rationalized by saying that if they did not practice on a baby who "doesn't matter" they would not know how to use the technique for a normal baby.

On the questionnaire, internists were asked to rate a number of professional considerations which would affect their treatment of a debilitated, chronically ill patient. "Opportunity to learn, practice, or teach new techniques" was rated among the top three out of six items by only 28 percent of the internists. The difference between residents and physicians was negligible. When asked about the influence of professional values upon their decisions to treat infants with congenital anomalies, 39 percent of the pediatricians ranked "Opportunity to learn, practice, or teach new techniques" among the top three out of six items.

Some members of the house staff claimed that there were fewer resuscitations at the end of the academic year (which runs from July 1 to June 30) than at the beginning. The performance of resuscitative procedures in order to practice the technique was said to produce this result. In fact, a study of the hospital records of all patients who died or who were successfuly resuscitated during an entire year showed that there were substantially fewer resuscitations in May and June than in the other ten months of the year (35 percent as compared to 53 percent). There was no relationship between month and number of major treatment or diagnostic procedures which were used on the patients.

Whether or not the patient had the right to refuse resuscitation was also a subject of controversy. Some informants thought that a patient should not be resuscitated if he had indicated that he did not wish to be resuscitated. Others disagreed. A case in which a retired nurse was resuscitated against her will was reported to have caused considerable controversy in one of the hospitals in which interviews were conducted. Two contradictory views of this event were described by a nurse and an intern:

> Recently a retired nurse was resuscitated on the private service and there's been a lot of controversy about that. There was a note in her handbag saying that she didn't want to be resuscitated. This has caused a lot of us to think about these things. I think that she shouldn't have been resuscitated. She had barely been able to walk for the last fifteen years and she was very old. She was 80 years old.

> Sometimes there is controversy between the nurses and the house staff. For example, there was an elderly former nurse who entered the hospital saying that she did not want to be resuscitated. However, she was resuscitated and now is doing well. Actually, I don't think that patients have the right to refuse resuscitation although some of the nurses think they do.

The survey results showed that the attitude of the patient had less influence upon the decision to resuscitate than it did upon the decision to treat (see

Table 4.7

Influence of Patient's Attitude upon Treatment and Resuscitation of Adult Patients with Physical Damage by Internists

PHYSICIAN BEHAVIOR	PATIENT'S PROGNOSIS			
	UNSALVAGEABLE[a]		UNCERTAIN[b]	
	PATIENT'S ATTITUDE TOWARD TREATMENT[c]			
	FAVORABLE	UNFAVORABLE	FAVORABLE	UNFAVORABLE
Percent who would treat actively	51	22	47	33
Percent who would re-suscitate	48	33	64	58
Number of cases	(430)	(479)	(479)	(430)

[a] Melanoma of the leg metastasized to the spinal cord.
Row 1: $z = 16.71$, $p < .01$; Row 2: $z = 7.78$, $p < .01$.
[b] Myocardial infarction combined with jaundice and history of lung cancer.
Row 1: $z = 5.98$, $p < .01$; Row 2: $z = 3.21$, $p < .01$.
[c] In the unsalvageable case, the patient requests to be treated actively or not to be treated actively. In the case where the prognosis was uncertain, the patient is described as being alternatively optimistic about the future or fatalistic about dying.

Table 4.7). The attitude of the infant's family also had less influence upon the decision to resuscitate than upon the decision to treat (see Table 4.8).[7]

Conclusion

Evidence has been presented which shows that for both internists and pediatricians the patient's capacity for social interaction is a significant factor in their decisions to withdraw treatment. In addition, both internists and pediatricians distinguish between different levels of treatment, being more ready to withdraw the "heroic" forms when patients are terminal or severely damaged or both.

In certain types of situations which the physican encounters frequently and which are visible to the medical profession and even to the general public, norms have emerged which permit the physician in effect to hasten death. Two examples of this are the prescription of narcotics to terminal patients in

Table 4.8

Influence of Family Attitude upon Treatment and Resuscitation of Salvageable Infants by Pediatricians

PHYSICIAN BEHAVIOR	SALVAGEABLE INFANTS WITH BRAIN DAMAGE[a]			
	CASE 1		CASE 2	
	FAMILY ATTITUDE TOWARD TREATMENT			
	FAVORABLE	UNFAVORABLE	FAVORABLE	UNFAVORABLE
Percent who would treat actively	58	33	59	44
Percent who would re- suscitate	17	13	22	11
Number of cases	(458)	(464)	(464)	(458)

[a] Columns 1 and 2: seizures with spasticity and hypertonia;
Columns 3 and 4: mongoloid with severe respiratory distress.

Family attitude: Row 1: col 1 vs. col 2: $z = 12.24$, $p < .01$
Row 2: col 1 vs. col 2: $z = 4.81$, $p < .01$
Row 1: col 3 vs. col 4: $z = 10.57$, $p < .01$
Row 2: col 3 vs. col 4: $z = 8.87$, $p < .01$

---

[7] Among the internists, the effect of age and social class variables is very similar with respect to both types of medical behavior. Among the pediatricians, the effect of socioeconomic status disappears in decisions to resuscitate.

pain and the termination of respirator treatment for the patient who has suffered irreversible brain death.

The physician's response to the patient who has already died appears to be closer to the traditional medical ethic than his treatment of dying patients. Although resuscitation procedures are not recommended for terminal patients, a substantial proportion of respondents indicated that they would resuscitate patients who had died of terminal illness. In fact, the proportions of internists who said that they would resuscitate moderately brain-damaged salvageable patients and physically damaged unsalvageable patients were higher than the proportions saying that they would actively treat these patients. Pediatricians, on the other hand, were less likely to say that they would resuscitate salvageable infants than that they would treat them actively.

In the following chapter, we will examine the actual records of patients who died in a university hospital to see whether the treatment which they received corresponded to the findings from the surveys.

Chapter 5: Decision-Making Viewed
Through Hospital Records*

A reasonable criticism of the type of data which have been presented in the previous chapters is that it may not reflect the actual behavior of physicians. In order to validate these findings, attempts were made to obtain information from hospital records concerning the treatment of critically ill patients. The principal problem in conducting such studies is to find suitable samples of cases. After much consideration, it was decided that the most appropriate way to validate the study of doctors' attitudes toward the treatment of critically ill adult patients was through: (1) Examination of the hospital charts for all patients who had died and all those who had been successfully resuscitated during a calendar year (1969) on the non-private[1] service of the major teaching hospital in which most of the interviews were conducted; (2) Observation of a sample of patients on this service during the course of their treatment.

In order to validate in part the study of decisions to perform pediatric heart surgery, the hospital charts of all cases of mongoloid children with heart defects who were seen and catheterized by pediatric heart surgeons at the

---

*Portions of material in this chapter appeared in the article: Diana Crane, "Decisions to treat critically ill patients: a comparison of social versus medical considerations," *The Milbank Memorial Fund Quarterly/Health and Society*, Winter 1975.

[1] On the non-private service, patients are cared for by interns and residents under the supervision of senior physicians.

same hospital during the period 1964–69 were studied. No attempt was made to validate the surveys of pediatricians and neurosurgeons.

Critically Ill Patients in the Hospital Records:
Research Design and Data Collection

A major problem in studying factors associated with death and resuscitations was to obtain a complete listing of patients who had experienced these events. The hospital provided a computer listing of the hospital record numbers of all patients who had died on its clinical service in 1969. In order to obtain a list of patients who had been successfully resuscitated, a complete list of patients on that service for whom resuscitation equipment had been utilized was obtained from the office supplying this equipment. Whether or not the patients had actually been resuscitated was checked in their hospital charts (including the physician's notes on the case and the notes prepared by nurses who had provided intensive nursing care). A few patients from the list of those for whom resuscitation equipment had been used had not been resuscitated. In these cases, it is likely that the patients had had a crisis which required use of equipment from a resuscitation cart but had not had a cardiac or respiratory arrest. In addition, a few patients on the list of deaths which the hospital provided had been resuscitated (according to their charts) but were not on the list of resuscitations. Usually these patients had been resuscitated in the emergency room. It seems likely that the sample is complete with respect to persons who died. It may be incomplete with respect to a few persons who were resuscitated and lived since resuscitations are not always recorded in hospital charts. For the same reason, it may also slightly underestimate the number of resuscitations which were performed upon those who died. The total number of cases in the sample was 286.

Since hospital records vary greatly in the amount of information which they provide about a patient, a number of other sources of information were also used. For all patients in the sample upon whom autopsies had been performed (46 percent of the sample), the clinical summaries of their cases which were compiled prior to the autopsy were consulted. Diagnoses were coded from these clinical summaries by a second-year medical student who had recently completed a pathology clerkship.[2] For the remaining patients, diagnoses were obtained from the hospital records and coded with the advice of the medical student. The diagnosis which was coded was the one which was provided on the patient's discharge summary and which probably repre-

---

[2] The author is grateful to Evelyn Roberts for her assistance in this matter and to Stephanie Garrett, R.N., for her assistance in the earlier phases of this segment of the study.

sents the final clinical opinion of the case. The records of 5 percent of the cases could not be located. For these cases, computer listings of the discharge summaries were used to code the diagnoses. Major diagnostic or treatment procedures which had been performed on the patient were defined as those which required the signed permission of the patient or a member of his family. They were coded on the basis of the presence of signed permission slips in the hospital chart for that patient *and* a record in the chart that the procedure had been carried out, such as the physician's notes or a formal record of the procedure itself.

Social variables such as age, sex, and race were available from the hospital's computer listing. Data on social class and the patient's living arrangements were coded from the charts and also from the admission slips which are filled out when a patient enters the hospital. Information about alcoholism, drug addiction, and psychiatric problems was coded from the hospital charts.[3]

The charts and autopsy records were also searched for evidence of degree of brain damage. If the patient had had a stroke, this was coded. If the chart said that he had sustained severe documented brain damage, this was also coded. If the chart indicated that there was a possibility of brain damage, this was coded as such.

In general, it must be understood in interpreting these data that a hospital chart is by no means a complete record of events and decisions which take place during the patient's stay in the hospital. The accuracy and consistency of the information obtained from charts concerning degree of brain damage, physical damage, and salvageability is open to question. It is with this qualification that the findings in the following section are presented.

Because of the difficulties in obtaining complete and accurate data from the hospital charts, an attempt was made to follow cases while they were being treated on the same non-private service. These data were collected by a nursing instructor[4] who was training students on this service. In connection with her teaching duties, it was necessary for her to be familiar with the histories and progress of the patients on the service. Using a record of admissions which is maintained on each of the floors of this service, she took every third patient admitted by each of the two interns on one of the floors of the service (and, if she had time, a similar series for interns on the other two floors of the service). If the patient did not have heart disease, cancer,

---

[3] It was found that it was *not* possible to code certain types of information from the hospital charts, such as physicians' perceptions of patients' life expectancies and families' attitudes toward patients.

[4] The author is grateful to Susan Daggett, R.N., for her assistance with this phase of the study. These patients were admitted to the non-private service between November and January, 1970–71.

a chronic respiratory, renal, or liver disease, or stroke (cerebrovascular accident), the patient was discarded and the next third admission was taken. Data were recorded concerning use of major diagnostic and treatment procedures, including resuscitation, and extent of mental and physical damage, doctor's perceptions of the patient's life expectancy, and social variables, such as age, race, and social class.

Treatment of Critically Ill Patients: Hospital Records versus Questionnaires

Fifty percent of the patients in the hospital records sample were resuscitated; only 11 percent of those who were resuscitated were discharged alive. Such statistics are not unusual. Most studies indicate that success rates for resuscitations (defined as percentage of patients discharged from the hospital) are less than 20 percent (Jung *et al.* 1968).

On the assumption that each resuscitation in the hospital records sample represents a decision by a member of the house staff of a prestigious hospital, these data will be compared with the behavior of those residents in the internal medicine survey who were located in prestigious medical settings.[5] In the first part of the subsequent analysis, an attempt will be made to compare cases in the two samples which are as much alike as possible. Afterwards, some general trends in the hospital records will be presented.

As Table 5.2A shows, of those who had cardiac or respiratory arrests on the first day of their hospital stay, 68 percent were resuscitated. Among those who had such arrests after their tenth day in the hospital, 33 percent were resuscitated. This confirms the impression obtained from the exploratory interviews that physicians tend to resuscitate patients when they do not know their medical histories. On the non-private service whose medical records were examined, patients were usually unknown to the house staff prior to admission. Since resuscitations which were performed after there had been sufficient time for an adequate evaluation of the patient are more likely to reflect the criteria which are used in evaluating critically ill patients, resuscitations which were performed during the first two days of the patient's hospital stay before a thorough assessment of the patient's condition could have been performed are not included in the first part of the following analysis.

---

[5] Prestige of the hospitals included in the sample was determined by the prestige of their medical school affiliations. The relative prestige of the latter was evaluated using the mean Medical College Achievement Test (MCAT) science scores of the medical students which they admitted in 1967. The top eight schools were considered as having high prestige since their scores were substantially higher than those of the other medical schools. This group included the medical school affiliation of the hospital where the exploratory interviews were conducted.

The number of cases in the hospital records sample in which the diagnoses closely resembled the diagnoses of patients described in the questionnaire was small. In addition, a substantial number of the patients in the hospital records sample who were resuscitated were resuscitated on the first or second hospital day (52 percent). On the whole, the decision-making patterns in the two samples were similar (see Table 5.1). In other words, in both samples, controlling for type of damage, salvageable patients were more frequently resuscitated than unsalvageable patients and, among the salvageable patients, those with physical damage more frequently than those with mental damage. The major exception was the high proportion of resuscitations among pa-

Table 5.1
Decisions to Resuscitate by Residents in Internal Medicine:
Survey[a] vs. Hospital Records

PATIENT'S PROGNOSIS AND TYPE OF DAMAGE[b]		PERCENT OF MEDICAL RESIDENTS	
		WHO WOULD RESUSCITATE: SURVEY	WHO DID RESUSCITATE: HOSPITAL RECORDS
Salvageable-Physical:		76 (75)	58 (17)
Salvageable-Mental:		45 (75)	27 (15)
Unsalvageable-Physical:	(i)	55 (27)	67 (6)
	(ii)	35 (48)	—
	(iii)	15 (75)	13 (16)
Unsalvageable-Mental:	(i)	—	33 (6)
	(ii)	—	17 (6)

[a] Subgroup of sample who were located in prestigious medical settings (see footnote 5).
[b] Row 1: chronic pulmonary fibrosis; cardiovascular and pulmonary diseases.
Row 2: stroke with moderate or severe brain damage.
Row 3: multiple sclerosis; multiple sclerosis and similar types of diseases.
Row 4: melanoma of the leg metastasized to the spinal cord.
Row 5: cancer of the esophagus; metastatic cancer (all types).
Row 6: multiple sclerosis and similar types of diseases combined with moderate or severe brain damage.
Row 7: metastatic cancer (all types) combined with moderate or severe brain damage.

tients with multiple sclerosis and similar types of diseases in both the survey and the hospital records sample. The subgroup of medical residents in the survey was not typical of the national sample of medical residents in this respect and it is interesting that a similar difference is found in the hospital records sample (although the number of cases is very small).

The data tentatively suggest that the survey respondents may have exaggerated their likelihood of resuscitating patients since the proportions of patients resuscitated in the hospital records sample is lower than in the survey. Since the study as a whole is concerned with the conditions under which treatment is withdrawn, these data suggest that it may actually be withdrawn to a greater extent than the survey results suggest. Alternatively, the lower rate of resuscitation in the hospital records study may be due to the fact that doctors were not available at the time some of the deaths occurred.

When the entire group of cases is examined, the relative priorities accorded to different types of illnesses are also evident. For the purposes of this analysis, chronic diseases were categorized into three types[6]: terminal diseases of extended duration such as metastatic cancer and uremia; slow-wasting diseases such as multiple sclerosis; and degenerative diseases such as cirrhosis of the liver, cardiovascular disease, and pulmonary disease.[7] These three types of diseases differ in terms of salvageability, the first type being the least salvageable and the third type the most salvageable. Within the first category, it appeared that physicians distinguished in terms of salvageability between diseases such as metastatic cancer and uremia, and conditions such as malignant hypertension and chronic renal failure. Again, in order to see the nature of the priorities which are accorded to these different types of illnesses, it is necessary to distinguish between the group which was resuscitated within the first two hospital days and the remainder (see Table 5.2B). The problem is complicated by the fact that these disease conditions frequently occur in combination with one another.

Although the numbers are small, it is clear that cases of metastatic cancer and uremia are not likely to be resuscitated. Since this is true both among those who died or were resuscitated early in their hospital stay and among the remaining cases, it appears that these conditions are easily identifiable,

---

[6] This set of categories was devised by Evelyn Roberts.

[7] The complete set of definitions is as follows: *Terminal Conditions, Extended Duration:* metastatic carcinoma, lethal non-metastatic carcinoma (e.g., oat cell, leukemia), uremia, malignant hypertension, chronic renal failure, progressive liver failure, acute yellow atrophy; *Slow-Wasting Diseases:* malignant cancer not proven to be metastatic, benign tumors, multiple sclerosis, myasthenia gravis, subacute hepatic necrosis, Hodgkins disease; *Degenerative Diseases:* cirrhosis, arteriosclerotic cardiovascular disease, emphysema and bronchitis, diabetes, history of cardiovascular accident, alcoholism. Various combinations of these conditions were also coded.

Table 5.2
Variables Related to Resuscitation in Hospital Records Study

A. Timing

	DAY OF CARDIAC OR RESPIRATORY ARREST[a]			
	1	2	3-10	OVER 10
Percent resuscitated	68 (88)	50 (26)	47 (86)	33 (81)

[a] $G = -.41$ (Goodman and Kruskal's gamma)

B. Type of Disease

	TYPE OF DISEASE[b]					
	TERMINAL EXTENDED: CANCER OR UREMIA, ALONE OR IN COMBI-NATION	TERMINAL EXTENDED: OTHER, ALONE OR IN COMBI-NATION	SLOW-WASTING	DEGEN-ERATIVE	COMBINA-TION OF SLOW-WASTING AND DEGEN-ERATIVE	OTHER
Deaths during first two days of hospital stay						
Percent resuscitated	17 (18)	85 (13)	73 (11)	80 (44)	72 (7)	78 (18)
Deaths after first two days of hospital stay						
Percent resuscitated	16 (31)	53 (17)	33 (9)	48 (71)	50 (14)	67 (12)

[b] Row 1: $G = .40$; Row 2: $G = .37$.

C. Brain Damage

	AMOUNT OF BRAIN DAMAGE[c]		
	NONE	POSSIBLE	SEVERE
Percent resuscitated	58 (115)	47 (118)	33 (39)

[c] $G = -.28$

and are not likely to be given this type of heroic treatment at any time. Among the remaining categories of conditions, no priorities are visible in the treatment of those who died or were resuscitated within two days after admission.

Among members of the group that were resuscitated later, priorities are discernible. The priorities appear to be allocated in terms of salvageability: metastatic cancer and uremia are least likely to be resuscitated; slow-wasting diseases are next, then degenerative diseases, combinations of these two and the second type of terminal extended disease (see Table 5.2B). Patients with the other conditions which included acute illnesses and strokes are most likely to be resuscitated.

Brain damage is a condition which cross-cuts these categories. When this was looked at separately, there was an inverse relationship between degree of brain damage and resuscitation (see Table 5.2C). It was also clear that patients with severe brain damage were more likely to die or to be resuscitated during the first two hospital days than later.[8]

The same set of priorities can be seen in the allocation of treatment or diagnostic procedures to the different types of chronic conditions although the relationship is not as strong (table not shown). The fact that length of hospital stay is correlated with number of procedures used[9] clouds the issue. This relationship is to be expected since the longer the patient stays in the hospital, the more opportunities there are to use major procedures on him.

Another way of assessing the priorities which are accorded these types of patients is through the comments which are written on the hospital charts by the interns and residents during the course of treatment. Very few residents and interns made comments which indicated their philosophy of treatment. The few comments which do appear are of some interest. The following comment documents a type of decision which, according to the data, is quite frequently made — the decision not to treat actively a patient with metastatic cancer:

> The plan is not to be at all vigorous in treating this cancer patient, and her hypercalcemia which is 17.6 is only being treated with hydration. The family realizes what is occurring and is in full agreement . . . Would continue only minimum supportive care.

A note in the records by an intern who also discussed the same patient in an interview reveals the ambivalence that is probably not untypical of young physicians in such cases. In the interview he described the patient as:

> . . . an 84-year-old emergency case. She had been lying at home comatose and incontinent for two weeks before her family brought her to the hospital.

---

[8] Sixty-seven percent of those with severe documented brain damage died or were resuscitated during the first two hospital days compared to 36 percent of those who had possible brain damage and 36 percent of those with no brain damage.

[9] Thirty-eight percent of those who stayed in the hospital for up to seven days had had a major diagnostic or treatment procedure compared to 75 percent of those who had stayed over 21 days in the hospital (N = 251).

We treated her with antibiotics and I.V. for two days. She remained unresponsive. The attending physicians wanted to stop everything. The residents wanted to dialyze her. This is a major procedure . . . The conflict here is that the younger physicians are more interested in technology. The residents have seen miraculous cures. You can't predict what kind of cure you'll get. Perhaps for every dramatic cure you get, there is the cost of putting people through unnecessary prolongation procedures.

In the patient's chart, he wrote:

Will not dialyze because although it only represents a slight increase in the intensity of our efforts, we must be willing to stop at some point when considering the rehabilitation potential of this 84-year-old patient and the severity of her disease.

A few hours later, he wrote:

At about 1:45 she stopped breathing entirely and had no detectable pulse. *Brief efforts at resuscitation were unsuccessful.* [Italics by the author.]

On the other hand, a patient dying from a very painful type of cancer, cancer of the esophagus, is described in the clinical summary of the autopsy records as receiving painful procedures which did not alleviate his discomfort:

Dysphagia was of such a degree that the patient would only tolerate liquids and these with significant burning pain . . . The possibility of a gastrostomy was raised but surgical opinion was that the patient would benefit little. An intra-esophageal tube was therefore recommended and a Davol tube was placed without difficulty by the ENT surgeons. Following this, swallowing was difficult and I.V. fluids were required. Pain in the throat was a notable feature . . . A barium swallow showed a fistulous tract beside the esophageal replacement tube, the termination of which was uncertain . . . Repeat esophagoscopy was performed, at which time the Davol tube was advanced to bridge the cardia. Post-operatively there was no X-ray evidence of pneumonia or perforation. Local irritation was still a feature. Three days later, after no further improvement, the patient was found dead at 8:00 a.m.

The autopsy revealed that:

[the Davol feeding tube] seemed to have gone into the submucosa and the muscularis mucosae at the level of the cardia and one can see that there must have been great difficulty inserting the tube since there is a big tumor nodule at the level of the cardia which probably forced the top of the tube from the esophageal lumen into the submucosa and musculares . . . The misplacement of the tube meant that the relieving function was not served.

Occasionally conflicts between staff or between staff and family members were evident from the records. The following series of notes describes a conflict between the intern in charge of a patient's care and a resident from another department who acted as a consultant on the case:

Intern's on-service note (February 1): This is the third hospital day for this unfortunate 55-year-old male with disseminated Ca [cancer] of the large bowel and hepatic metastases. He underwent exploratory laparotomy in January at which time the above was noticed as well as entrapment of the left ureter which apparently could not be freed . . . Last night he underwent retrograde study which showed the left ureter to be completely occluded and the right to have almost total occlusion. I have talked to Dr. _____, the GU resident who saw the patient and he states that after much discussion they have decided not to perform a *nephrotomy* because of the patient's underlying condition and the complexity of the procedure. This is a difficult decision in this patient and although it is likely that he may die soon of his Ca we think that there are a few more months of relatively useful life left and the patient could be benefited by a draining procedure. If this is not done he will certainly die soon from renal failure.

Note by GU resident (February 1): The only feasible type of diversion for this man would be an R nephrotomy. (This is a major procedure.) I do not feel this is indicated. With metastases to the liver, his survival at best can be measured in months—regardless of what he looks like today. I might add that life with a nephrotomy is in itself decidedly unpleasant.

Intern's note (February 2): . . . Urologists will not do diversion procedure but Dr. _____ will talk to them re this. Have put patient on an acute renal failure regimen . . . Will try to get urologists to reconsider.

Intern's note (February 6): Patient is gradually but definitely going down the tubes . . . Urologists have finally decided not to give patient diversionary procedure.

The following note describes an 83-year-old female patient who was actively treated against the wishes of her family:

Patient now afebrile and is on Methicillin therapy for probable pneumonia. In view of her deteriorating clinical status . . . the patient has been started on peritoneal dialysis. The decision to dialyze her was made because it is felt that she has a potentially reversible acute process superimposed upon a chronic renal disease. This decision is supported by Dr. _____, Dr. _____, Dr. _____, and the hospital administrator and lawyer were consulted prior to dialysis in view of the family's refusal to sign the permission form.

This patient died in the hospital without being resuscitated nineteen days later. Refusals of treatment by patients and their families were relatively infrequent on this service. Nurses who were in charge of the various floors of the service claimed that such refusals occurred rarely. Only one instance of a refusal of treatment occurred among the 96 cases which were followed on this service. The interviews suggested that refusals of treatment were more common on the private service but no data were collected to substantiate this hypothesis.

Non-Private Service Patients: Observations of Treatment

The non-private service whose records are the subject of the analysis being presented in this chapter treats approximately 5000 patients per year. The 286 deaths and resuscitations represent therefore only 6 percent of the total patient population. These are of course the patients who are unquestionably "critically ill." Observations of a random sample of patients who were admitted to the service were undertaken in part to see if the results would vary from those obtained on the basis of an analysis of the hospital charts. Since the latter are often incomplete, it is possible that observations of patients during the course of their treatment yields more accurate information and hence different results from those described above.

The patients in the random sample were not as ill as those in the hospital records sample. Only 5 percent were resuscitated and only 6 percent died, compared to 50 percent resuscitated and 94 percent dead in the sample of deaths and resuscitations. When their diseases were rated as minor, moderate or major by the nurse-observer, 5 percent of the patients had minor illnesses only, 53 percent had moderate illnesses, and 38 percent had major illnesses.[10] Seventy-one percent of the sample were considered by those in charge of their care to have a life expectancy of over a year. Forty-eight percent had received some type of diagnostic or treatment procedure compared to 48 percent of the other sample. However, many patients in the hospital records sample were not on the service long enough to have had such procedures performed. Forty-three percent of the hospital records sample stayed in the hospital more than a week compared to 61 percent of the random sample. Among those in the hospital records sample who stayed more than a week, 66 percent had received a major procedure. Fifty-three percent of those in the random sample who had stayed more than a week had received such a procedure.

Medically their conditions were also somewhat different. In the random

---

[10] A minor illness was one which was temporary with complete recovery possible and no residual damage (e.g., pneumonia). A moderate illness was one which involved acute exacerbation with residual damage (e.g., acute renal failure with kidney damage or a slowly progressive terminal cancer). A major illness was one which involved a threat to life. The patient could die and will have definite residual damage if he lives. The possibility of survival is tenuous even if he survives an acute episode (e.g., outpatient with uremia who cannot be dialyzed or a rapidly progressing terminal cancer).

sample there were many more cases of degenerative diseases than in the hospital records sample (68 percent compared to 46 percent) and fewer cases of slow-wasting diseases (4 percent compared to 15 percent). These differences are due in part to the nature of the sampling used in selecting the random sample. Only 8 percent of the random sample had suffered brain damage compared to 56 percent of the hospital records sample, but about the same proportions were deviant (30 percent). The random sample was somewhat younger than the hospital records sample.

Again, there was no relationship between deviance and the use of treatment or diagnostic procedures (see Chapter 3 for a discussion of this relationship in the hospital records sample). However, while there was a strong inverse relationship between age and the use of treatment and diagnostic procedures in the hospital records sample, this relationship was direct in the random sample. There was no apparent reason for this difference in the findings in the two samples. Patients with terminal conditions in the random sample were much more likely to have received major procedures than in the hospital records sample (72 percent compared to 37 percent). This is probably due to the fact that these patients in the random sample had a longer life expectancy than those in the hospital records sample and could therefore be expected to benefit from such procedures. Thirty-eight percent of the terminal patients in the random sample were estimated by staff to have a life expectancy of over a year, 29 percent a life expectancy of six months to a year, and 29 percent a life expectancy of less than six months. While about the same proportions of each of these three groups received major procedures, even those whose life expectancy was less than six months were probably more likely to be able to benefit from such procedures than those in the hospital records sample. Another reason that the figure for the hospital records sample is not higher may be that some of the terminal patients may have been thoroughly worked up before — in some cases, not long before — and hence did not need to have certain procedures repeated.

On the whole the data gathered by observations of patient care are consistent with the findings of the data gathered from the hospital records. It suggests that the latter method is adequate for such studies provided that the data collected are relatively precise and of sufficient importance to be routinely entered on the patient's chart.

Mongoloid Children with Heart Defects: Hospital Records

The survey of pediatric heart surgeons showed very clearly that these surgeons are unwilling to operate upon mongoloid children unless the parents are very anxious to have the operations performed (see Table 3.6). Even then many surgeons say that they would not be likely to perform such operations. It is therefore of interest to examine hospital records of mongoloid children with heart defects in order to find out how frequently operations are performed upon these children.

A complete listing was obtained of cases of mongoloid children who were catheterized[11] between 1964 and mid-1969 by the pediatric cardiology department of the teaching hospital in which most of the exploratory interviews were conducted. The records of these 33 cases were searched by a pediatric nurse who had had experience both in pediatric cardiology and with mongoloid children.[12] A variety of medical and social variables were coded.

Three types of comparisons are appropriate for this group of cases. The first is with the entire group of children excluding mongoloids who were catheterized during the same period in the same setting.[13] One would assume that non-mongoloid children would routinely receive surgery if their heart defects required it. For example, the survey shows that surgeons are very likely to operate upon children with severe physical defects in addition to a heart defect (see Table 3.7).

Secondly, the proportion of operations performed upon mongoloid children seen by the clinic at the teaching hospital can be compared with survey responses regarding such cases by surgeons located in teaching hospitals which were major units of a medical school's teaching program. The third type of comparison is within the mongoloid group itself. Under what conditions does a mongoloid with heart defects receive surgery? Can the decision to operate be explained primarily in terms of medical variables or in terms of social variables?

In analyzing these relationships, the special characteristics of this group of mongoloid children have to be taken into consideration. Of those for whom the information was available, 87 percent of the parental marriages were intact, 91 percent of the children were cared for by their own mothers, and 89 percent were living with their natural fathers. Only one child was living in an institution. The families were relatively large (21 percent had five or more children). Data on father's occupation were available for only a fraction of the group but 55 percent were able to pay for medical treatment out of private medical insurance or other private resources. On the other hand, 55 percent of the children were treated by residents rather than by attending phy-

---

[11] Catheterization is a diagnostic procedure for heart ailments.

[12] I am grateful to Tony Winner, R.N., M.A., for her assistance with this study.

[13] A pediatric cardiologist who was interviewed in connection with the study suggested that comparison with non-mongoloid children might in fact be misleading since the heart lesions of mongoloid children are typically more severe than those of normal children and for this reason they often receive more extensive treatment.

sicians, suggesting that, while these families are not poor, they are not affluent either. The group was largely white (82 percent).

The group of children was distributed fairly evenly over three categories representing severity of mongolism: 36 percent required custodial care, 33 percent were capable of self-care, and 18 percent were in an intermediate category, being incapable of self-care, but attending a special school (this information was not available for the remaining 12 percent). There was, however, a strong inverse correlation (G = —.85) between the child's age and the severity of his mongolism, younger children being more severely affected. This relationship is probably due to the fact that severe mongoloids are likely to be institutionalized as they grow older and as a result less likely to receive this type of medical attention. This group of children tended to have fairly severe heart conditions: 48 percent suffered from both heart failure and pneumonia, 39 percent suffered from one of these, and 3 percent suffered from neither (information was unavailable for 9 percent).

Among 1,292 non-mongoloid children who were catheterized at the same hospital during the same period, 43 percent had had heart operations. Thirty-nine percent of the mongoloid group received surgery. In evaluating these figures, it is necessary to point out that a sizable proportion of the non-mongoloid children did not have diagnoses similar to those of the mongoloid children. Of the non-mongoloid children with diagnoses similar to those of the mongoloid children,[14] 65 percent received operations. These statistics summarize decisions which were made in an organizational setting where there was a very clear departmental policy that mentally retarded children should receive exactly the same medical care as normal children. It is also important to note that the mongoloid children with one exception were not institutionalized. The latter did not receive an operation.

The questionnaire asked surgeons about their decisions to operate upon mongoloid children with two types of cardiac defects: tetralogy of Fallot and atrio-ventricular canal. Only one case of the former appeared in the mongoloid sample. However, atrio-ventricular canal was the most frequently occurring diagnosis in this group (42 percent of the cases). Among the 14 cases of atrio-ventricular canal, 29 percent had had surgery. In the survey, 54 percent of the surgeons at comparable hospitals said that they would usually perform such an operation upon a mongoloid child when the parents favored the operation. When the child was described as being institutionalized the figure was 13 percent. Since only one of the children in this group was institutionalized and the parents of the remaining children had presumably sought treatment for them, it seems reasonable to assume that they favored surgery. This sug-

---

[14] I.e., atrio-ventricular canal, ventricular septal defect, atrial septal defect, patent ductus arteriosus, tetralogy of Fallot, and Eisenmenger syndrome.

gests that these operations are performed under the conditions stated in the questionnaire somewhat less frequently (31 percent of the cases where the child was not institutionalized) than the questionnaire results suggest. In the sample of non-mongoloid children, there were 14 whose primary diagnosis was atrio-ventricular canal. All of these children received operations.

A child with patent ductus arteriosus combined with rubella syndrome and developmental retardation was also described on the questionnaire. Fifty-seven percent of the surgeons at comparable hospitals said that they would operate on such a child. In the mongoloid group all of the six children with this defect received operations. This figure tends to confirm the survey results. Since the number of cases is so small, it would not be appropriate to conclude that this type of operation is performed more frequently than the survey results suggest. Among the normal children with this defect, 53 percent received operations.

Within the mongoloid group itself, there was no correlation between severity of heart disease and performance of surgery. This was surprising, since exploratory interviews had suggested that these operations tend to be performed in order to facilitate the management of the child's condition (see Chapter 3). Type of diagnosis did make a difference: all of the children with patent ductus arteriosus received operations compared to 30 percent of the children with other types of defects.

Severity of mongolism was not correlated with performance of surgery, but, since there was an inverse correlation between the former variable and the child's age, severity of mongolism and performance of operations was examined among older children only. Again there was no relationship. There was, however, a strong inverse relationship between age and performance of surgery ($G = -.58$), and some indication that heart disease was more severe in younger children.

There was also a strong inverse relationship between number of siblings and performance of surgery. Fifty percent of those who had no siblings or only one sibling received surgery compared to 30 percent of those with two or three siblings and 14 percent of those with four or five siblings. There was also a strong inverse correlation between sib order of the child and surgery (see Table 5.3). Sixty-three percent of those who were first-born received surgery, compared to 43 percent of those who were second-born, and 38 percent of those who were in later sib positions. This suggests that parents put less pressure upon surgeons to operate when they have other children.[15]

Although this sample of mongoloid children with heart defects is very

---

[15] There was no relationship between performance of surgery and sex of patient. Children whose families were covered by Medicaid rather than private medical insurance were more likely to receive surgery (58 percent compared to 22 percent).

Table 5.3
Sibling Characteristics and the Decision to Operate upon Mongoloid
Children with Cardiac Defects

A. Number of Siblings

| | NUMBER OF SIBLINGS IN CHILD'S FAMILY[a] | | |
	NONE TO ONE	TWO TO THREE	OVER THREE
Percent of	50	30	14
operations performed	(8)	(10)	(7)

[a] $G = -.51$

B. Sibling Order of Child

| | SIBLING ORDER OF CHILD[b] | | |
	1	2	OVER 2
Percent of	63	43	38
operations performed	(8)	(7)	(11)

[b] $G = -.47$

small, the findings appear to indicate that social variables play a more important role than medical variables in determining whether or not such operations are performed. This confirms the findings of the questionnaire but at the same time the data suggest that even in a hospital where there was a strong normative bias in favor of operating upon these children, these operations occur less frequently than the questionnaire results would indicate.

Conclusion

Examination of the records of the treatment which critically ill patients received in a university hospital suggests that physicians are less likely to use major procedures than they indicated on the questionnaires. For example, the proportion of patients resuscitated in the hospital records sample is lower than the proportion of physicians who said that they would resuscitate comparable patients on the questionnaire. In the same hospital where the pediatric service was very much in favor of treating mentally retarded children, the proportion of mongoloid children who received cardiac surgery was lower than the questionnaire results would suggest.

Although no attempt was made to validate the results of the pediatric survey, the recent study by Duff and Campbell (1973) indicates that in the special-care nursery of at least one university hospital, treatment is generally withheld from severely damaged children after their cases have been carefully evaluated.

How should the findings reported in this chapter be interpreted? On the one hand, the lower rate of attempted resuscitation in the hospital records sample may simply reflect the unavailability of medical personnel at the exact time when death occurred (resuscitation must be begun immediately since the brain is damaged if more than four minutes elapse without oxygen). On the other hand, the data may reflect a real disparity between the attitudes and the actual behavior of physicians in the treatment of critically ill patients. This in turn suggests that there may be a conflict between the official medical ethic in this area and the pressures which physicians face in actual practice. In describing their attitudes some physicians pay lip service to the traditional ethic which in practice they find to be inappropriate.

Part II: Sources of Variation Among Physicians: Some Organizational, Social, and Cultural Variables

Chapter 6: Context for Decision-Making: The Hospital Setting

Having identified the criteria which physicians use in deciding to treat critically ill patients, we will attempt in this and in subsequent chapters to identify the characteristics of physicians which are associated with preferences for conservative norms concerning patient care, on the one hand, and for more permissive norms on the other. A number of variables will be examined in this and in the subsequent chapter, including organizational setting, professional and social values, and personal characteristics of the physician, such as social class origin and religious affiliation. In a sense, we are asking whether the physician is autonomous in making these decisions or whether his decisions are influenced by his organizational affiliations or by ethical orientations which predated his medical training.

Type of Hospital Setting and Quality of Patient Care: A Review of the Literature

That hospital environment is an important influence upon the behavior of physicians has been thoroughly documented in recent years. At least three different types of hospital environments have been studied. The first distinction is between teaching hospitals and non-teaching hospitals. The latter constitute the overwhelming majority (79 percent) of all hospitals (Goss 1970, p. 265). Among teaching hospitals, there are those which are associated with medical schools and those which are not. For the most part, studies of these hospital environments have examined the relationship between type of setting and quality of patient care.[1] A number of studies have shown that quality of patient care is superior in teaching hospitals compared to non-teaching hospitals (Goss 1970). Some of these studies also show that teaching hospitals affiliated with medical schools give superior care to that given by teaching hospitals which are not affiliated with medical schools (Goss 1970, p. 264).

What factors underlie these differences? Trussell *et al.* (1962, reviewed by Goss 1970, p. 261) concluded that social control is stronger in teaching settings and produces better patient care. Kendall (1963) in her analysis of learning environments in affiliated and non-affiliated teaching hospitals provides considerable evidence that social control is greater in the former. For example, house staff were more likely to report that their work was evaluated or reviewed by senior physicians in affiliated than in non-affiliated hospitals. She suggests that faculty in the non-affiliated hospitals have fewer opportunities for such activities because they are themselves less actively involved in hospital activities. Physicians in affiliated hospitals were also found to place more emphasis upon medical research while physicians in unaffiliated hospitals were more concerned with patients and problems of medical practice.

Intensive field studies by Mumford (1970) and Miller (1970) of university and community hospitals provide additional documentation for Kendall's findings. Mumford, for example, shows how the two types of hospitals develop different orientations toward medicine in their house staffs. She describes in detail the socialization process which produces on the one hand physicians concerned with specialization and advancing scientific knowledge, and on the other, physicians who are concerned with the patient's psychosocial needs as much as his medical problems. Both studies show how the scientific orientation of the affiliated hospital contributes to more skillful handling of the technical aspects of patient care.

Roemer and Friedman (1971) argue that the variable which affects the quality of the patient care provided by a hospital is not medical school affiliation but the structure of the hospital's medical staff organization. The hospital whose organization is highly structured by firm leadership and by clearly specified policies and regulations provides better care than one where physicians are allowed a great deal of freedom in their hospital activities. Their data show, however, that university hospitals tend to have this type of highly structured medical organization as do many non-university hospitals.

While quality of patient care is likely to be higher in hospitals with medical school affiliations than in those without such affiliations, the relationship between quality of patient care and the variables being studied in this book remains to be specified. One would expect that quality of care would be related

---

[1] Quality of patient care was measured in terms of outcome (i.e. death rates) and process measures such as diagnostic procedures, therapeutic procedures, and justification for hospitalization.

to duration and intensity of treatment but this need not reflect differences in values concerning the allocation of treatment. In other words, treatment accorded critically ill patients in these different types of hospital settings could vary in two ways: (1) the priorities accorded patients who differ in terms of physical or mental damage and in terms of salvageability could vary or (2) similar priorities could be used in all types of hospitals, but within each type of critically ill patient, the proportions of physicians treating actively in different types of hospitals could vary. In this chapter, we will attempt to ascertain which of these possibilities is the correct one. Finally, it is possible that the tendency to be consistently active in different types of cases is found more frequently in some hospital settings rather than others. A discussion of a wide range of factors associated with activism defined in this manner appears at the end of Chapter 7.

Medical School Affiliation and the Care of Critically Ill Patients

Only the effects of environments of teaching hospitals can be examined here. Hospitals which are the *major* teaching units of medical schools can be compared with hospitals that play less important roles in medical teaching (i.e. that are used for *limited* purposes or for *graduate* training only) and with those that are not associated with medical schools. Hospital settings can also be characterized in terms of the prestige of the medical schools with which they are associated. Medical schools like other institutions can be ranked in terms of prestige which in turn is likely to reflect differences in quality. Such stratification systems can be viewed as organizational sets (Caplow 1964, Crane 1970): two or more organizations of the same type, each of which is continuously visible to every other, and continually comparing its own with others' performances on relevant criteria. Any organization set has a small group of leaders, a small group of second-rank but solidly established competitors and a large subset whose members are considered marginal and of progressively poorer quality. The higher a given organization's prestige, the more influence it has upon the standards of achievement in the set as a whole and the greater its ability to exemplify those standards.

In this study, the Medical College Achievement Test (MCAT) science scores of medical students entering these schools have been used as a measure of the relative prestige of these institutions. Since the mean scores of students entering eight of these schools were substantially higher than those entering the remaining schools, it seemed likely that hospitals affiliated with these schools constituted an elite. In this prestige structure, hospitals affiliated with the remaining schools probably constitute a second level of prestige while the bottom level is comprised of hospitals not affiliated with medical schools which include those which offer internships and residencies (such

108 *Sources of Variation Among Physicians*

as those in the samples being examined here) and the very large group of hospitals which do not.[2]

There was no indication that physicians in hospitals with different types of medical school affiliations used different types of priorities in allocating treatment to critically ill patients. Hospitals closely affiliated with medical schools and hospitals without such affiliations allocated care on the basis of salvageability and type of damage as described in Part I of this book. However, in some of these categories, higher proportions of physicians in closely affiliated hospitals treated such patients actively. In other words, if one examined the selection of priorities by physicians in any one of these types of hospitals, the allocations were in general similar to those described previously. If one compared the proportions of physicians treating actively in different types of hospitals, in some cases the proportions of physicians treating actively were higher in the closely affiliated hospitals.

Among the neurosurgeons, it was clear that a larger number of surgeons at closely affiliated (major) hospitals were more likely to operate upon unsalvageable patients than were surgeons at the other types of hospitals (see Table 6.1) except in the case of a relatively simple and highly effective procedure (see Table 6.1, Row 2).[3] But within the category of unsalvageable patients, the distinction between level of treatment accorded to patients with physical or mental damage was maintained (Table 6.1, Rows 1 and 2 versus 3).

Among the medical residents, similar relationships appeared (table not shown). The same priorities were maintained, but in dealing with two of the unsalvageable patients in the case histories, the proportion of residents at the closely affiliated hospitals who were treating actively was higher than at less closely affiliated hospitals. In the case of the third unsalvageable patient, the proportion of active physicians in all types of hospitals was low, probably because that type of condition is exceedingly painful. These relationships are more pronounced when the prestige of the hospital's medical school affiliation and the medical residents' treatment decisions are examined (see Table 6.2). Among the pediatric residents, a relationship between prestige of hospital affiliation and percentage of active physicians appears in the treatment of

---

[2] This type of analysis was conducted for the samples of internists and pediatricians only. In the neurosurgery and pediatric heart surgery samples, the names of the hospitals with which the surgeons were affiliated were not known so that measures of prestige could not be used. The surgeons were asked to indicate on the questionnaires the type of medical school affiliation of the hospital in which they performed the majority of their operations but they were not asked to name the hospital.

[3] The procedure involved removal of a metastatic tumor from the base of the spine.

Table 6.1
Percent of Neurosurgeons "Usually Operating"
by Type of Medical School Affiliation of Hospital
in Which the Majority of Their Operations Are Performed

PATIENT'S PROGNOSIS — TYPE OF DAMAGE[a]	TYPE OF MEDICAL SCHOOL AFFILIATION OF SURGEON[b]				
	MAJOR	LIMITED	GRADUATE	NONE	No TEACHING
Unsalvageable: Physical damage	61	45	54	41	48
Unsalvageable: Physical damage	77	73	76	71	83
Unsalvageable: Mental damage	33	17	25	19	20
Total number of cases	142	171	68	111	153

[a] Row 1: solitary metastatic brain tumor affecting physical capacities only; $G = .18$, $p < .02$.

Row 2: tumor metastatic from kidney to thoracic epidural space; $G = .14$, n.s.

Row 3: solitary metastatic brain tumor affecting mental capacities; $G = .20$, $p < .01$.

In this and in subsequent tables, G is Goodman and Kruskal's gamma.

[b] Columns 2 and 3 and columns 4 and 5 were grouped for computation of gamma.

Table 6.2
Percent of Medical Residents Who Would Treat Very Actively
by Prestige of Their Hospitals' Medical School Affiliation

PATIENT'S PROGNOSIS — TYPE OF DAMAGE[a]	PRESTIGE OF PHYSICIAN'S CURRENT HOSPITAL AFFILIATION		
	HIGH	LOW	NONE
Unsalvageable: Severe physical damage	18 (116)	21 (409)	24 (225)
Unsalvageable: Moderate physical damage	49 (89)	36 (256)	24 (145)
Unsalvageable: Moderate physical damage	52 (27)	27 (143)	26 (80)

[a] Row 1: cancer of the esophagus; $G = -.01$, n.s.

Row 2: melanoma of the leg metastasized to the spinal cord; $G = .32$, $p < .01$.

Row 3: multiple sclerosis; $G = .32$, $p < .05$.

salvageable and unsalvageable patients with mental damage (see Table 6.3).[4] These types of relationships do not appear among either the internists or the pediatricians.[5]

Mumford (1970), on the basis of field studies, found that residents in a hospital closely affiliated with a medical school were less sensitive to their patients' wishes than residents in a community hospital. In the present study, medical residents in closely affiliated hospitals appeared to be more rather than less responsive to their patients' wishes. Larger numbers of residents at university hospitals were active in the case of the unsalvageable patient who wished to be actively treated than in the case of the unsalvageable patient who did not want to be actively treated. But in *both* instances the proportion of residents treating very actively at the university hospitals is substantially higher than at the other types of hospitals.

Similarly the proportion of residents at prestigious hospitals who were

Table 6.3
Percent of Pediatric Residents Who Would Treat
Mentally Damaged Patients Very Actively
by Prestige of Their Hospitals' Medical School Affiliation

PATIENT'S PROGNOSIS — TYPE OF DAMAGE[a]	PRESTIGE OF PHYSICIAN'S CURRENT HOSPITAL AFFILIATION		
	HIGH	LOW	NONE
Salvageable-mental			
Social status high-			
Family attitude low	73	47	39
	(15)	(166)	(62)
Social status low-			
Family attitude high	70	60	50
	(40)	(126)	(66)
Unsalvageable-mental[b]	33	13	8
	(15)	(166)	(62)

[a] Rows 1 and 2: mongoloid with severe respiratory distress: $G = .28$, $p < .05$; $G = .28$, $p < .05$.

Row 3: anencephaly; $G = .38$, $p < .05$.

[b] Since the proportions treating very actively are so small for this case, the percentages used for this and subsequent comparisons represent those respondents whose scores fell into the lowest third of possible scores (low scores represent high activism).

[4] Among the medical residents this type of relationship occurred in the response to the case history concerning the severely brain-damaged salvageable patient. Fifty-two percent of the residents located in prestigious hospitals indicated that they would treat such a patient very actively compared to 14 percent in hospitals with no prestige.

[5] Among the internists, there was, however, a relationship between prestige of hospital affiliation and active treatment of the salvageable case with physical damage.

responsive to the patient's demand for active treatment was larger than in less prestigious settings (see Table 6.4). The difference between the proportions treating very actively when the unsalvageable patient did not want to be treated actively and when he did want to be treated actively is 36 percent among residents in prestigious settings compared to 23 percent among residents in the least prestigious hospitals (see Table 6.4). They were, however, less likely to say that they would resuscitate these patients than residents in less prestigious hospitals. Residents at affiliated hospitals were also more responsive to the wishes of the patient whose salvageability was uncertain in

Table 6.4
Percent of Medical Residents Who Would Treat Very Actively
by Prestige of Their Hospitals' Medical School Affiliation and
Social Characteristics of Patients

A. Patient Attitude

PRESTIGE OF PHYSICIAN'S CURRENT HOSPITAL AFFILIATION	PATIENT'S PROGNOSIS, TYPE OF DAMAGE, AND ATTITUDE			
	UNSALVAGEABLE-PHYSICAL[a] PATIENT ATTITUDE			
	HIGH	LOW	DIFFERENCE	z[b]
High	64 (53)	28 (36)	36	3.27, p < .01
Low	49 (128)	21 (138)	28	4.67, p < .01
None	37 (62)	14 (83)	23	3.29, p < .01
PRESTIGE OF PHYSICIAN'S CURRENT HOSPITAL AFFILIATION	SALVAGEABLE UNCERTAIN-PHYSICAL[c] PATIENT ATTITUDE			
	HIGH	LOW	DIFFERENCE	z
High	53 (36)	36 (53)	17	n.s.
Low	42 (138)	29 (128)	13	2.17, p < .05
None	43 (83)	42 (62)	1	n.s.

[a] Melanoma of the leg metastasized to the spinal cord.

[b] In this and in subsequent tables in this chapter and in Chapter 7, z indicates the difference between proportions in two independent samples (Blalock 1960, pp. 175–178). For purposes of this analysis, these distributions were treated as dichotomous variables, since comparisons were being made between the proportions of very active physicians and the remaining members of the sample. The probabilities shown are for one-tailed tests of significance.

[c] Myocardial infarction combined with jaundice and history of lung cancer.

B. Age and Social Class

PRESTIGE OF PHYSICIAN'S CURRENT HOSPITAL AFFILIATION	PATIENT'S PROGNOSIS, TYPE OF DAMAGE, AND SOCIAL CHARACTERISTICS			
	SALVAGEABILITY: UNCERTAIN-PHYSICAL[d]			
	AGE			
	45 YRS	75 YRS	DIFFERENCE	z
High	39 (36)	41 (27)	2	n.s.
Low	47 (138)	22 (143)	25	5.00, $p < .01$
None	29 (83)	11 (80)	18	3.00, $p < .01$
PRESTIGE OF PHYSICIAN'S CURRENT HOSPITAL AFFILIATION	SALVAGEABILITY: UNCERTAIN-PHYSICAL[e]			
	SOCIAL CLASS			
	HIGH	LOW	DIFFERENCE	z
High	53 (36)	56 (27)	3	n.s.
Low	42 (138)	29 (143)	13	2.17, $p < .05$
None	43 (83)	30 (80)	13	1.63, $p = .05$

[d] Dyspnea and hypotension combined with possibility of lung cancer.

[e] Myocardial infarction combined with jaundice and history of lung cancer.

the allocation of treatment but were not more likely to resuscitate such a patient. Finally, there was some indication that residents at prestigious hospitals were less affected by the socioeconomic characteristics (age and social class) of their patients (see Table 6.4) in their decisions to treat, than were physicians in less prestigious settings.

Pediatric residents at closely affiliated hospitals were more active in the situation where the parents wanted the mongoloid child to be treated than they were when the parents did not. The proportion of residents at the unaffiliated hospitals who were very active when the parents favored treatment was the same as the proportion of residents who were very active at the closely affiliated hospitals when the parents did not favor treatment (table not shown). However, pediatric residents at prestigious hospitals were active whether or not parental attitude was in favor of treating this case and were considerably more active than physicians at less prestigious hospitals (see Table 6.3). Pediatric residents at all types of hospitals were affected by the socioeconomic characteristics of the patients in the case histories when the family's attitude toward treatment was unfavorable. The combinations of these variables with family attitude variables may have given them different meanings than in the internal medicine cases.[6]

The survey showed that medical residents at prestigious hospitals were more responsive to a terminal patient's request for vigorous treatment than residents in less prestigious settings. Why should residents at prestigious hospitals be more responsive to the patients' desires for treatment than residents at less prestigious hospitals? Observations of ward rounds at a hospital which was affiliated with a prestigious medical school for graduate training only suggested that the house staff was too demoralized to respond effectively to the psychosocial needs of their patients. The majority of the house staff were foreigners from non-English speaking countries, a characteristic which did not facilitate this type of interaction. The following field notes by the writer describing ward rounds[7] which were held on two occasions in this hospital convey the impression described above:

Day 1: Dr. A. had had the previous evening off. He was fifteen minutes late in arriving. Dr. B. wanted to wait for him but Dr. C. wanted to start at 8:30 so they started . . .

There was a long discussion between Drs. B. and C. over the diagnosis of a middle-aged Negro whose infection was in doubt. Dr. D. told me that they were debating over whether or not to believe the lab tests. He said that about 25 percent of the time the lab tests were wrong. In this case, the lab tests showed that the man had an infection but the doctors could not find a site for the infection. (Dr. E. had told me yesterday that the lab had recently switched to a new system of reporting results and that that had produced some inaccuracy and confusion.)

Dr. E. (the senior resident) was not present. Dr. A. had mentioned yesterday that Dr. E. had some personal problem and had not been on rounds for about three weeks until yesterday.

Dr. A. gave a number of "orders," i.e. he said "let's do this" or "get that" (referring to tests). He complained because Dr. F. left the group for a while. The group combined talking to the patients and talking about them in their presence.

With an 80-year-old woman whose arm was partially paralyzed, Dr. B. pulled her up by her hands so that they could examine her back. She said, "Don't pull me," obviously in pain. They left her in much distress, although when they arrived she had been smiling contentedly.

---

[6] There were no relationships between type of hospital affiliation and decisions to operate among the pediatric heart surgeons.

[7] The rounds to be described here are so-called "work" rounds in which the house staff examines the patients and prepares its program for their treatment for that day. These rounds are different from rounds in which cases are formally presented to attending physicians for teaching purposes (see Miller 1970).

Day 2: Official rounds for the day were not held by mutual agreement between Dr. A. and Dr. B. Dr. B., Dr. G. and a medical student made "unofficial" rounds. Neither Dr. B. nor Dr. G. were wearing white coats or white trousers. Dr. G. was wearing a rather dirty pair of jeans.

The group visited four patients in a dreary ward which did not seem very clean. One was a chronic alcoholic. Dr. G. said that most of their patients were chronic alcoholics. Dr. B. appeared to be begging Dr. G. to undertake some type of treatment for the man. "Please do it this afternoon," he said.

The next patient was a young black schizophrenic who was lying in a wheelchair with his legs propped up on a chair. He had one arm in a cast. Dr. B. complained that Dr. G. had not taken an hematocrit on the man for several days so he had nothing to compare with the present hematocrit. There was much searching through the man's chart for some test which Dr. G. could not find. Dr. G. said to me: "Dr. B. is always like this." Dr. B. said that he was responsible for the patients. He seemed to be very impatient with Dr. G. The medical student seemed completely detached and somewhat disgusted.

While the group was examining a fourth patient, the black fell out of his wheelchair and was then lifted into the bed.

The ward seemed to be somewhat demoralized. Dr. B. and company received little respect from the nurses or the patients. A nurse listened briefly to one segment of the rounds and then disappeared. Dr. B. muttered briefly at one point: "We need rounds today."

Effects of Hospital Settings: Some Explanations

It is not clear from these findings whether differences in behavior of house staff in these different types of hospitals are due to characteristics of the hospital settings or to normative standards of medical performance which are maintained in these hospitals. There was some indication that prestigious hospitals differed from less prestigious ones on a number of variables. For example, medical residents and internists working in prestigious hospitals tended to be associated with larger hospitals than those working in less prestigious hospitals. Pediatric residents and pediatricians in prestigious hospitals reported larger numbers of decisions similar to those described in the case histories than their counterparts in less prestigious hospitals. In all four samples, physicians affiliated with unprestigious hospitals were located primarily in church or private institutions. Physicians affiliated with hospitals with some or high prestige were most likely to be associated with public hospitals, and, to a lesser extent, with private hospitals and were least likely to be associated with religious hospitals.[8]

There was some indication that medical residents in government hospitals were more likely to be active in the treatment of patients than those in private or religious hospitals. In the same sample, size of hospital and to a lesser extent the number of critical decisions faced by the residents in an average month were associated with more active treatment of patients. This was not generally the case among the pediatric residents. Since characteristics of the hospital setting other than prestige do not have consistent effects upon the behavior of the house staff, it seems likely that standards of performance associated with prestigious hospitals rather than working conditions influence the attitudes of house staff in those hospitals.[9]

It is possible that the stratification system among medical schools is such that it reinforces the development of distinct subcultures in these medical specialties which transmit different standards of medical performance. The correlation between the prestige of the respondent's medical school and the prestige of the hospital in which he was currently practicing was very high.

---

[8] The gamma coefficients are as follows:

	Prestige of Current Hospital Affiliation	
	Medical Residents	Internists
Size of hospital (number of beds)	.37[c]	.46[c]
Physician's monthly case load	−.07	.07[b]
Number of "critical" decisions per month	.11	.15
Hospital control[a]	.37[c]	.37[c]
	Pediatric Residents	Pediatricians
Size of hospital (number of births per year)	−.12[b]	−.15[c]
Physician's monthly case load	.09	.11[c]
Number of "critical" decisions per month	.29[c]	.30[c]
Hospital control[a]	.46[c]	.45[c]

[a] Government, private, religious.
[b] Chi square significant at the .05 level.
[c] Chi square significant at the .01 level.

[9] Variables such as board certification and quality of nursing care were not related to level of treatment.

This was also the case for the prestige of the hospital where the respondent had served his internship and the prestige of his hospital's medical school affiliation.[10] For medical residents and pediatric residents, relationships similar to those described in the previous section were found when one examined the effects of prestige of internship and of the prestige of the medical schools which the residents had attended upon these types of medical decisions. Among the medical residents, these relationships tended to be stronger and to be found in a larger number of the case histories. Again these relationships are not found among physicians.

Treatment of critically ill patients by *physicians* did not appear to vary consistently by type or prestige of the medical school affiliation of the hospital with which they were associated. Prestige of the hospital settings in which these physicians were trained also did not seem to exert an influence upon their decisions to treat critically ill patients. Since such differences did appear among *residents* in these settings, it is necessary to explain the absence of similar findings among physicians.

Physicians versus Residents: Two Medical Cultures?

How can the lack of variation in the behavior of physicians in different hospital settings be explained? There are actually three types of physicians who practice in these settings: (1) full-time staff physicians who do all their work in a single hospital and (2) part-time staff physicians (also called private physicians) who care for patients in two or more hospitals. Both full-time and part-time physicians have private patients and supervise house staff who are participating in the care of those patients. (3) A final category (attending physicians) consists of physicians from either of these groups who for a period of time are assigned to a ward with special responsibilities for teaching house staff.

The lack of variation in the behavior of private physicians in different types of hospital settings may be due to the fact that these physicians are less involved in these settings than full-time staff or attending physicians or residents and, as a result, they are less responsive to social pressures in these settings.

---

[10] Goodman and Kruskal's gamma coefficients (all chi squares significant at .01 level) are:

	Prestige of Current Hospital Affiliation	
	(1) by Prestige of Medical School	(2) by Prestige of Internship
Internists	.52	.85
Medical residents	.66	.75
Pediatricians	.21	.56
Pediatric residents	.86	.75

Although physicians in internal medicine and pediatrics were asked to respond to the questionnaires in terms of their practices in hospitals which were named in the covering letters they received, it is possible that they did not do so and that their responses do not, therefore, reflect the effects of these settings. However, adding a variable composed of the physician's hospital status (full or part-time) and the proportion of patients treated in the hospital by the part-time physician did not change the lack of relationship between prestige of hospital affiliation and the physician's treatment decisions.

Another interpretation of the differences between the attitudes of physicians and residents in these settings is that there are in effect two medical cultures in these hospitals. One of these cultures is located in the non-private service; its members are house staff and attending physicians who tend to be full-time staff. The other culture consists of the part-time physicians who practice on the private service of these hospitals. There may be considerable conflict between the house staff and these physicians. The interviews which were conducted in the university hospital provided considerable evidence of such conflict in that particular setting.[11] Medical residents gave examples of private physicians who did not want their patients to be treated as actively as the house staff thought desirable:

A lot of times there are controversies . . . Private physicians like to give supportive care and not vigorous therapy. They say "let's just try to keep the person alive for two months." The house staff and the consultants believe in vigorous therapy . . . Older physicians are less interested in trying new things and in learning. Now we have to fight for our rights to do these things . . . In order to make the private service a good internship, the hospital has had to give us more power. This has meant that there is a lot of fighting with senior physicians. Traditionally, the power had been given to the private men and they had kept us from being aggressive. Now, sometimes we win and sometimes we don't. For example, Dr. X is not vigorous with diagnostic tests and won't permit one-tenth of the usual diagnostic tests to be done on his patients. He wants to save the patients' money. He has made such a fuss about this that the staff has been instructed to bend with him, but there is going to be trouble. Last year the house staff circulated a petition saying that they wouldn't treat his patients but it never got to the right people.

In turn, part-time physicians resented the independence of the house staff and felt that decisions were being made concerning their patients of which they did not approve:

The house staff always wants to do more tests and to pursue every abnor-

---

[11] This problem was mentioned spontaneously by interviewees; the conflict was not suspected initially by the author.

mality. We prefer to leave certain things unexplored, in order to spare the patient cost and discomfort. That is, if it makes no difference to the welfare of the patient . . . The house staff will start your patient on antibiotics without saying anything about it. You may disagree. Usually this can be worked out on an individual basis but if I anticipate the house staff will move too fast, I usually tell them. I don't often have conflicts with them. You need their help so you try to cooperate as best you can.

Two internists who responded to the questionnaire described a similar type of conflict between house staff and part-time physicians:

[The case histories] are answered in the spirit of the *institution*. They are *not* my decisions, since the house staff will *force* these procedures on *any* patient. The circumstances are such that the physician has no choice. I admit patients with these problems to other hospitals if I can. [Italics by the respondent.]

In answering the questions above, the writer was constantly faced with the dilemma of putting down what he would like to do personally, or voting for certain procedures which would be unavoidable in a hospital situation. We are constantly pressured to carry out diagnostic and therapeutic procedures because of established customs and expectations.

Mumford's study suggests that these two cultures are more likely to be in conflict with one another in the closely affiliated hospital.[12] In the community hospital, on the other hand, she found only one "culture," that of the part-time physicians whom the house staff seek to emulate. However, interviews by the author at a hospital which was affiliated with a prestigious medical school for graduate training only suggested that in hospitals of this sort there is also conflict. In these hospitals, it is the part-time physicians who put pressure on the house staff to treat more actively than they otherwise would. A medical resident who was interviewed made the following comment:

Usually the private physicians want to use exhaustive measures to keep patients alive whereas the house staff would be willing to do the necessary things . . . Sometimes the residents will argue that it is not useful to put certain patients in the intensive care unit. But the private physician will argue that if the patient is kept on the floor, no one will care for him. There are constant arguments between the house staff and the private physician.

Residents have a reputation among physicians for being very active in the treatment of patients. A number of physician-informants commented upon this, not always approvingly, implying that such "heroics" were the result of poor judgment. Our questionnaire data bear this out insofar as residents in

---

[12] The strains between medical practitioners and medical educators have been thoroughly documented by Kendall (1965).

both pediatrics and internal medicine were significantly more active than physicians in their treatment of most of the patients described in the case histories. Again, their selections of priorities were similar but within each category they were more likely to indicate that they would use very active treatment.[13] They were also somewhat more likely to indicate that they would resuscitate these patients.[14]

However, mainly in hospitals affiliated with medical schools were residents more likely to be very active in their treatment of patients than were physicians. In hospitals without such affiliations, the proportions of very active residents and physicians were generally about the same. This type of relationship also appeared when the decisions of residents were compared to those of physicians with prestige of hospital controlled (see Table 6.5). In other

Table 6.5

Percent of Physicians and Residents Who Would Treat Very Actively by Prestige of Their Hospitals' Medical School Affiliation

A. Internal Medicine

PRESTIGE OF CURRENT HOSPITAL AFFILIATION	PROGNOSIS AND TYPE OF DAMAGE OF PATIENT			
	SALVAGEABLE — PHYSICAL DAMAGE[a]			
	PHYSICIANS	RESIDENTS	DIFFERENCE	z[b]
High	67 (121)	77 (116)	10	1.66, p < .05
Low	51 (308)	69 (409)	18	9.00, p < .01
None	55 (231)	71 (225)	16	3.47, p < .01
PRESTIGE OF CURRENT HOSPITAL AFFILIATION	SALVAGEABLE — MODERATE MENTAL DAMAGE[c]			
	PHYSICIANS	RESIDENTS	DIFFERENCE	z
High	22 (80)	33 (89)	11	n.s.
Low	19 (182)	38 (266)	19	4.75, p < .01
None	30 (147)	26 (145)	−4	n.s.

---

[13] The residents were more active than the physicians with respect to the following cases: internal medicine questionnaire: 2, 5, 6, 7; pediatric questionnaire: A1a, B1b, 2, 3, 4.

[14] Residents were more likely than physicians to say that they would or might resuscitate the following types of patients: internal medicine questionnaire: 2, 5, 6; pediatric questionnaire: B1b, 2, 3, 4.

Table 6.5 Cont'd

PRESTIGE OF CURRENT HOSPITAL AFFILIATION	SALVAGEABLE — SEVERE MENTAL DAMAGE[d]			
	PHYSICIANS	RESIDENTS	DIFFERENCE	z
High	20 (41)	52 (27)	32	2.78, p < .01
Low	8 (126)	11 (143)	3	n.s.
None	11 (84)	14 (80)	3	n.s.

PRESTIGE OF CURRENT HOSPITAL AFFILIATION	UNSALVAGEABLE — PHYSICAL DAMAGE[e]			
	PHYSICIANS	RESIDENTS	DIFFERENCE	z
High	35 (80)	49 (89)	14	1.82, p < .05
Low	21 (182)	36 (266)	15	3.75, p < .01
None	29 (147)	24 (145)	−5	n.s.

PRESTIGE OF CURRENT HOSPITAL AFFILIATION	UNSALVAGEABLE — PHYSICAL DAMAGE[f]			
	PHYSICIANS	RESIDENTS	DIFFERENCE	z
High	17 (41)	52 (27)	35	3.24, p < .01
Low	17 (126)	27 (143)	10	2.00, p < .05
None	23 (84)	26 (80)	3	n.s.

[a] Chronic pulmonary fibrosis.
[b] The probabilities shown are for one-tailed tests of significance.
[c] Stroke with moderate brain damage.
[d] Cerebral atrophy with severe brain damage.
[e] Melanoma of the leg metastasized to the spinal cord.
[f] Multiple sclerosis.

B. Pediatrics

PRESTIGE OF CURRENT HOSPITAL AFFILIATION	PROGNOSIS AND TYPE OF DAMAGE OF PATIENT			
	SALVAGEABLE — PHYSICAL DAMAGE[a]			
	PHYSICIANS	RESIDENTS	DIFFERENCE	z[b]
High	38 (40)	58 (55)	20	2.00, p < .05
Low	50 (262)	55 (292)	5	n.s.
None	50 (144)	59 (128)	9	n.s.

Table 6.5 Cont'd

PRESTIGE OF CURRENT HOSPITAL AFFILIATION	SALVAGEABLE — MENTAL DAMAGE[c]			
	PHYSICIANS	RESIDENTS	DIFFERENCE	z
High	48 (40)	71 (55)	23	2.30, p < .05
Low	45 (262)	52 (292)	7	1.75, p < .05
None	39 (144)	45 (128)	6	n.s.

PRESTIGE OF CURRENT HOSPITAL AFFILIATION	SALVAGEABLE — MENTAL DAMAGE[d]			
	PHYSICIANS	RESIDENTS	DIFFERENCE	z
High	40 (40)	49 (55)	9	n.s.
Low	40 (262)	47 (292)	7	1.75, p < .05
None	38 (144)	42 (128)	5	n.s.

PRESTIGE OF CURRENT HOSPITAL AFFILIATION	UNSALVAGEABLE — PHYSICAL DAMAGE[e]			
	PHYSICIANS	RESIDENTS	DIFFERENCE	z
High	19 (27)	32 (25)	13	n.s.
Low	17 (139)	35 (82)	18	3.00, p < .01
None	17 (65)	53 (38)	36	4.00, p < .01

PRESTIGE OF CURRENT HOSPITAL AFFILIATION	UNSALVAGEABLE — MENTAL DAMAGE[f]			
	PHYSICIANS	RESIDENTS	DIFFERENCE	z
High	15 (13)	33 (15)	18	3.00, p < .01
Low	11 (123)	13 (166)	2	n.s.
None	5 (79)	8 (62)	3	n.s.

[a] Myelomeningocele.
[b] The probabilities shown are for one-tailed tests of significance.
[c] Mongoloid with severe respiratory distress.
[d] Seizures with spasticity and hypertonia.
[e] Hypoplastic left ventricle (resident non-respondents excluded).
[f] Anencephaly.

words, as the interviews suggested, the tendency of residents to treat very actively appears to be the function of a particular type of medical setting.[15]

Why should residents in unaffiliated hospitals tend to be no more active than physicians in the same hospitals and less active than residents in affiliated hospitals? The answer may lie in the different medical subcultures which appear to exist in different types of hospitals. Unlike regular internists, "attending" physicians in that specialty were more likely to be active in their treatment of patients when they were associated with prestigious hospitals. As was reported above, Kendall (1963) has found that residents in unaffiliated hospitals are less adequately supervised than residents in affiliated hospitals. She suggests that this is due to the fact that chiefs of service and attending physicians perform their roles as supervisors on a part-time basis in unaffiliated hospitals. As a result, the standards of performance are lower than in closely affiliated hospitals.

The emphasis upon doing everything possible for the patient which is found in many prestigious hospital settings appears to have as a consequence the fact that critically ill patients receive active treatment regardless of their chances of resuming normal social roles. This is seen most clearly in the attitudes of residents in prestigious hospitals toward the treatment of a severely mentally damaged adult or infant (see Table 6.5). It also means, however, that patients are likely to receive active treatment in these settings regardless of their age or social class statuses (see Table 6.4). On the other hand, the emphasis on active treatment does not have the consequence, as might be anticipated, that the wishes of the patient are ignored (see Table 6.4).

The standards of the part-time physician appear to lie somewhere in between the two poles: they are less active than the residents in affiliated hospitals but not less active than residents in unaffiliated hospitals, perhaps in both cases out of concern for the welfare of the patients whose interests they represent.[16]

---

[15] Medical residents at prestigious hospitals were not, however, systematically more active than either physicians or residents in less prestigious settings. For example, in the case of a very painful type of cancer, cancer of the esophagus, medical residents at prestigious hospitals were less active than physicians in the same type of hospital and less active than residents in hospitals with no prestige.

[16] On the assumption that the characteristics of the typical patient in a hospital might be an important component in the overall atmosphere of the hospital and hence in its effect upon physician behavior, an attempt was made to measure the social class level of the patient population in the hospitals included in the internal medicine and pediatric samples. The hospitals were asked to estimate the proportion of their total admissions or discharges in 1970 (or 1969 if the 1970 records were incomplete) which were paid for by Medicaid or Medicare. Percentages ranged from 20 percent to over 70 percent. Unfortunately this information was not available for all hospitals in the sample, so that this information could not be coded for between 13 and 18 percent of the various samples.

Colleague Consensus and Decision-Making in Surgery

In the preceding analysis, it has been assumed that physicians make decisions about critically ill patients entirely alone. The use of questionnaire surveys requires such an assumption but, in order to make replies more realistic, the internists and pediatricians were asked to indicate how they would make their decisions in specific medical settings.[17] Some respondents indicated in comments on the questionnaires that their behavior varied in different hospital settings and that in any particular setting it was influenced by other members of the staff. One internist commented:

> All the cases described above would have multiple consultations and only rarely would a single practitioner make the decision regarding life or death "on his own."

In this and the following sections an attempt will be made to indicate how a medical department actually does influence the types of decisions which its staff makes. How do norms concerning the treatment of patients develop in these settings? How are young physicians socialized in this respect?

Since surgical procedures are so clearly defined, it is probably easier to develop a policy concerning the utilization of such procedures than it is to develop a policy concerning the many and varied kinds of treatments used by internists and pediatricians. Interviews with surgeons suggested that surgical departments develop policies concerning the applicability of surgical procedures in certain types of cases. Pediatric cardiologists also made frequent references to the existence of policies concerning pediatric heart surgery in their department:

> In _____ Hospital the head of the department had made a policy that mongoloid children were not to have open heart surgery. However, here it is frequently done.

> There are two general categories that provoke discussion. One is the severely mentally retarded child who is not even trainable. The usual decision is to

---

In general, physicians associated with hospitals with relatively poorer patient populations (i.e. those for whom over 60 percent of the patients were paid for by public rather than private insurance) tended also to be associated with hospitals closely affiliated with medical schools, and with hospitals controlled by local or state governments. There was some indication that physicians in the hospitals with relatively poorer patient populations were more active than those in hospitals where patients were able to pay their own hospital bills through private insurance. However, these relationships appeared to be due to the fact that hospitals with poorer patient populations tend to be closely affiliated with medical schools rather than to the effect of the patient population itself. Physicians in these hospitals are more likely to be performing supervisory or teaching roles while residents are expected to treat patients very actively.

[17] The covering letter which was sent to respondents included the name of a hospital with which they were affiliated. They were asked to reply to the questions in terms of their practice in that hospital.

ignore this factor completely. This is by executive fiat. It comes up periodically and is ignored. This is because of a departmental ruling.

Children with mental retardation are treated the same way as any others. This is a very clear policy here. Anyone who vocally disagrees with it would be in trouble.

It was clear that not everyone in the department agreed with this policy although members believed that everyone followed it. A physician informant said:

The house officers rarely go against the mainstream. If they disagree with the majority of the physicians, they generally do what the majority says.

The pediatric heart surgeons took a different point of view. The following remark was fairly typical of their attitude:

You talk about these things with other physicians. There is give and take and this has some effect. You come to your point of view gradually and it may change as you get older. There is nothing formalized about the whole thing.

The practice of reviewing surgical decisions in the presence of all staff members, either before or after the operations are performed, contributes to the development of a consensus of opinion. In the university hospital where the interviews were conducted, the pediatric heart surgeons and cardiologists debated their surgical decisions before the operations took place. Apparently, the attitudes of the pediatric heart surgeons who belonged to the department of surgery predominated over those of the cardiologists who belonged to the department of pediatrics since, as we saw in the previous chapter, non-mongoloid children with diagnoses similar to those of mongoloid children were much more likely to receive operations (65 percent compared to 39 percent).

The neurosurgeons discussed their decisions after the operations had been performed. This probably reduced the amount of social control which the department exerted over its members' decisions. A neurosurgeon described his perception of the group's influence:

There is a gentleman's agreement. Nothing is written, or stated as policy. But there is an understanding which everyone has. It's a dynamic thing. It waxes and wanes. You're exposed to it in training and it's modified over time. It's an unwritten law. It's an agreement about how these cases should be handled. You find this gentleman's agreement in any group. In other institutions they might have different standards but they would all agree among themselves.

On the other hand, such meetings probably have a significant influence upon the quality of treatment and play an important role in the socialization of residents, as the following quote from a neurosurgeon informant indicates:

All deaths are presented at a weekly meeting. They are discussed and criticized. All the interesting cases are presented and they are selected by the residents, so you can't hide a case. You don't get house privileges unless you treat properly and there is a constant check on your performance although this is not the purpose of the conference. The essential purpose of the conference is to expose the residents to the thinking of the senior staff, but a secondary benefit is the constant watch on treatment.

In an attempt to assess the effect of departmental policy upon surgical decision-making, both neurosurgeons and pediatric heart surgeons were asked to indicate whether the majority of their colleagues in the department in the hospital where they performed the majority of their operations were in favor, not in favor, or had no consensus concerning two operations. In each case, colleague consensus appeared to be a strong influence upon surgical decision-making (see Table 6.6). The percentages of those who said that they would perform the operation when their colleagues were reported to be in favor of it were much greater than when they were reported to be not in favor or when there was no consensus.[18] It can be argued, of course, that the surgeons' perceptions of their colleagues' attitudes are biased by their own attitudes toward the cases in question and that these findings reflect no more than that, although comments from the interviews do provide some substantiation for the survey data.

In only one of the four cases was there a relationship between type of consensus and type of medical school affiliation.[19] In other words, policies of this sort are apparently not found more consistently in one kind of department rather than in another. In fact the similarities between these different types of departments in the proportions of respondents saying that their departments were in favor, not in favor, or lacked consensus, were striking.

Coser (1962), in her comparative study of the social organization of a surgical ward and a medical ward, found that in the former major decisions concerning patient treatment were made by the senior physicians. There was

---

[18] The neurosurgery question concerning colleague consensus did not specify the type of brain damage which had ensued as a result of one of the conditions (solitary metastatic brain tumor) although the case history questions did. Responses to both case history questions are compared with the relevant "consensus" question (see Table 6.6A).

Table 6.6 shows the distributions of responses to versions of the case histories where the parental situation was unfavorable (i.e. absence of financial resources or parental attitude negative). When the responses to versions of the case histories where the parental attitude is favorable are run against colleague consensus, the correlations are equally high.

[19] Neurosurgeons who were associated with hospitals which had major affiliations with medical schools were more likely to report consensus among their colleagues in favor of operating upon patients with solitary metastatic brain tumor.

Table 6.6
Percent of Surgeons "Usually Operating" by Colleague Consensus
on That Type of Operation

A. Neurosurgeons (N = 650)[a]

PATIENT'S PROGNOSIS — TYPE OF DAMAGE	TYPE OF COLLEAGUE CONSENSUS		
	IN FAVOR	NO CONSENSUS	NOT IN FAVOR
Salvageable: Physical damage	67 (356)	31 (179)	12 (97)
Unsalvageable: Physical damage	67 (388)	30 (159)	8 (86)
Unsalvageable: Mental damage	31 (388)	13 (159)	2 (86)

[a] Row 1: newborn myelomeningocele; G = .71,[b] p < .01.
Row 2: solitary metastatic brain tumor; G = .74, p < .01.
Row 3: solitary metastatic brain tumor; G = .63, p < .01.

B. Pediatric Heart Surgeons (N = 207)[a]

PATIENT'S PROGNOSIS — TYPE OF DAMAGE	TYPE OF COLLEAGUE CONSENSUS		
	IN FAVOR	NO CONSENSUS	NOT IN FAVOR
Salvageable: Physical damage	78 (142)	51 (45)	46 (13)
Salvageable: Mental damage	31 (64)	0 (73)	3 (66)

[a] Row 1: atrio-ventricular canal combined with urogenital anomaly; G = .53.[b]
Row 2: atrio-ventricular canal combined with mongolism; G = .84.[b]
[b] Parental situation: unfavorable (see footnote 18).

no sharing of decision-making among different levels of staff and no delegation of authority on important matters. Coser interpreted this type of behavior on the part of the surgical staff to be the result of the nature of the decisions which they were sometimes required to make, decisions which demanded fast action in the face of emergencies. On the medical floor, on the other hand, she found much more delegation of authority. The intern and resident were encouraged to make decisions although in doing so they weighed information from a variety of sources.

The findings reported here suggest that there may be more consensus involved in the making of surgical decisions than Coser indicated. However, the spirit of her analysis is confirmed by our data in that surgical wards appear to develop fairly clear-cut policies which exert an influence over individual decisions. As a result such decisions may give the impression of being almost arbitrary. As we shall see, social control is exerted in a different fashion on medical and pediatric wards.

Departmental Policy and Decision-Making in Internal Medicine

In the university hospital where interviews were conducted, the internists, both house staff and physicians, almost unanimously denied the existence of any informal policy or guidelines in their department concerning the treatment of critically ill patients. A few suggested that the policy of the department was to be as active as possible in every case. Several suggested that it would be impossible to develop guidelines concerning this type of medical care:

It's not possible. Each case must be evaluated on its own merits.

Guidelines have a tendency to rigidify, and not to allow for specific situations. People speak out about allowing people to die. If you try to make it more specific, you may put a house officer under tremendous strain.

Many were even reluctant to admit that other physicians had influenced their approach to these problems. Most members of the house staff denied that the chief resident had had any influence upon them in this respect. They also denied that they had received any advice about these types of patients from senior staff or visiting physicians. One resident said:

We rarely discuss patients like that with the attendings. They are never around when you have to make these kinds of decisions.

An intern replied to this question:

Very little. No one is interested in the dying patient.

The attending physicians were also ambivalent about giving advice, as this comment by a physician informant suggests:

If an intern or resident asks your advice concerning the care of a terminal patient, do you (a) tell him what you would do if you were caring for the patient? (b) tell him that he must learn to make such decisions on his own? It depends on the problem. If the question is rhetorical, then you don't answer it. Occasionally the question is asked as an entertainment and you are not receptive. If a house officer is really looking for information I give it. If I have no strong feelings, I don't say anything about it. The house officers here are very independent.

Some members of the house staff suggested that they did acquire a point of view toward these cases from one another:

> The idea of being very active regarding resuscitation is handed down from resident to intern. It's not official.

Another intern said:

> I suppose unconsciously you learn something from the residents but nothing specific.

Occasionally it was evident that an individual could identify a role model, a senior physician who had influenced his views in this area, but for the most part they appeared to be extremely individualistic in their approach to patient care, as is suggested by this comment by a resident:

> I've talked over policies with respect to letting people die, but I've never consciously adopted other people's ideas regarding to resuscitate or not to resuscitate. I think the decision to resuscitate or not to resuscitate is like politics or religion. You're not influenced by what other people say.

An intern said:

> I wouldn't allow anyone to tell me what to do. My patients are my patients.

They were also asked whether they would comment if a colleague made a decision of which they disapproved, such as an inappropriate resuscitation. Most of those interviewed indicated that they would not comment in such an instance. They appeared to take the view that it was inappropriate to comment about another physician's patient. A resident made the following comment:

> If it's an intern on my case, I'll discuss it. I wouldn't say anything if it wasn't my case. But if I felt strongly about it, I might talk to the other resident. There's a hierarchy of power here. It's a political situation.

The system of rounds rather than departmental meetings in medicine also contributes to the individualism of patient care. There are several different types of rounds. One type is the work round which is conducted by the house staff without the assistance of senior physicians, usually early in the morning. These rounds which are attended by all interns and residents on a ward and an assortment of medical students, nurses, and technicians consist of a review of the status of each patient on the floor. New patients are presented to the others by the house officers who are responsible for their care. This type of activity obviously serves to make each one aware of the decision-making of the others but since these groups are constantly breaking up and being re-formed as the house officers rotate from one floor to another and from one type of service to another, it is difficult for set "policies" to emerge. Not infrequently, this system leads to sharp changes in policies toward individual patients whose course of treatment spans two different rotations. Decisions made by an earlier team may be reversed entirely by a subsequent group.

Another type of rounds consists of the formal presentation of cases to attending physicians (Miller 1970). Here again the fact that a single senior physician is involved in each presentation, and control over the proceedings is largely in the hands of relatively junior staff members, prevents the development of an official policy through this route.

Finally, the chief resident who supervises the interns and residents makes informal rounds in the evenings during which each case is discussed. Although they were reluctant to admit it, these meetings probably did contribute to the development of some consensus toward patient care among the house staff. One intern who said that the chief resident had influenced him a great deal said:

> He is aware of each patient and has a general idea of their course. He sees us every day and discusses our problems.

The absence of sharp controversies among them concerning patient care was probably due to this factor.

Departmental Policy and Decision-Making in Pediatrics

The pediatric physicians and residents who cared for infants in the premature nursery also denied the existence of policies or guidelines but there appeared to be more conflict in this setting than on the medical service. A physician informant said:

> There's no policy. The individual decisions are made by the house officers. Sometimes there are very heated debates about whether or not a child should have been resuscitated.

Others indicated that the policy was to be very vigorous but that there was by no means unanimous agreement on this. A pediatric fellow commented:

> The chairman of the department is very vigorous. His attitude would be to resuscitate every child regardless of the situation. However, this view is not held by the vast majority of the house staff and they would not do it.

The house staff were critical of the senior physicians for not having provided guidelines in these difficult cases. They obtained advice about medical management but not about how vigorous they should be with particular infants. One intern informant said:

> There is no policy. This is a big deficit in the nursery. These people never work with the house staff. Nobody will really state a hard opinion. Everybody is anxious about the whole problem. They won't give us any guidelines.

Do you think such policies are advisable? I think there should be guidelines. Even if they just discussed it so it could be gotten out in the open so you know where you are, it would be a help . . . I think the attending staff here have shirked their responsibilities.

Another intern said:

You don't see too much of the faculty. It's principally the house staff that does the clinical care. In the nursery the interns function more on their own than almost anywhere else in the hospital.

The advice which they did receive was often not very helpful. A resident said:

Most professors have a very idealistic viewpoint. The longer they are away from day to day patient care, the more they cite the textbook approach rather than what is actually practical. In other words, they tell you what should be done rather than what is good for the family and they don't consider what the family would have to go through to have something accomplished or what would be the relative outcome in terms of the amount of difficulty to the patient involved in getting it done.

An intern said:

It's very difficult to get out of the older physicians what we should do. We often put cases to them which are philosophically loaded. We talk about practical maneuvers which are contingent on moral issues. Their answers are always very unsatisfactory. The moral issues really have to be solved by the individual who is making the decisions.

Another resident said:

They are further away from patient care than they realize. We ask for advice but come away with empty feelings.

Others said that the views of the attending staff differed greatly. At times, the advice of a senior physician could be a liability rather than an asset. One resident suggested that house staff were reluctant at times to ask for consultations concerning a child who had serious problems for fear that this would limit their choices of therapy for the child. He described an example of such a case:

The child would have had a more rapid demise if so many consultants hadn't been involved. If they put something on a chart, then you tend to do it for legal reasons. If there's any legal issue raised, then it could be difficult if you hadn't done what had been on the chart.

On the other hand, the house staff frequently mentioned that they obtained valuable advice from one another. An intern said:

The greatest single influence on us is the collective influence of the residents who are senior to us. We work most closely with them.

A resident said:

The most important influence are the senior residents who are really facing these problems and who are most familiar with the operation of the hospital and with what the senior staff thinks.

Their respect for each other's decisions was such that one informant reported that if a colleague left a patient in his care he would carry out his wishes for the patient rather than his own. This did not seem to be the case among the internists where policy toward an individual patient could change when the house staff changed on a service.

Conflicts concerning patient care occurred on both the non-private medical service and in the premature nursery but in the latter setting the conflicts seemed to be sharper, more prolonged, and less easy to resolve. A number of factors were probably responsible for these differences. The inherent ambiguity of the decisions in the premature nursery was undoubtedly a factor. It was more difficult to ascertain whether or not an infant had suffered brain damage. Even the diagnosis of mongolism can be difficult to make with certainty in the newborn. By comparison, the diagnosis of cancer can frequently be made relatively easily and unambiguously. Even brain damage is easier to ascertain in an adult. The cultural conflict is also sharper in dealing with newborns since American society places a high value on the newborn child. Letting an infant die appears to go against a very widely held value even when the child would be incapable of living up to the expectations which his parents have for him. Finally, it seemed that in this setting there was no one with sufficient authority to act as an arbiter in making these decisions. The senior staff seemed to have abdicated this role perhaps through lack of interest or apathy, perhaps through genuine uncertainty about how these questions should be resolved. Even the chief resident did not concern himself with the premature nursery very much. One resident commented:

The chief resident makes rounds once a week. How much he's involved depends on how much you want to involve him. He's supposed to come on Fridays at 1 o'clock but he doesn't always do it ... We have a more independent existence from the chief resident than any other area in pediatrics.

For whatever reason, it appeared that conflicts about the treatment of certain infants had involved considerable bitterness and had not been satisfactorily resolved. Since most of the house staff were interviewed in connection with this study, it was possible to obtain information about certain conflicts from a number of different points of view. For example, an intern said of one case: "We fought about Baby _____ every day or two. There was very clear disagreement." This particular conflict involved a controversy between two interns and the resident who was in charge of the premature nursery for a month.[20] One of the interns described the medical facts of the case as follows:

> The patient was born at another hospital. The mother had had premature separation of the placenta so that the baby had been without oxygen for several minutes. When it was born, it had seizures which means that it was without oxygen for a while. It was referred here with constant seizures and anoxia.

> We made heroic efforts and incubated it. This means long watching and waiting over it and we pulled it through. The studies showed brain damage. There was a controversy. Some doctors felt that we should continue, even if the baby was brain-damaged. Others felt we shouldn't. He was kept alive. *Why did they take the attitude that he should be kept alive?* I'm not sure if they made a conscious decision. Perhaps they were unwilling not to do something and in effect, kill the child . . . they feel they must preserve life at all costs.

Another intern gave his version of the case:

> There was pressure by the resident to keep him alive . . . I couldn't be a hundred percent sure of my prognosis, but I felt certain that he was going to be a severely retarded, unwanted child. I wanted Baby _____ to die but I was not allowed to let him die. He had a flat E.E.G. measured twice before I made this decision or rather as I was making this decision. This was one of the contingencies that I took into consideration. The E.E.G. was essentially flat. The child had had a combination of seizures and other social factors, the strongest being that the family told me that they didn't want it. I knew that the child would have serious problems if it did live. There was the young unmarried mother and grandparents who didn't want to care for the child.

The intern who took over the case from this intern commented:

> My own feeling at the time that I received the patient was that he should not have been resuscitated vigorously. Eventually he was discharged severely damaged. He will live. The mother was quite angry with me that he was saved when I saw her in the clinic later. She had not wanted the child to live. She was quite an intelligent woman.

It appeared that this child was actively treated as a result of the strong convictions of the resident who was in charge of the premature nursery at the time. During the period when the child was being treated in the nursery, this resident commented:

---

[20] The pediatric interns and residents spent approximately one month in the premature nursery during the course of their year's training.

Baby X was a challenge. His outlook is completely unpredictable. But you can give odds that he has a 50-50 chance of being a functional human being and about 20 percent chance of being severely retarded. He was not born here and may very probably have suffered damage at birth. Then he had seizures. However, a fair percentage of children who have seizures do well. I thought it was a treatable illness but I was bucking the interns all the way. They didn't want to do anything. That's how I got very involved with the child.

In a staff meeting one morning, he commented that he had a personal commitment to that baby. The nurses in the nursery did not share his enthusiasm for the child. One nurse said:

Baby _____ is in a constant state of epilepsy. We expect him to have brain damage. He acts as if he has brain damage. The resident is very interested in this child. He prolonged the child's life. He wants it to get better. However, the mental condition of the child will be poor. Many of us who have seen this before are not enthusiastic. We do what he says but our heart and soul are not in it. But we do what we are told.

She suggested that the attitude of the nurses toward the child could affect the kind of nursing care it receives:

These children take a lot of nursing time and it means that we neglect well babies . . . If there is a choice between feeding or giving a medication to one of these children or to giving it to a well baby I try to give it to both of them but sometimes I find that I can't give it to both at the same time. In my mind, if this one is not going to make it and this one is going to make it, then I tend to give it to the latter.

Another controversy was described by a resident who also disagreed with the philosophy of the interns who were working with him.

There is one case that really upset me. This was a 1200 gram premie who had apneic spells and was distended. He went into arrest. The interns called me after half an hour during which time they attempted to resuscitate the child. I was upset because they hadn't called me before. They were about to quit on him and pull out the tube. I hadn't been consulted on this. With vigorous resuscitation, the baby was brought back. He had multiple cardiac arrests and it later turned out that he had a ruptured stomach. He was operated on and put on the respirator. After three or four weeks he died. I couldn't have been vigorous enough in voicing my objections to what they had done. I felt that they weren't being vigorous enough with that child. I felt that that child had a chance.

One of these interns also mentioned the case in an interview. He said that he had been about to pronounce that infant dead when the resident intervened:

The resident made vigorous attempts to resuscitate him and succeeded. Then they operated and removed the child's stomach. The child had numerous cardiac arrests and severe infection. The chances of the child being mentally normal were one out of 5000. Even the resident would see it that way, I think.

Conclusion

It appears that priorities concerning the treatment of critically ill patients are similar in hospitals which are closely affiliated with medical schools and in those which are not. However, the proportions of physicians who would treat such patients very actively in these different types of hospitals varies depending upon specialty and rank (resident versus physician). Relatively little variation except in the treatment of unsalvageable patients was found among neurosurgeons. However, residents in internal medicine and pediatrics who were associated with closely affiliated hospitals and with prestigious hospitals tended to be more active than their counterparts in other types of hospitals. Contrary to findings from previous studies, residents in internal medicine who were located in prestigious hospitals were more sensitive to the wishes of the patient and less sensitive to his socioeconomic and age characteristics.

In both internal medicine and pediatrics, similar proportions of physicians were active in these different types of settings but information from the interviews suggested that there are two cultures in these hospitals, that of the house staff and the attending physicians and that of the private physicians. The culture of the hospital staff varies depending upon the type of hospital affiliation while that of the physicians, on the whole, does not. Therefore residents tend to be more active than physicians in prestigious hospitals because the culture in these hospitals maintains higher standards of medical performance, while residents in unaffiliated hospitals are no more active and sometimes less active than physicians due to inadequate supervision by attending physicians.

It appears that this emphasis upon high standards of treatment leads to the aggressive treatment of some types of patients who are unlikely to be able to resume their social roles. However, in hospitals where standards of treatment are lower, it is possible that patients who could be returned to normal existence do not receive sufficient care. The higher morale of residents in prestigious hospitals is probably an important factor in their greater sensitivity to the wishes of the patient. Presumably, the standards of such prestigious medical services could be adjusted to take into account the social potential of the critically ill patient in the determination of the level of treatment.

It also appears that the kind of socialization which young physicians receive concerning the treatment of critically ill patients varies considerably from one medical specialty to another. In surgical departments, difficult decisions are discussed by all the members. The majority of surgeons in both surgical specialties reported that there was consensus among members of their departments concerning the desirability of performing specific types of operations. Under these conditions one would predict that young physicians would be criticized if their decisions deviated from the norms established by the departments to which they belong.

In internal medicine, the process of socialization appears to be delegated by the senior physicians to the senior residents whose activities in this area are most intensive. The role of the attending physicians who go on rounds with the house staff is attenuated by the fact that they perform this role for only one month at a time. In addition, individualism appears to be the norm. Young physicians tend to disclaim that they are influenced by older physicians in these matters. The relative absence of controversy among them, however, seems to suggest that intensive contact with a small group of senior residents does lead to the development of a fairly consistent point of view toward these problems, at least in the prestigious department in which these interviews were conducted. The absence of this kind of contact in less prestigious hospitals may explain the differences which were described above. As was indicated there, however, it appears that all physicians internalize certain norms concerning the priorities to be allocated to different categories of patients, depending upon salvageability and type of damage.

Senior physicians apparently played virtually no role in the socialization of residents concerning the activities of the premature nursery. Since other premature nurseries were not studied, it is not known how frequently this type of situation occurs in such settings.[21] Its consequences were obvious: increased conflict and controversy among the house staff which were in turn exacerbated by the ambiguities inherent in the kinds of cases which they handled.

Freidson (1970, p. 89), reviewing recent research on socialization and the performance of physicians, concluded that the medical setting is the more important variable. The organization of the immediate work environment is more likely to influence the physician's behavior than the type of education which he has received. It is likely that the behavior of the physicians who were observed in this study would be different if the organizational variables were altered. However, it also seems likely that the kinds of environments which these young physicians subsequently entered were not unlike the environments described here. In other words, it seems fair to conclude that most

---

[21] Unlike the nursery described here, some premature nurseries are under the direction of neonatalogists who presumably provide the kind of social control which was lacking in this setting.

departments of surgery are like those described here, close-knit and homogeneous in terms of this kind of decision-making. It also seems plausible that departments of internal medicine in general are likely to be much more heterogeneous than surgical departments in this respect, decision-making being highly individualistic. The extent to which premature nurseries in general resemble the one described here is not known.

Chapter 7: The Active Physician:
Cultural Influences Upon Medical Decisions

In previous chapters, the influence of medical institutions upon medical decision-making has been examined. In this chapter, we will expand the range of variables considered in order to study the role of cultural influences. It is possible that cultural institutions play important roles in shaping the attitudes of physicians toward the treatment of critically ill patients. In spite of the professionalization of medical practice, one would expect that attitudes and values acquired through religious socialization would affect physicians' decisions concerning patients. In a rapidly changing society, one would also expect to find generational differences in attitudes toward these matters. Variations in the values held by members of different social classes have been found in many areas and might be expected here. Religion is probably the most important of these variables since all the major religious faiths prescribe appropriate behavior toward sick persons. This variable will be given the most attention in the following pages in which I will examine how these non-medical variables influence the behavior of physicians in different types of medical settings.

In addition to examining cultural influences affecting specific decisions, I will also look at the factors associated with a tendency toward activism. While in general, as we have seen, the physician takes social factors into account in defining the treatable patient, there is considerable variability in the behavior of physicians in these samples. Is it possible to identify the characteristics of physicians who tend to be more rather than less active in the treatment of these patients, who appear to be using physiological rather than social criteria in defining the treatable patient?

137

Religious Prescriptions toward Dying, Death and the Newborn

While it is clear that religious organizations shape the attitudes of their followers toward crucial events such as birth and death, little is known about the effect of religious affiliation on medical practice.[1] Few studies have examined the intersection between the two institutions in modern societies. In recent years, however, religious faiths in modern societies have increasingly found it necessary to take positions concerning the treatment of dying patients.

Western religions, such as Judaism and Christianity, take the viewpoint that illness is treatable by means of human rather than divine intervention. These religions advocate activism toward the treatment of illness. Religions which prescribe activism in the treatment of all illness have difficulty dealing with the critically ill patient. At what point, if at all, is it appropriate to cease being active? It might even be argued that it is the activism of Western religions which has produced the problem of euthanasia. In such activist traditions, it is not sufficient simply to withdraw treatment or neglect the patient. Something active, in other words, euthanasia, is necessary to deal with the patient's "problem," his "terrible death," so that it will proceed faster than it otherwise might. The "problem" of euthanasia is thus uniquely Western. It would not occur to those with a fatalistic attitude toward life and death.

Official policies of Western churches vary on the issue of termination of care. The Episcopal Church, for example, has taken a strong stand against euthanasia (Mann 1970, pp. 99–100). However, a leading Episcopal theologian, Joseph Fletcher, has long been a persistent advocate of euthanasia, particularly by withdrawal of medical treatment.

Official Catholic policy is clearly in favor of the withdrawal of treatment in hopeless cases. Pope Pius XII in the 1950s expressed the view that there is no need for the physician to employ extraordinary means to preserve life. He even appeared to sanction the use of one practice that is close to euthanasia, the administration of drugs to relieve pain in sufficient doses to induce respiratory arrest. While the new ethical and religious directives for Catholic health facilities state that "euthanasia in all forms is forbidden," they also state that (Department of Health Affairs, United States Catholic Conference, 1971, p. 8):

> It is not euthanasia to give a dying person sedatives or analgesics for the alleviation of pain, when such a measure is judged necessary, even though they may deprive the patient of the use of reason or shorten his life.

Even orthodox Judaism, which is probably more activist in its orientation toward medical care generally than any other religious faith, is permissive on

---

[1] Freeman *et al.* (1972), a review of research on medical sociology which deals largely with the United States, contains no references to religion whatsoever in the subject index.

this issue. The leading Jewish authority on this subject, Rabbi Imanuel Jakobovits, indicates that Jewish tradition appears to sanction withdrawal of medical treatment in cases of incurable patients "in acute agony," since "artificial" prolongation of life is not sanctioned. In general, however, Jewish religious tradition appears to emphasize the prohibition of all acts which would tend to hasten death (Jakobovits 1962, p. 122).

Non-Western religions such as Islam, Buddhism, and Hinduism tend to be fatalistic in their approach to physical illness.[2] While Islam contains strands of activism and of fatalism toward these matters, the predestinarian elements in Islam have tended to predominate in recent years, with the result that illness tends to be viewed in countries where this faith is widespread as "God's will" rather than as a problem which can be solved by human intervention. Buddhism also has contradictory implications for medical care. It stresses humanitarianism, but does not emphasize the importance of treating illness *per se*. Illness is seen as only one aspect of human suffering. Hinduism also contains some ideas which are favorable to the development of medical institutions but these tend to be contradicted by the strong fatalistic elements which produce apathy toward medical care.

Glaser (1970) suggests that fatalistic attitudes affect the treatment of the dying in less developed countries, where nurses and other auxiliary personnel are not motivated to work hard to save dying adult patients or sick children. However, Glaser argues that these attitudes should not affect the behavior of physicians since modern medicine is an international social system, which prescribes similar values and behaviors wherever it is practiced. This system is powerful enough to counteract religious influences in particular settings.

Are those who profess non-Western religions, such as Islam, Hinduism, and Buddhism, less active in their treatment of critically ill patients than followers of Western religions? The presence of substantial numbers of Asian residents in the samples of pediatricians and internists permits this hypothesis to be tested in this study. Among the followers of Western religions, one would expect that Jews would be most active in their treatment of patients and Catholics least active since the official pronouncements of a former spiritual leader of that faith have sanctioned withdrawal of therapy. However, since tendencies toward approval of the withdrawal of therapy are to be found in both Protestantism and in Judaism, such differences may not be discernible.

An alternative hypothesis would suggest that the values of the medical profession predominate here and that religious differences will have minimal effects (Glaser 1970). Knutson's study (1968) of attitudes of graduate stu-

---

[2] I am indebted to the discussion by Glaser (1970) for much of the material in this and in the subsequent paragraph.

dents in public health toward medical practice in connection with body transplants provides some support for Glaser's view. He found that ethical judgments were unrelated to religious identification, although he suggested that beliefs about a human soul and the sanctity of the body act as intervening variables in the relationship of religious identification to ethical judgments.

Finally it can be argued that religious faith is not the significant variable but that the important factor is religiosity, regardless of religious faith. Babbie (1970), who examined the relative influence of scientific and religious orientations upon ethical decisions by doctors, concluded that the relevant dimensions are not science and religion *per se* but the types of morality which each of these institutions represents. Traditional religion is associated with traditional morality which emphasizes free will and the ability of the individual to influence events. The new social morality associated with a commitment to science and to scientific research regards individuals as being influenced by environmental factors which are beyond their control. Commitment to one of these types of morality as reflected by their religiosity was associated with attitudes toward mercy-killing of a deformed infant; those committed to the new social morality were more sympathetic toward mercy-killing. Babbie suggests that physicians affiliated with traditional religions vary in their acceptance of this new social morality (as indicated by their attitudes on such an issue), Jews being most willing to accept it, Protestants next, and Catholics least.

The relevant hypotheses can be summarized as follows:

(1) Religious affiliation will have no influence upon decisions to treat critically ill patients; the values of the medical profession will predominate.

(2) If religious affiliation does make a difference: (a) Jews will be more active than Protestants who in turn will be more active than Catholics; (b) followers of Western religious faiths will be more active in the treatment of such patients than followers of non-Western faiths.

(3) Religiosity which reflects commitment to traditional or liberal moral philosophies will have more of an effect upon decisions to treat such patients than religious affiliation *per se*.

Unfortunately, the nature of the data will not permit a definitive testing of all of these hypotheses or of their relative importance. At best, we can suggest which of these hypotheses appear to be most fruitful.

Religious Affiliation and Religiosity in the Four Medical Specialties

The six samples differed considerably in the religious backgrounds of their members although not in terms of religiosity (see Table 7.1).[3] Over one-half

---

[3] The questions were (a) In what religious denomination were you raised? (b) If you have changed your religion, please indicate your new faith. (The new faith

the neurosurgeons and two-thirds of the pediatric heart surgeons were Protestant (mainly liberal Protestants). In the other four samples the three major religious faiths were more evenly represented. The two samples of residents contained small proportions who had been reared in Asian religions. In all six samples, the percentages who indicated that they had not been reared in any religious faith was 7 percent or less. However, all six samples were fairly evenly divided between the proportions indicating that religion was important or unimportant. Religion was most important to the pediatricians and least important to the neurosurgeons (see Table 7.2).

In all the samples (except the pediatric heart surgeons), the Catholics were the most religious, the Protestants next, and the Jews least religious. Among the pediatric heart surgeons, religiosity was about equally distributed among the three faiths, with the Protestants being slightly less religious than either the Catholics or the Jews. Among the pediatric and medical residents, those who had been reared in Asian religions were less religious than the Catholics but more religious than the Protestants or the Jews.[4] Age was unrelated to religiosity except among the pediatricians.

Among the pediatricians, religious affiliation was unrelated to prestige of hospital affiliation. Among the internists, Jews were most likely and liberal Protestants least likely to be affiliated with highly prestigious hospitals. Among the pediatric and medical residents, Jews and Protestants were most likely to be located in prestigious hospitals, while Catholics and those of Asian faiths were more likely to be training in hospitals with no medical school affiliation.

In general, similar patterns appeared when religious affiliation was compared to type of hospital affiliation. As indicated in the previous chapter, information concerning prestige of hospital affiliation was not available for the surgical samples. There was no relationship between religious affiliation and type of hospital affiliation in either of these samples. In the physician and resident samples, Catholics were most likely and Jews least likely to be affiliated with religiously controlled hospitals. There was some indication that the more religious physicians were likely to be located in religious hospitals.[5]

---

was coded if respondents had changed their religion; most had not done so.) (c) In general, how important would you say that your religion is to you? (Check one of the following.) 1. Extremely important. 2. Fairly important. 3. Fairly unimportant. 4. Not at all important. This last question was first used in Babbie's study (1970).

[4] In each sample, some respondents who indicated that they had not been reared in any religious faith and had not adopted one since childhood, indicated that religion was important to them. Presumably, these individuals were referring to private rather than organized religion. Spray and Marx (1968) also found that some of the nonbelievers in their sample indicated that religion was important to them.

[5] Religious affiliation will be treated as an ordinal variable in this chapter since the findings which are presented below suggest that different religious groups can be

Religion, Religiosity, and the Adult Patient

There are two ways of examining the effects of religious variables upon treatment decisions. The first way is to examine the relative proportions of members of different religious faiths who say that they would actively treat specific cases. The second approach is to characterize physicians in terms of

ranked in a consistent fashion in terms of their attitudes toward the treatment of critically ill patients. The gamma coefficients for religious affiliation (Catholics, Jews, and liberal Protestants) by type of hospital affiliation were —.07 for neurosurgery and —.04 for pediatric heart surgery. The gamma coefficients for the other samples were as follows:

Medical Residents

	Prestige of Hospital	Hospital Control	Religious Affiliation[a]	Religiosity
Prestige of Hospital	—	.37[e]	—.24[e]	—.18[e]
Hospital Control[b]		—	—.46[e]	—.16[e]
Religious Affiliation			—	—.15[e]
Religiosity				—

Internists

	Prestige of Hospital	Hospital Control	Religious Affiliation[a]	Religiosity
Prestige of Hospital	—	.37[e]	.10[e]	—.09[d]
Hospital Control[b]		—	.17[e]	—.21[e]
Religious Affiliation			—	—.19[e]
Religiosity				—

Pediatric Residents

	Prestige of Hospital	Hospital Control	Religious Affiliation[c]	Religiosity
Prestige of Hospital	—	.46[e]	—.25[e]	—.24[d]
Hospital Control[b]		—	—.24[e]	—.19[d]
Religious Affiliation			—	.24[d]
Religiosity				—

their tendency to treat actively as shown by the consistency of their behavior toward several cases and measured by a scale of activism based on their responses to several cases (see Chapter 2). Is activism in this sense related to religious variables? The second type of activism will be examined at the end of this chapter.

In general, the evidence concerning the tendency of members of different religious faiths toward active treatment of individual cases was complex. Among the neurosurgeons, there were no differences by religious affiliation. Among the internists, Jews tended to be most active, as anticipated, but liberal Protestants[6] rather than Catholics were the least active with respect both to decisions to treat and to decisions to resuscitate (see Table 7.3). However, among the residents there were few differences by religious affiliation with respect to treatment. There was some indication that Asians were least active in decisions to treat, but members of the other three religious

		Pediatricians		
	Prestige of Hospital	Hospital Control	Religious Affiliation[c]	Religiosity
Prestige of Hospital	—	.45[e]	—.05	—.15[e]
Hospital Control		—	.08[e]	—.14
Religious Affiliation			—	.39[e]
Religiosity				—

[a] Catholics, Asians, Jews and liberal Protestants for medical residents, and Jews, Catholics and liberal Protestants for internists (order reflects degree of activism as shown in Table 7.3).

[b] Government, private, religious.

[c] Catholics, Asians, Jews and liberal Protestants for pediatric residents, and Catholics, Jews and liberal Protestants for pediatricians (order reflects degree of activism as shown in Table 7.8).

[d] Chi square significant at .05 level.

[e] Chi square significant at .01 level.

[6] Glock and Stark (1965, pp. 120–121) identified four groups of Protestants: liberals consisting of Congregationalists, Methodists, and Episcopalians; moderates consisting of Disciples of Christ and Presbyterians; conservatives consisting of American Lutherans and American Baptists; and fundamentalists consisting of Missouri Synod Lutherans, Southern Baptists and sects such as Assemblies of God, the Church of Christ, the Church of the Nazarene, the Foursquare Gospel Church. In the present study, the liberal and moderate denominations were grouped together as liberal Protestants and the conservative and fundamentalist as conservative. The latter are excluded from the analysis since the number of cases was too small in relation to the number and variety of denominations and sects included in this category.

Table 7.1
Religious Affiliation by Specialty
(in percentages)

PHYSICIAN'S SPECIALTY	CATHOLIC	JEW	TOTAL PROTESTANT	RELIGIOUS AFFILIATION PROTESTANT LIBERAL	CONSERV.	UNSPEC.	ASIAN[a]	OTHER; NO ANS.	NONE	TOTAL
Neurosurgeons	18	14	53	35	8	10	—	10	4	650
Internists	16	38	39	28	4	7	—	4	3	660
Medical residents	25	28	33	19	8	6	6	5	3	750
Pediatric heart surgeons	13	12	66	48	7	11	—	6	1	207
Pediatricians	24	28	40	26	6	7	—	3	4	447
Pediatric residents	23	22	34	17	8	9	9	6	7	475

[a] In this and subsequent tables, Asian includes Buddhists, Hindus, and Moslems.

Table 7.2
Commitment to Religion by Specialty
(in percentages)

PHYSICIAN'S SPECIALTY	PHYSICIAN'S RATING OF HIS RELIGIOUS COMMITMENT					
	EXTREMELY IMPORTANT	FAIRLY IMPORTANT	FAIRLY UNIMPORTANT	NOT AT ALL IMPORTANT	NO ANS.	TOTAL
Neurosurgeons	18	33	23	20	6	650
Internists	22	35	26	17	1	660
Medical residents	20	34	28	17	1	750
Pediatric heart surgeons	20	37	25	17	1	207
Pediatricians	23	38	18	19	2	447
Pediatric residents	18	41	23	15	3	475

affiliations did not behave consistently in this area. Generally, among the residents, Catholics, Jews and Asians were most active and liberal Protestants least active regarding decisions to resuscitate (see Table 7.3).

Differences among members of the various religious faiths also appeared when the social characteristics of the patients were varied. For example, among the internists, there was some indication that Jews and Protestants were less responsive and Catholics more responsive to age and social class variables (see Table 7.4AB). On the whole, these differences were found in both decisions to treat and in decisions to resuscitate. Among the residents, Catholics also appeared to be most sensitive to these variables. Among physicians, Jews were most sensitive to the patient's attitude toward a terminal illness (see Table 7.4C). When the prognosis was uncertain, Protestants were most likely to indicate that they would be influenced by the patient's attitude. Among residents, Protestants were most sensitive to this variable in the case of a terminal illness, and Catholics and Asians when the prognosis was uncertain. These findings are summarized in Table 7.5.

Table 7.3
Percent of Internists and Medical Residents Who Would Begin
Resuscitation by Religious Affiliation

A. Brain Damage in Salvageable Patients

CHARACTER- ISTIC OF PATIENT[a]	PHYSICIANS			RESIDENTS			
	RELIGIOUS AFFILIATION			RELIGIOUS AFFILIATION			
	JEWISH	CATHOLIC	LIBERAL PROTESTANT	JEWISH	CATHOLIC	ASIAN	LIBERAL PROTESTANT
Moderate brain damage	49 (66)	50 (49)	29 (64)	43 (53)	67 (81)	53 (35)	31 (43)
Severe brain damage	28 (83)	13 (44)	11 (76)	19 (46)	26 (79)	41 (29)	6 (34)

[a] Row 1: stroke with moderate brain damage; $\chi^2 = 11.98$, df $= 2$, p $< .01$ (physicians); $\chi^2 = 35.98$, df $= 3$, p $< .01$ (residents).

Row 2: severe cerebral atrophy; $\chi^2 = 17.56$, df $= 2$, p $< .01$ (physicians); $\chi^2 = 26.56$, df $= 3$, p $< .01$ (residents).

B. Physical Damage in Salvageable and Unsalvageable Patients

CHARACTER-ISTIC OF PATIENT[a]	PHYSICIANS			RESIDENTS			
	RELIGIOUS AFFILIATION			RELIGIOUS AFFILIATION			
	JEWISH	CATHOLIC	LIBERAL PROTESTANT	JEWISH	CATHOLIC	ASIAN	LIBERAL PROTESTANT
Salvage-able-physical	70	60	50	72	73	72	62
	(220)	(127)	(192)	(146)	(237)	(94)	(126)
Unsal-vageable-physical: Severe (i)	20	22	11	10	18	18	9
	(220)	(127)	(192)	(146)	(237)	(94)	(126)
Moderate (ii)	43	38	29	41	42	42	45
	(137)	(83)	(116)	(100)	(158)	(65)	(92)
Moderate (ii)	44	40	30	47	38	50	15
	(83)	(44)	(76)	(46)	(79)	(29)	(34)

[a] Row 1: chronic pulmonary fibrosis; $\chi^2 = 27.15$, df $= 2$, p $< .01$ (physicians); $\chi^2 = 13.44$, df $= 3$, p $< .01$ (residents).

Row 2: cancer of the esophagus; $\chi^2 = 12.98$, df $= 2$, p $< .01$ (physicians); $\chi^2 = 22.81$, df $= 3$, p $< .01$ (residents).

Row 3: melanoma of the leg metastasized to the spinal cord; $\chi^2 = 8.36$, df $= 2$, p $< .05$ (physicians); $\chi^2 = 1.60$, df $= 3$, n.s. (residents).

Row 4: multiple sclerosis; $\chi^2 = 4.83$, df $= 2$, n.s. (physicians); $\chi^2 = 28.86$, df $= 3$, p $< .01$ (residents).

Table 7.4
Percent of Internists and Medical Residents Who Would Begin Resuscitation
by Social Characteristics of Patients and Religious Affiliation of Physicians

A. Social Class

	CHARACTERISTICS OF PATIENT			
RELIGIOUS AFFILIATION	UNSALVAGEABLE — SEVERE PHYSICAL DAMAGE[a] SOCIAL CLASS			
	LOW	HIGH	DIFFERENCE	z[b]
Physicians				
Jewish	12	22	10	2.00, $p < .05$
	(71)	(66)		
Catholic	11	31	20	2.22, $p < .05$
	(34)	(49)		
Liberal Protestant	14	13	−1	n.s.
	(52)	(64)		
Residents				
Jewish	12	7	−5	n.s.
	(47)	(53)		
Catholic	9	25	16	3.20, $p < .01$
	(77)	(81)		
Asian	9	15	6	n.s.
	(30)	(35)		
Liberal Protestant	10	12	2	n.s.
	(49)	(43)		
	SALVAGEABILITY UNCERTAIN — PHYSICAL DAMAGE[c] SOCIAL CLASS			
	LOW	HIGH	DIFFERENCE	z
Physicians				
Jewish	58	64	6	n.s.
	(83)	(66)		
Catholic	77	71	−6	n.s.
	(44)	(49)		
Liberal Protestant	61	68	7	n.s.
	(76)	(64)		
Residents				
Jewish	55	52	−3	n.s.
	(46)	(53)		
Catholic	59	74	15	3.00, $p < .01$
	(79)	(81)		
Asian	62	79	17	n.s.
	(29)	(35)		
Liberal Protestant	68	58	−10	n.s.
	(34)	(43)		

[a] Cancer of the esophagus.
[b] The probabilities shown are for two-tailed tests of significance.
[c] Myocardial infarction combined with jaundice and history of lung cancer.

B. Age

RELIGIOUS AFFILIATION	CHARACTERISTICS OF PATIENT			
	SALVAGEABLE — PHYSICAL DAMAGE[d]			
	AGE			
	35 YRS.	65 YRS.	DIFFERENCE	z
Physicians				
Jewish	66	63	−3	n.s.
	(66)	(71)		
Catholic	62	39	−23	−2.30, $p < .05$
	(49)	(34)		
Liberal Protestant	46	41	−5	n.s.
	(64)	(52)		
Residents				
Jewish	57	86	29	5.80, $p < .01$
	(53)	(47)		
Catholic	76	53	−23	−3.83, $p < .01$
	(81)	(77)		
Asian	72	60	−12	n.s.
	(35)	(30)		
Liberal Protestant	63	63	0	n.s.
	(43)	(49)		

	SALVAGEABILITY UNCERTAIN — PHYSICAL DAMAGE[e]			
	AGE			
	45 YRS.	75 YRS.	DIFFERENCE	z
Physicians				
Jewish	71	62	−9	n.s.
	(66)	(83)		
Catholic	66	59	−7	n.s.
	(49)	(44)		
Liberal Protestant	56	49	−7	n.s.
	(64)	(76)		
Residents				
Jewish	66	59	−7	n.s.
	(53)	(46)		
Catholic	74	55	−19	−3.80, $p < .01$
	(81)	(79)		
Asian	83	59	−24	−2.40, $p < .05$
	(35)	(29)		
Liberal Protestant	86	49	−37	−5.29, $p < .01$
	(43)	(34)		

[e] Dyspnea and hypotension combined with possibility of lung cancer.
[d] Chronic pulmonary fibrosis.

Table 7.4 Cont'd

C. Patient Attitude

RELIGIOUS AFFILIATION	CHARACTERISTICS OF PATIENT			
	UNSALVAGEABLE — MODERATE PHYSICAL DAMAGE[t] PATIENT ATTITUDE			
	LOW	HIGH	DIFFERENCE	z
Physicians				
Jewish	31	53	22	3.67, p < .01
	(66)	(71)		
Catholic	38	39	1	n.s.
	(49)	(34)		
Liberal Protestant	25	36	11	n.s.
	(64)	(52)		
Residents				
Jewish	36	46	10	2.00, p < .05
	(53)	(47)		
Catholic	36	50	14	2.33, p < .05
	(81)	(77)		
Asian	47	40	−7	n.s.
	(35)	(30)		
Liberal Protestant	19	63	44	6.29, p < .01
	(43)	(49)		
	SALVAGEABILITY UNCERTAIN — PHYSICAL DAMAGE[g] PATIENT ATTITUDE			
	LOW	HIGH	DIFFERENCE	z
Physicians				
Jewish	62	64	2	n.s.
	(71)	(66)		
Catholic	67	71	4	n.s.
	(34)	(49)		
Liberal Protestant	55	68	13	n.s.
	(52)	(64)		
Residents				
Jewish	60	52	−8	n.s.
	(47)	(53)		
Catholic	52	74	22	4.40, p < .01
	(77)	(81)		
Asian	51	79	28	2.55, p < .05
	(30)	(35)		
Liberal Protestant	58	58	0	n.s.
	(49)	(43)		

[t] Melanoma of the leg metastasized to the spinal cord.
[g] Myocardial infarction combined with jaundice and history of lung cancer.

Table 7.5

Summary of Level of Significance of Findings Concerning Willingness to Begin Resuscitation by Salvageability and Social Characteristics of Patients[a]

A. Internists

RELIGIOUS AFFILIATION	SALVAGEABILITY AND SOCIAL CHARACTERISTICS					
	UNSALV.; SOCIAL CLASS	SALV. UNCERTAIN; SOC. CLASS	SALV.; AGE	SALV. UNCERTAIN; AGE	UNSALV.; PAT. ATTIT.	SALV. UNCERTAIN; PAT. ATTIT.
Jewish	.05	n.s.	n.s.	n.s.	.01	n.s.
Catholic	.05	n.s.	.05	n.s.	n.s.	n.s.
Liberal Protestant	n.s.	n.s.	n.s.	n.s.	n.s.	n.s.

B. Medical Residents

RELIGIOUS AFFILIATION	SALVAGEABILITY AND SOCIAL CHARACTERISTICS					
	UNSALV.; SOCIAL CLASS	SALV. UNCERTAIN; SOC. CLASS	SALV.; AGE	SALV. UNCERTAIN; AGE	UNSALV.; PAT. ATTIT.	SALV. UNCERTAIN; PAT. ATTIT.
Jewish	n.s.	n.s.	.01	n.s.	.05	n.s.
Catholic	.01	.01	− .01[b]	− .01[b]	.05	.01
Asian	n.s.	n.s.	n.s.	− .05[b]	n.s.	.05
Liberal Protestant	n.s.	n.s.	n.s.	− .01[b]	.01	n.s.

[a] In all cases, damage to patient is physical.

[b] Minus signs indicate that the tendency is to treat younger patients more actively than older ones.

Religiosity. Religiosity was unrelated to decisions to treat critically ill patients except in neurosurgery. Among the neurosurgeons, those who were less religious were clearly less active in dealing with terminal patients than those who were more religious.[7] There were no differences by religiosity with respect to salvageable patients. In the internal medicine samples, relationships between religiosity and decisions to treat or resuscitate were due to the uneven distribution of religious faiths on this variable. These relationships disappeared when religious affiliation was controlled.

---

[7] The gamma coefficients were as follows: unsalvageable physical (age 40): .14, p < .05; unsalvageable mental (age 40): .10, n.s.; unsalvageable physical (age 65): .13, p < .05; unsalvageable mental (age 65): .19, p < .01.

Narcotics Decision. In the decision to incur high risk to the patient in the prescription of narcotics, there was a strong relationship between absence of religiosity and willingness to take such a risk among both the internists and the medical residents (see Table 7.6B). Kirkpatrick's findings (1949) concerning the relationship between absence of religious faith and humanitarianism may be relevant here. It is possible that the less religious physicians are more sensitive to the sufferings of such patients. The religious physicians may be more inclined to believe that such suffering is of spiritual benefit to the patient. On the other hand, a comparable difference does not occur in decisions to treat or resuscitate terminal cancer patients, so it is possible that this decision has a special meaning and may be a reflection of conservatism-liberalism rather than humanitarianism.

Religious affiliation is also related to the decision to incur high risk to the patient in the prescription of narcotics (see Table 7.6A). Catholics and Asians are least likely and Jews and liberal Protestants most likely to be willing to incur high risk to the life of the patient in such a situation. When religious background and importance of religion are examined in relation to

Table 7.6
Narcotics Decision by Religious Variables
(percent willing to incur high risk to life of patient)

A. Religious Affiliation[a]

| SPECIALTY | RELIGIOUS AFFILIATION | | | |
	JEWISH	LIBERAL PROTESTANT	CATHOLIC	ASIAN
Internists	47	43	31	—
Medical residents	35	38	25	17

[a] Row 1: $\chi^2 = 8.19$, df = 2, p < .05.
Row 2: $\chi^2 = 31.21$, df = 3, p < .01.

B. Religious Commitment[a]

| SPECIALTY | RELIGIOUS COMMITMENT | | | |
	EXTREMELY IMPORTANT	FAIRLY IMPORTANT	FAIRLY UNIMPORTANT	NOT AT ALL IMPORTANT
Internists	40	35	47	55
Medical residents	23	23	33	41

[a] Row 1: G = −.24, p < .01.
Row 2: G = −.24, p < .01.

Table 7.6 Cont'd

C. Religious Affiliation and Citizenship[a]

| SPECIALTY | RELIGIOUS AFFILIATION AND CITIZENSHIP | | | | | |
	WEST. CITIZ. LIB. PROT.	WEST. CITIZ. JEWISH	WEST. CITIZ. CATHOLIC	WEST. CITIZ. CONS. PROT.	EAST. CITIZ. EAST. RELIGION	EAST. CITIZ. WEST. RELIGION
Medical residents	38	35	27	23	17	7

[a] $\chi^2 = 50.05$, df $= 5$, p $< .01$.

this decision, it appears that the latter is the more important variable among the internists (table not shown). Religious Catholics are less likely to take such a risk than either nonreligious Catholics or religious members of other faiths. On the other hand, among the Jews, only those who say that their religion is extremely important to them are relatively reluctant to take such a risk in spite of the strong prohibitions in that faith against such behavior. The more religious liberal Protestants are also less likely to be willing to engage in this type of behavior and this would seem to be in line with the position taken by the Episcopal Church.

Among the medical residents, religious affiliation is affected by citizenship. It appears that among Western members of Western religions,[8] liberal Protestants and Jews are most willing to take this type of risk (see Table 7.6C). Compared to Western members of Western religions, Asian members of Western religions, and members of Eastern religions are much less likely to take this type of risk.

Respirator Decision. The effects of religious faith and religiosity of respondents are much less noticeable in the decision to turn off the respirator when brain death has occurred (see Table 7.7). In general, Jews are least likely and liberal Protestants most likely to say that they would turn off the respirator. Controlling for citizenship among the residents did not affect these relationships (table not shown).

Table 7.7
Respirator Decision by Religious Affiliation
(percent willing to turn off respirator)

| SPECIALTY | RELIGIOUS AFFILIATION[a] | | | |
	CATHOLIC	JEWISH	LIBERAL PROTESTANT	ASIAN
Neurosurgery	73	61	72	—
Internists	57	57	76	—
Medical residents	68	67	84	63

[a] Row 1: $\chi^2 = 3.90$, df $= 2$, n.s.
Row 2: $\chi^2 = 30.87$, df $= 2$, p $< .01$.
Row 3: $\chi^2 = 36.54$, df $= 3$, p $< .01$.

[8] Western members of Western religions included citizens of European countries as well as Americans. The behavior of Europeans was similar to that of Americans in this area.

Summary. To summarize, among the neurosurgeons it appears that religious affiliation has little effect upon decisions to treat critically ill patients. Religiosity affects only decisions to treat terminally ill patients.

Among the internists, Jews and Catholics tend to be most active and liberal Protestants least active in their decisions to resuscitate most cases. Catholics appear to be more sensitive to social class and age distinctions than Jews and Protestants.

Finally, Jews are among those most likely to be willing to hasten the death of a terminally ill patient in pain, but are least likely to say that they would turn off the respirator when the criteria for brain death have been met. The behavior of conservative Protestants tended to be inconsistent, perhaps due to their small numbers in the sample or alternatively due to inconsistencies in the positions toward these issues taken by the various sects which were included in this category. Religiosity has relatively little effect on internists' decisions to treat critically ill patients but is related to the decision to hasten the death of a terminal patient in pain.

The explanation for these differences did not appear to lie in the evaluations of members of these various religions of the relevance of social characteristics and attitudes of patients. There was some indication that Protestants placed a higher value upon the patient's "desire to die" than members of other religions and a clear indication that members of Eastern religions ranked this characteristic of the patient very low. This probably explains the latter's lack of response to the terminal patient's attitude toward his treatment. Asian citizens who were members of Western religions also gave a low rank to this item.

An alternative explanation lies in the role of the hospital environment. The physician may be more likely to behave in accordance with his religious beliefs in some types of hospital environments rather than in others. When the religious affiliation of the hospital in which the medical resident practiced was examined in relation to his religious affiliation, it appeared that Catholic residents were less likely to treat or to resuscitate these types of patients in religious (presumably Catholic) hospitals, and most likely to do so in government (non-federal) hospitals. (The numbers of Jewish and liberal Protestant residents affiliated with religious hospitals were too small to make a similar analysis for these faiths.) This pattern did not occur among Catholic physicians.

Since government hospitals were more likely to have close affiliations with medical schools, the activism of the Catholic residents in these settings is not surprising. An alternative explanation would be that these findings are simply a function of the differential distribution of physicians by religious affiliation in different types of hospitals. When the effects of religious affiliation were compared with those of hospital affiliation among the residents, religious affiliation was related to their decisions to resuscitate while hospital affiliation was related to decisions to treat.[9] In other words, prestigious hospital settings have most effect upon decisions to use various types of treatments, presumably to raise the patient's level of functioning while religious affiliation has most influence upon decisions which affect the patient when he has died or is close to death. Among the physicians, religious affiliation was related to decisions to resuscitate and to a lesser extent to decisions to treat these patients. The relationships between hospital prestige and their decisions both to treat and resuscitate were weak or negative in most cases.

Although Catholics were more willing to risk respiratory arrest in prescribing narcotics to a terminally ill patient in pain in hospitals which were closely affiliated with medical schools, in each setting they were less likely to do so than Jews. The behavior of the latter group, on the other hand, was not affected by the hospital environment. They were equally likely to take such a risk in all four types of settings. The decision to turn off the respirator was not affected by hospital environment.

The relationship between religiosity and the decision to risk respiratory arrest in the prescription of narcotics remained when hospital affiliation was controlled. Within each category of hospital affiliation the less religious physicians were more likely to take such a risk.[10]

Interpretation. Perhaps the strongest conclusion which can be drawn from these findings is that the medical and religious cultures are quite separate in this area. In a small and relatively homogeneous specialty like neurosurgery,

---

[9] The gamma coefficients for medical residents were as follows:

	Willingness to Resuscitate:		*Willingness to Treat:*	
	Religious Affiliation[a,b]	Hospital Prestige[a]	Religious Affiliation[a,b]	Hospital Prestige[a]
Salvageable-physical damage	.12[d]	.13	.10[d]	.14
Salvageable-moderate brain damage	.38[d]	.18	.24[d]	.28[c]
Salvageable-severe brain damage	.37[d]	.01	—.13[d]	.46[d]
Unsalvageable-moderate physical damage (cancer)	—.03	—.04	—.10[c]	.29[d]
Unsalvageable-moderate physical damage (multiple sclerosis)	.22[d]	.09	—.16[d]	.24[d]
Unsalvageable-severe physical damage	.26[d]	—.10	.23[d]	.11

[a] Includes Catholics, Asians, Jews, and liberal Protestants only.
[b] Based on weighted data.
[c] Chi square significant at .05 level.
[d] Chi square significant at .01 level.

[10] Since there was no relationship between religiosity and the decision to turn off the respirator, the introduction of the variable, hospital affiliation, has no effect.

which has less than 2000 members in the United States (Congress of Neurological Surgeons, 1969), this separation is complete. Behavior in this area is influenced by professional values; religious values have no effect.

In a large and more heterogeneous specialty such as internal medicine, religious affiliation accounts for some differences in behavior but these appear to be largely the result of cultural rather than religious influences *per se*. There are three reasons for believing that this is the case: (1) the relationship between religiosity and religious affiliation; (2) the absence of evidence that physicians in these samples are responding to prescriptions pronounced by leaders of religious faiths; and (3) differences in the behavior of physicians of the same religion but from different cultural backgrounds as indicated by citizenship.

Among members of each of the three major religious affiliations, Jewish, Catholic and liberal Protestant, the level of religiosity was different. Catholics were the most religious and Jews the least. On this basis, if religious affiliation were the important factor, one would expect that religiosity would be related to the variables under study. In other words, the less religious respondents from different religious backgrounds would behave in a similar fashion. In general, this does not appear to be the case. Instead, members of each faith have fairly distinct patterns of behavior in this area.

It is also clear from these data that members of these faiths are not responding to prescriptions pronounced by their religious leaders. For example, although Catholicism is the only faith in which religious leaders have indicated that such behavior might be permissible, religious Catholics are *less* likely than nonreligious Catholics to be willing to risk respiratory arrest in prescribing narcotics for a terminally ill cancer patient. On the other hand, the Jews whose religion has strong sanctions against such behavior are among those who are most likely to say that they would behave in this manner. Among the internists, only the most religious Jews are less likely to say they would do this. Among the medical residents, there is no difference between the most religious and the least religious Jews in this respect.

More difficult to explain is why these different religio-cultural backgrounds should produce different degrees of sensibility to social class, age grading, and patient attitude. One possible interpretation may be that members of these different groups have different images of the social world. We will discuss this further in a later section of this chapter. First, we will examine comparable data concerning pediatrics and pediatric heart surgery.

Religion, Religiosity and the Infant

In the treatment of newborn infants, one would expect Catholics to be most active since the Catholic religion prescribes that every attempt should be made to protect a new life from the point of conception onwards. In this area, the Catholic Church takes a very different position from its attitude toward the dying patient. The other two major faiths do not make this differentiation between the beginning and the end of life.

Among the pediatric heart surgeons, however, the liberal Protestants were the most likely to say that they would operate on brain-damaged children, although the percentage differences were not large.[11] Catholics were most likely to say that they would operate on physically damaged children but in only one of the four cases was the percentage difference as high as 15 percent. In every case but one the least religious pediatric heart surgeons were the most likely to say that they would operate but the percentage differences exceeded 15 percent in only two instances, both involving the treatment of brain-damaged children (Cases 1b and 6b of pediatric surgery questionnaire). Again there were no differences among neurosurgeons on either of these variables in the treatment of cases involving newborns.

Proportions of Active Pediatricians. Among the pediatricians, the proportions of active physicians were highest among the Catholics and lowest among the liberal Protestants in the treatment and resuscitation of salvageable infants (see Table 7.8). Among the residents, Catholics and Asians were most likely to be active and Protestants least likely to be active in resuscitating salvageable infants but there were no significant differences in their treatment of these children. These same religious variations also appear among the pediatric residents in the decision to resuscitate the unsalvageable infant with physical damage. Among the residents, only Asian Catholics and members of Asian religions say that they would be likely to resuscitate an anencephalic infant (unsalvageable-mental damage) (see Table 7.12B). There were, however, no religious differences in responses to this case among the physicians. Among the residents, Jews were most active in their treatment of unsalvageable infants. Controlling for religious affiliation, the less religious residents were less likely to say that they would resuscitate the salvageable infants. This type of finding did not occur in the other samples.

Social Variables. The Protestants and Asians were the only subgroups among both the residents and the physicians whose decisions to treat or to resuscitate a severely physically damaged child (a patient with a myelomeningocele) were not affected by the economic situation of the infant's parents. Jews and Catholics were most influenced by this variable (see Table 7.9). In decisions to treat a mongoloid infant, liberal Protestants were most influenced by family attitude with respect to decisions to treat while Jews were most influenced by this variable with respect to decisions to resuscitate (table not shown).

---

[11] In no case were they as large as 15 percent.

Table 7.8
Percent of Pediatricians and Pediatric Residents Who Would Begin
Resuscitation by Religious Affiliation

A. *Brain Damage in Salvageable and Unsalvageable Patients*

CHARACTER- ISTIC OF PATIENT[a]	PHYSICIANS			RESIDENTS			
	RELIGIOUS AFFILIATION			RELIGIOUS AFFILIATION			
	CATHOLIC	JEWISH	LIBERAL PROTESTANT	CATHOLIC	ASIAN	JEWISH	LIBERAL PROTESTANT
Salvage- able: Mental damage							
(i)	18 (113)	18 (128)	9 (114)	21 (129)	22 (75)	19 (78)	9 (70)
(ii)	13 (113)	13 (128)	12 (114)	29 (129)	23 (75)	16 (78)	10 (70)
Unsalvage- able: Mental damage	2 (68)	3 (55)	3 (50)	3 (67)	3 (42)	0 (38)	0 (40)

[a] Row 1: mongoloid with severe respiratory distress; $\chi^2 = 10.93$, df $= 2$, p $< .01$ (physicians); $\chi^2 = 15.99$, df $= 3$, p $< .01$ (residents).

Row 2: seizures with spasticity and hypertonia; $\chi^2 = .15$, df $= 2$, n.s. (physicians); $\chi^2 = 29.53$, df $= 3$, p $< .01$ (residents).

Row 3: anencephaly; $\chi^2 = .64$, df $= 2$, n.s. (physicians); $\chi^2 = 7.70$, df $= 3$, p $< .01$.

B. *Physical Damage in Salvageable and Unsalvageable Patients*

CHARACTER- ISTIC OF PATIENT[a]	PHYSICIANS			RESIDENTS			
	RELIGIOUS AFFILIATION			RELIGIOUS AFFILIATION			
	CATHOLIC	JEWISH	LIBERAL PROTESTANT	CATHOLIC	ASIAN	JEWISH	LIBERAL PROTESTANT
Salvage- able: Physical damage	36 (113)	29 (128)	17 (114)	42 (129)	31 (75)	25 (78)	27 (70)
Unsalvage- able: Physical damage	16 (45)	18 (73)	12 (64)	38 (62)	33 (33)	25 (40)	17 (30)

[a] Row 1: myelomeningocele; $\chi^2 = 21.07$, df $= 2$, p $< .01$ (physicians); $\chi^2 = 21.66$, df $= 3$, p $< .01$ (residents).

Row 2: hypoplastic left ventricle; $\chi^2 = .96$, df $= 2$, n.s. (physicians); $\chi^2 = 12.67$, df $= 3$, p $< .01$ (residents).

Table 7.9

Percent of Pediatricians and Pediatric Residents Who Would Treat Very Actively[a] by Social Characteristics of Patients and Religious Affiliation of Physicians

SOCIAL CLASS OF PATIENT'S FAMILY	PHYSICIANS			RESIDENTS			
	RELIGIOUS AFFILIATION						
	CATHOLIC	JEWISH	LIBERAL PROTESTANT	CATHOLIC	ASIAN	JEWISH	LIBERAL PROTESTANT
High	72	61	47	72	48	70	66
	(68)	(55)	(50)	(68)	(42)	(38)	(40)
Low	52	32	47	39	59	34	58
	(45)	(73)	(64)	(62)	(33)	(40)	(30)
Difference	20	29	0	33	11	36	8
z	2.86,	4.83,		4.71,	.98,	5.14,	1.14,
	$p < .01$	$p < .01$		$p < .01$	n.s.	$p < .01$	n.s.

[a] Salvageable physical: myelomeningocele.

Respirator Decision. In the samples of internists liberal Protestants were most likely and Jews and Catholics least likely to say that they would turn off the respirator after brain death had occurred. Catholic pediatric residents were as likely as liberal Protestant pediatric residents to be willing to turn off the respirator (see Table 7.10). When the distribution was controlled by citizenship, Western Catholics were most likely to say that they would turn off the respirator. Western Jews were less likely to say that they would do so

Table 7.10

Respirator Decision by Religious Variables (percent willing to turn off respirator)

A. Religious Affiliation[a]

SPECIALTY	RELIGIOUS AFFILIATION			
	CATHOLIC	ASIAN	JEWISH	LIBERAL PROTESTANT
Pediatric heart surgeons	78	—	61	72
Pediatricians	59	—	67	68
Pediatric residents	78	77	66	79

[a] Row 2: $\chi^2 = 5.09$, df = 2, $p < .10$.
Row 3: $\chi^2 = 14.53$, df = 3, $p < .01$.

Table 7.4 Cont'd

B. Religious Affiliation and Citizenship[a]

SPECIALTY	RELIGIOUS AFFILIATION AND CITIZENSHIP						
	W. CITIZ. CATHOLIC	W. CITIZ. CONS. PROT.	W. CITIZ. LIB. PROT.	E. CITIZ. EAST. REL.	E. CITIZ. CATHOLIC	W. CITIZ. JEWISH	E. CITIZ. LIB+CONS. PROT.
Pediatric residents	88	80	79	77	67	66	53

[a] $\chi^2 = 41.60$, df = 6, p < .01.

than Eastern Catholics or members of Eastern religions (see Table 7.10B). There were no differences by religiosity.

In spite of considerable differences between religious and nonreligious hospitals in terms of prestige and medical school affiliation (see Chapter 6, footnote 8: the religious hospitals were lowest in prestige and least likely to be closely affiliated with medical schools), behavior of members of the different religious groups did not appear to be affected in any consistent manner by hospital environment as measured by hospital control.

Again, among the pediatric residents, religious affiliation was related to decisions to resuscitate while hospital prestige had more effect upon decisions to treat these types of patients.[12] Among the pediatricians, religious affiliation was related to some of the decisions to resuscitate and to treat while hospital prestige was not related to either.

Interpretation. It is clear from the behavior of the pediatricians that there is a separation between the religious and medical cultures in this area. Pediatricians were asked whether they would be likely to use an "intravenous injection of a lethal dose of potassium chloride or a sedative drug" upon a three-day old anencephalic infant. In the entire sample of 922 physicians only four (three residents and one physician) said that they would be likely to perform such an act and 15 said that they might do so. In other words, a total of 19 (2 percent) out of 922 physicians said they would or might perform such an act. The only comparable data for clergy known to the author are from a study by Meister (1971) who interviewed 50 Catholic, Jewish, and Protestant clergymen in the Baltimore metropolitan area.[13] To the question

---

[12] The gamma coefficients for pediatric residents were as follows:

	Willingness to Resuscitate:		Willingness to Treat:	
	Religious Affiliation[a,b]	Hospital Prestige[a]	Religious Affiliation[a,b]	Hospital Prestige[a]
Salvageable-physical damage	.23[d]	—.14	.00	—.06
Salvageable-brain damage (mongolism)	.23[d]	—.02	—.09[c]	.31[d]
Salvageable-brain damage (seizures)	.35[d]	.00	—.07	.11
Unsalvageable-physical damage	.31[d]	—.23	.11[c]	—.08
Unsalvageable-brain damage	.73[d]	.58	—.05[d]	.37[c]

[a] Includes Catholics, Asians, Jews and liberal Protestants only.
[b] Based on weighted data.
[c] Chi square significant at .05 level.
[d] Chi square significant at .01 level.

[13] Meister drew a random sample from lists of religious institutions and lists of clergy faculty in local seminaries and colleges. The Jewish group included clergy

"Is euthanasia of monsters[14] permitted?," 42 percent (21 out of 50) of these clergymen answered yes. In this sample of 50 clergymen residing in a single city, more individuals are willing to permit "euthanasia of monsters" than in a national sample of 922 pediatricians.

On the other hand, there may be a difference between sanctioning others to perform such an act and willingness to perform it oneself. Babbie (1970, p. 163) asked a sample of physicians who were teaching in medical schools whether they would be sympathetic to the case of a physician who was being tried for murder for having complied to a mother's request to let her baby die at birth if it exhibited deformities caused by ingestion of thalidomide during pregnancy. Two-thirds of his sample indicated that they would be sympathetic to such a case. However, this does not indicate that these physicians would have been willing to perform such an act themselves. There is also a considerable difference between letting a baby die and killing it with an injection of poison.

While Babbie found that sympathy toward an individual in such a situation was inversely related to religiosity, the few respondents in the present study who said that they would or might perform an act of euthanasia upon an anencephalic infant tended to be more rather than less religious. Jews were underrepresented and only one person without any religious background was included in this group. It appears that the factors associated with this type of behavior are different from those associated with the decision to administer a high dose of narcotics to a terminal cancer patient.

Finally, the pediatric sample provides additional evidence that cultural rather than religious attitudes influence behavior in this area. Again, although members of the various religious faiths differed considerably in religiosity, there were characteristic patterns of behavior associated with each faith. In addition, Asian followers of Western religions behaved differently in some instances from their Western counterparts which also suggests that cultural rather than religious variables are at work. In the following section we will attempt to define more precisely the cultural attitudes associated with the various religious groups.

Cultural and Religious Attitudes Toward the Medical Role

It seems more appropriate on the basis of the evidence presented above to interpret the behavior of these physicians as being related to their member-

---

from Conservative, Orthodox, and Reform denominations. The Protestant group included Methodists, Baptists, and Presbyterians. Both academic and "pulpit" clergy were included.

[14] A lay term for infants born with severe congenital anomalies, including anencephaly.

ship in ethnic rather than religious groups. For example, the behavior of Catholic physicians in this area is in part a reflection of Catholicism as an organized religion but is also a reflection of the attitudes and behavior of American Catholics as an ethnic group. Similar statements apply to Jews and liberal Protestants. Durkheim's analysis of religion (1951) suggests some of the ways in which the nature of these religious communities could affect attitudes in this area.

The following characterizations represent an attempt to develop ideal types from an accumulation of inconsistent and sometimes contradictory data. The Catholic physician's behavior in this area appears to be characterized by a concern for the preservation of life. This concern for the preservation of life is seen in the relative reluctance of Catholic internists to risk respiratory arrest in the administration of narcotics to a terminal cancer patient (see Table 7.6). Similarly, Catholic physicians (but not Catholic residents and Catholic surgeons) are reluctant to turn off the respirator after brain death has occurred (see Tables 7.7 and 7.10A).[15] Catholic residents and to a lesser extent physicians are especially likely to say that they would resuscitate brain-damaged patients (see Tables 7.3A and 7.8A). The Catholic physician tends to respond more than physicians from the other two groups to social class and age differences among patients (see Tables 7.4AB and 7.9).

The Jewish physician also has a strong concern for the preservation of life but in his approach to these issues he places more emphasis upon the individual and less upon the individual's place in the social structure. He is less concerned by social class and age differences in the adult patient than the Catholic physician (see Table 7.4AB). His humanitarian concern for the patient is seen most clearly in his attitude toward the administration of narcotics to the terminally ill cancer patient (see Table 7.6). On the other hand, his concern for the patient is not affected by the fact that the individual has suffered brain damage, and as a result he is more reluctant than members of other religious groups to turn off the respirator after brain death has occurred (see Tables 7.7 and 7.10AB). He is also relatively active in the treatment of moderately and severely brain-damaged patients (see Table 7.3A).

The liberal Protestant physician appears to place a value on human life that is relatively independent of social, economic and age considerations (see Tables 7.4 and 7.9). He is least concerned with the preservation of life and is generally less active than members of the other two groups. His concern for the preservation of life tends to be affected by the adult patient's personal attitude (see Table 7.4C). He is negatively affected by brain damage which possibly represents to him the negation of personality (see Tables 7.3A and

---

[15] This is not the case for Catholic neurosurgeons and pediatric heart surgeons for reasons which will be discussed below.

7.8A). Support for this interpretation of the liberal Protestant's orientation toward these issues comes not only from the attitudes of the liberal Protestant internists and pediatricians but also from the attitudes of surgeons. These two specialties are predominantly liberal Protestant in membership and it appears that the attitudes which these specialists express derive from the liberal Protestant orientation toward these issues. They are relatively unconcerned with socioeconomic differences (see Table 7.11B), but strongly affected by patient attitude and family attitude (see Tables 3.6 and 7.11D) in cases involving brain damage. They are also much less active in the treatment of brain damage than physiological damage (see Table 7.11A). Their attitudes are also relatively unaffected by the ages of their patients (see Table 7.11C).

Following Durkheim's analysis of these three religious faiths, it is possible that the same factors which influence the tendencies of members of different religious faiths to commit suicide influence the attitudes of physicians belonging to these faiths toward the preservation of life. For example, the emphasis which Catholic physicians appear to place upon the preservation of life is another effect of characteristics of that faith which also produce the relative absence of propensity to commit suicide which is found among Catholics in general. Durkheim suggests that this can be attributed not to the religious

Table 7.11

Percent of Surgeons Usually Operating by Social Characteristics of Patients and Religious Affiliation of Physicians

A. Brain Damage

CHARACTERISTIC OF PATIENT[a]	NEUROSURGERY			
	RELIGIOUS AFFILIATION			
	CATHOLIC	JEWISH	PROTESTANT	
			LIBERAL	CONSERVATIVE[b]
Salvageable:				
Mental	53	57	57	50
Physical	90	84	91	88
Unsalvageable:				
Mental	15	22	23	22
Physical	43	50	51	44
Total	118	90	229	50

[a] Rows 1 and 2: cerebral hematoma; Row 1: $\chi^2 = .40$, df $= 2$, n.s.;
Row 2: $\chi^2 = 2.79$, df $= 2$, n.s.
Rows 3 and 4: solitary metastatic brain tumor; Row 3: $\chi^2 = 3.07$, df $= 2$, n.s.;
Row 4: $\chi^2 = 2.01$, df $= 2$, n.s.
[b] Omitted from chi square analysis.

Table 7.11 Cont'd

CHARACTERISTIC OF PATIENT[a]	PEDIATRIC HEART SURGERY			
	RELIGIOUS AFFILIATION			
	CATHOLIC	JEWISH	PROTESTANT	
			LIBERAL	CONSERVATIVE
Salvageable:				
Mental	11	17	22	20
Physical	93	83	85	80
Salvageable:				
Mental	48	54	60	60
Physical	93	100	93	93
Total	27	24	100	15

[a] Row 1: mongolism — tetralogy of Fallot.
Row 2: urogenital anomaly — tetralogy of Fallot.
Rows 3 and 4: rubella syndrome — patent ductus arteriosus.

B. Social Class

SOCIAL CLASS OF PATIENT[a]	NEUROSURGERY				PEDIATRIC HEART SURGERY			
	RELIGIOUS AFFILIATION							
	CATHOLIC	JEWISH	PROTESTANT		CATHOLIC	JEWISH	PROTESTANT	
			LIB.	CONSERV.[b]			LIB.	CONSERV.
High	46	49	51	54	96	83	92	93
Low	44	49	48	52	93	79	83	80
Total	118	90	229	50	27	24	100	15

[a] Neurosurgery: salvageable physical: newborn myelomeningocele; Row 1: $\chi^2 = .89$, df $= 2$, n.s.; Row 2: $\chi^2 = .58$, df $= 2$, n.s.
Pediatric heart surgery: salvageable physical: urogenital anomaly — tetralogy of Fallot.
[b] Omitted from chi square analysis.

beliefs *per se* but to the fact that the religious community is well integrated and does not encourage individual interpretation of religious beliefs.

Similarly, the solidarity of the Jewish religious community which derives from its minority status in society both protects the individual against suicide and predisposes the physician toward the preservation of life. On the other hand, the emphasis upon the religious community in Catholicism and Judaism rather than upon the individual may explain the relative lack of concern of these physicians with brain damage in the critically ill patient. In other words, the individual remains a member of the religious community whether or not he is still capable of behaving autonomously.

C. Age

AGE OF PATIENT[a]	NEUROSURGERY			
	RELIGIOUS AFFILIATION			
	CATHOLIC	JEWISH	PROTESTANT	
			LIBERAL	CONSERVATIVE[b]
Unsalvageable: Physical				
Age 40	43	50	51	44
Age 65	35	40	51	54
Unsalvageable: Mental				
Age 40	15	22	23	22
Age 65	8	13	17	12
Total	118	90	229	50

[a] Solitary metastatic brain tumor.
Row 1: $\chi^2 = 2.01$, df $= 2$, n.s.
Row 2: $\chi^2 = 9.30$, df $= 2$, p $< .01$.
Row 3: $\chi^2 = 3.07$, df $= 2$, n.s.
Row 4: $\chi^2 = 5.35$, df $= 2$, n.s.
[b] Omitted from chi square analysis.

D. Family Attitude

ATTITUDE OF PATIENT'S FAMILY[a]	NEUROSURGERY				PEDIATRIC HEART SURGERY			
	RELIGIOUS AFFILIATION							
	CATHOLIC	JEWISH	PROTESTANT		CATHOLIC	JEWISH	PROTESTANT	
			LIB.	CONSERV.			LIB.	CONSERV.
High	44	47	47	46	63	50	62	47
Low	31	31	33	28	11	17	22	20
Total	118	90	229	50	27	24	100	15

[a] Neurosurgery: salvageable mental: mongoloid hydrocephalic; Row 1: $\chi^2 = .24$, df $= 2$, n.s.; Row 2: $\chi^2 = .19$, df $= 2$, n.s.
Pediatric surgery: salvageable mental: mongoloid — tetralogy of Fallot.

The propensity of Protestants both toward suicide and toward the withdrawal of medical treatment can be explained in terms of the much greater emphasis in that religion upon freedom of thought and individual interpretation of religious beliefs. The importance of the latter to the Protestant physician can also be seen in his responsiveness to the attitudes of the patient and his family and in his relative unwillingness to treat the brain-damaged patient.

In addition, the emphasis upon hierarchy in the Catholic Church may perhaps be reflected in the Catholic physician's use of social class and age differences in differentiating between critically ill patients. The Jewish physician's humanitarian concern for the individual, particularly in the administration of narcotics to the terminal patient in pain, cannot, however, be explained in terms of this type of interpretation.

Table 7.12A
Percent of Medical Residents Who Would Treat Very Actively
by Religious Affiliation and Citizenship

CHARACTERISTIC OF PATIENT[a]	RELIGIOUS AFFILIATION AND CITIZENSHIP				
	W. CITIZ. JEWISH	W. CITIZ. LIB. PROT.	W. CITIZ. CATHOLIC	E. CITIZ. CATHOLIC	E. CITIZ. EAST. REL.
Unsalvageable: Moderate physical damage					
Patient attitude high	50 (45)	61 (46)	84 (43)	10 (23)	28 (24)
Patient attitude low	25 (53)	30 (39)	31 (51)	15 (16)	41 (33)
Difference	25	31	43	−5	−13
z[b]	5.00, $p < .01$	4.43, $p < .01$	5.38, $p < .01$	n.s.	n.s.
Salvageability uncertain: Physical damage					
Patient attitude high	41 (53)	47 (39)	57 (51)	55 (16)	58 (33)
Patient attitude low	29 (45)	27 (46)	39 (43)	22 (23)	38 (24)
Difference	12	20	18	33	20
z	2.40, $p < .05$	3.33, $p < .01$	2.57, $p < .05$	2.20, $p < .05$	n.s.
Unsalvageable: Severe physical damage					
Social class high	27 (53)	16 (39)	38 (51)	61 (16)	32 (33)
Social class low	23 (45)	22 (46)	3 (43)	30 (23)	15 (24)
Difference	4	−6	35	31	17
z	n.s.	n.s.	5.83, $p < .01$	1.94, $p < .06$	n.s.

Salvageable: Physical damage					
Age 35	71	67	81	100	76
	(53)	(39)	(51)	(16)	(33)
Age 65	88	82	60	39	71
	(45)	(46)	(43)	(23)	(24)
Difference	17	15	−21	−61	−5
z	4.25,	2.50,	−3.00,	−4.36,	n.s.
	$p < .01$	$p < .05$	$p < .01$	$p < .01$	

[a] Rows 1 and 2: melanoma of the leg metastasized to the spinal cord.

Rows 3 and 4: myocardial infarction combined with jaundice and history of lung cancer.

Rows 5 and 6: cancer of the esophagus.

Rows 7 and 8: chronic pulmonary fibrosis.

[b] The probabilities shown are for two-tailed tests of significance.

Table 7.12B
Percent of Pediatric Residents Who Would Begin Resuscitation by Religion and Citizenship

CHARACTERISTIC OF PATIENT[a]	RELIGIOUS AFFILIATION					
	W. CITIZ. JEWISH	W. CITIZ. LIB. PROT.	W. CITIZ. CATHOLIC	E. CITIZ. PROT.	E. CITIZ. CATHOLIC	E. CITIZ. EAST. REL.
Salvageable: Physical damage	26	30	29	35	52	28
Salvageable: Mental damage	19	9	9	25	46	23
Salvageable: Mental damage	16	11	15	25	46	25
Number of cases	(70)	(58)	(48)	(19)	(58)	(73)
Unsalvageable: Physical damage	28	18	13	0	44	31
Number of cases	(35)	(31)	(27)	(15)	(26)	(41)
Unsalvageable: Mental damage	0	0	0	0	11	3
Number of cases	(35)	(27)	(21)	(4)	(32)	(32)

[a] Row 1: myelomeningocele; $\chi^2 = 23.17$, df = 5, $p < .01$.
Row 2: mongoloid with severe respiratory distress; $\chi^2 = 67.88$, df = 5, $p < .01$.
Row 3: seizures with spasticity and hypertonia; $\chi^2 = 57.14$, df = 5, $p < .01$.
Row 4: hypoplastic left ventricle; $\chi^2 = 17.43$, df = 5, $p < .01$.
Row 5: anencephaly; $\chi^2 = 33.19$, df = 5, $p < .01$.

Still another orientation toward these issues appears in the behavior of the Asian members of the two samples of residents. Like the Catholics, the Asians are concerned with the preservation of life. This is seen particularly in their willingness to resuscitate infants (see Table 7.12B). They were much more active in this respect than Western residents. The only pediatric residents who said that they would resuscitate an anencephalic infant were Asian (see Table 7.12B). Like their Western Catholic counterparts, the Eastern Catholic medical residents were more sensitive to social class and age distinctions than members of other religious faiths (see Table 7.12A). This is indicated in a striking fashion in the proportions of members of these groups who were willing to treat very actively a middle-class patient suffering from terminal cancer and a truck driver with the same illness (see Table 7.12A, Rows 5 and 6). Members of this group were least likely to treat actively a cancer patient who requests active treatment (see Table 7.12A, Row 1). They were, however, more responsive to the attitudes of a patient whose diagnosis was uncertain, but he and his counterpart were presented as middle-class patients (the social class level of the terminal cancer patients was not specified). These kinds of differences were not found among the pediatric residents.

In general, the survey data do not suggest that Asian residents are likely to be fatalistic in their treatment of critically ill patients. In fact, in some situations, they are more active than Western physicians.

There is no way of knowing from these data whether these physicians would behave in a similar fashion in their countries of origin. For the most part, these countries could be characterized as less developed.[16] Interviews with foreign residents suggested that they would be less likely to treat these types of patients actively in their own countries. One resident commented:

> If I were in Iran my answers to some of the above questions would undoubtedly differ, due to economical and medico-legal situations which are not the same as here.

A Note on Age, Social Class, and Sex Differences

Age Differences. Generational differences in attitudes toward critically ill patients might reasonably be anticipated. Since new medical technology is continually being developed, each generation of physicians learns a new set of medical techniques. Presumably this affects their perceptions of medical priorities. There are also studies which show that there are generational differences between physicians in the quality of medical practice. Younger physicians are better physicians because their training is more recent. In a

---

[16] "Eastern" residents came from the following countries: India, Korea, Pakistan, Philippines, Taiwan, Thailand, and the Middle East, excluding Israel.

previous chapter, we showed that younger physicians are more likely to be aware of the necessity of distinguishing between chronic and acute illnesses in the treatment process.

Table 7.13

Percent of Internists with High Scores on Activism Scales
by Professional Age of Physician

ACTIVISM SCALE[a]	PROFESSIONAL AGE (YEAR OF M.D.)				
	BEFORE 1930	1930–39	1940–49	1950–59	1960–65
Resuscitation	48	44	35	31	41
Heroic operations	9	24	35	40	28
Heroic treatment	21	28	27	25	8
Total number of cases	32	114	194	232	87

[a] For construction of these scales, see pp. 173–174.
[b] G's are the following: Row 1: .09, $p < .01$; Row 2: −.15, $p < .01$; Row 3: .18, $p < .01$.

There was some indication that younger internists, but not younger pediatricians, were more likely to treat patients actively than were older physicians. However, it appears that these relationships do not reflect differences in attitudes but in medical expertise. A scale representing use of heroic operations was inversely related to age but scales representing willingness to begin resuscitation and to use heroic treatment showed that older rather than younger physicians were more likely to be active.[17] These data suggest that older physicians may be less active in the treatment of chronically ill patients because they are less familiar with the latest medical techniques and not because they are less inclined to treat these patients actively. This impression is confirmed by the data concerning neurosurgeons. There were no age differences except with respect to two operations (on a newborn with a myelomeningocele and on a newborn hydrocephalic). Medical thinking with respect to the former condition has changed considerably in recent years (J. M. Freeman 1972), and this is reflected in the attitudes expressed by surgeons from different age groups.[18]

---

[17] For a description of the construction of these scales, see pp. 173–174.
[18] Since age was not related to type of hospital affiliation among the surgeons, these differences cannot be attributed to the fact that the younger surgeons were more likely to be located in hospitals which are closely affiliated with medical schools.

Similarly, younger internists and neurosurgeons, particularly those who received their medical degrees during the 1960s, were more willing to turn off the respirator after brain death had occurred. On the other hand, internists who had obtained their degrees before 1930 were much more willing than other physicians to incur high risk to the patient in the prescription of narcotics.

There did not appear to be differences between age groups in their responses to social class, age, and brain damage but younger internists appeared to be more responsive to the attitudes of the terminal cancer patient. This was also reflected in their ranking of characteristics of the patients that would influence their decisions to treat. Younger internists were more likely to give a high rank to the patient's "desire to die" than older physicians. They were also less concerned by the patient's potential usefulness than older physicians. Younger physicians were consistently more active than older physicians on the cases used in that sample.[19]

In general there was some indication that physicians who had received their medical degrees before 1930 were less active in the treatment of brain damage, less sensitive to patient and family attitudes, and more sensitive to social class variables than younger physicians but since this group is so small in all four samples, it is difficult to be sure. It is possible that there was a marked shift in medical attitudes which began in the 1930s and continued after the second World War.

Social Class. It is difficult to anticipate relationships between social class origin of physicians and attitudes toward the treatment of chronically ill patients. While it is clear that social classes in the United States are associated with distinctive values, attitudes, and life styles, it is not clear how attitudes in this area would be affected. In addition, physicians from lower-class families are obviously upwardly mobile and during the process of a lengthy educational experience have probably assumed the values, attitudes, and life styles of the upper middle class. As a result one would expect the effects of social class origin to be rather slight.

In these samples, as in other studies which have examined social class origins of physicians (for example, Adams 1953, More 1960, Schumacher 1961), the respondents were predominantly from upper-middle-class parentage.[20] Almost 40 percent of the internists and neurosurgeons (47 percent of the pediatric surgeons) came from professional backgrounds. Among

---

[19] Age was not related to prestige of hospital affiliation in this sample.

[20] Social class origin was measured on the basis of the father's occupation which was classified into four categories using a scale developed by Warner (1960). The four categories consisted of professionals, semiprofessionals, skilled workers, and semiskilled and unskilled workers.

the pediatricians, this figure was slightly less than one third. Less than 6 percent in any of the samples were sons of semi-skilled or unskilled workers.

On the other hand, the correlation between social class origin of physician and the prestige of the hospital with which the physician was affiliated was low. Unlike the sharp differentiation which appears to exist in the legal profession in terms of the opportunities available to lower-class lawyers (Carlin 1966, p. 32), the lower-class physician (but not resident) was somewhat more likely to be associated with a prestigious hospital.

Since the proportion of lower-class respondents was small in all four specialties, it is difficult to generalize. There was some indication in the sample of internists that physicians from lower-class origins were more likely to treat patients actively than other physicians. This inverse relationship between social class and activity was also noticeable among the pediatric residents and the surgical samples.

Sex Differences. Finally one might expect differences by sex on certain variables. For example, one might expect that female physicians would be more sensitive to patient and family attitude than male physicians. Substantial numbers of female physicians were found only in the two resident samples and in the pediatrician sample. A tendency for female medical residents to be less active in the treatment of patients than their male counterparts disappeared when hospital setting was controlled.[21] There was no indication that female physicians were more sensitive to patient or family attitude or to the notion of a precious pregnancy.

The Active Physician

Until now, we have examined physicians' attitudes toward each case separately in order to determine the factors associated with an emphasis upon one type of patient characteristic rather than another. In this section, we will examine the factors associated with a general tendency to treat actively regardless of the characteristics of the patient.

An appropriate measure of activism for the internists was a set of scales representing their willingness to begin resuscitation, to recommend heroic operations, and to utilize heroic treatment for several cases rather than for a single case. As described in Chapter 2, the scales were developed on the basis of correlations between responses to the items included as determined from the results of a factor analysis. Heroic operations included appendectomies and small bowel resections. Heroic treatments included the use

---

[21] Sex was related to type of hospital affiliation in the medical resident sample ($G = .33$, $p < .01$).

of the endotrachial tube, respirator, tracheostomy, resuscitation, and antibiotics. The resuscitation items were drawn from six out of the seven internal medicine cases (case 3 was not included). The heroic operation and heroic treatment items were drawn from cases 1, 2, 5 and 6, and 1, 2, and 3 respectively.[22]

Some of the strongest correlations between these scales and other variables were those between the scales and the decision to leave the respirator

Table 7.14

The Active Physician: Correlations[a] Between Characteristics of Physicians and Activism Scale Scores[b]

CHARACTERISTIC OF PHYSICIAN	SPECIALTY							
	INTERNAL MEDICINE						PEDIATRICS	
	RESIDENTS			PHYSICIANS			RESIDENTS	PHYSICIANS
	RES.	OPS.	TREAT	RES.	OPS.	TREAT	RES.	RES.
Prestige of med. school	—	—	.23	—	—	—	—	—
Number of hosp. beds/births	—	.27	—	—	—	—	—	—
Social status of hospital patients	—	—	—	—	—	—	−.22	—
Religious affil.[c]	—	—	.21	.25	.20	.29	.36	—
Religiosity	—	—	—	—	—	—	.24	—
Relig. affil. and citizenship[d]	—	—	.20	—	—	—	.46	—
Sex (male)	.25	.26	.28	—	—	—	—	—
Respirator decision	—	.25	.24	—	—	—	.32	.32
Narcotics decision	—	—	.24	—	—	.30	—	—

[a] Goodman and Kruskal's gamma. Only variables with at least one correlation of .20 or above are shown in this table (see footnote 24). All chi squares are significant at the $p < .05$ level or beyond.

[b] Resuscitation, heroic operations, and heroic treatment.

[c] For computation of gamma, the order of the religious variables was as follows: *Medical residents:* Asian, Catholic, Jewish, liberal Protestant; *Internists:* Jewish, Catholic, liberal Protestant; *Pediatric residents:* Catholic, Asian, Jewish, liberal Protestant; and *Pediatricians:* Catholic, Jewish, liberal Protestant.

[d] For computation of gamma, the order of the variables was as follows: *Medical residents:* Eastern Catholics, Eastern religions, Western Catholics, Western Jews, Western liberal Protestants; *Pediatric residents:* Eastern Catholics, Eastern Protestants, Eastern religions, Western Catholics, Western Jews, Western liberal Protestants.

[22] See copies of questionnaires in Appendix 2. The following items were included in these scales: *Resuscitation Scale:* 18, 28, 47, 58, 68, 78; *Heroic Operations Scale:* 24, 25, 55, 66, 67; *Heroic Treatment Scale:* 16, 17, 18, 26, 27, 36, 37.

running and the decision not to increase the narcotics dosage for a terminally ill patient in pain (see Table 7.14). Since both of these items are indications of a strong orientation toward activism in the treatment of patients, this suggests that the scales are a valid measure of activism.

The proportions of very active physicians in these two samples were low. For example, the percentages with such scores[23] on the resuscitation scale which was based on responses to six out of seven cases were 12 percent among the residents and 14 percent among the physicians. On the heroic operations scale which was based on responses to four cases, 23 percent of the residents and 17 percent of the physicians had such scores. The comparable figures for the heroic treatment scale which was based on responses to three cases were 7 percent and 8 percent respectively.

Surprisingly, the correlations between these scales and the organizational affiliations of the internists were low. Gamma coefficients above .20 also occurred seldom and inconsistently between the scales and the characteristics of their hospital affiliations such as size, type of hospital control, etc.[24]

For example, being affiliated with larger hospitals (in terms of number of hospital beds) was associated with a tendency to perform heroic operations among the residents but not among the physicians. These findings suggest that the effects of organizational variables upon the responses of physicians to these types of patients are differentiated in terms of salvageability and type of damage and are not conducive to a general tendency toward activism.

Among the personal characteristics of the internists, the only variables which were consistently related to activism were religious affiliation, and religious affiliation combined with citizenship. The liberal Protestants were the least active. Among the physicians, the Jews were consistently the most active. Among the residents, the Asians were the most active as measured by the resuscitation and heroic treatment scales, while the Jews were most active on the heroic operations scale.

Only one measure of activism was available from the data on pediatricians. It included items drawn from three cases involving the use of bag-breathing to maintain respirations, the decision to place an infant upon a respirator,

---

[23] "Very active" meant positive responses to 5 or 6 items out of 6 items for the resuscitation scale, 4 or 5 out of 5 items for the heroic operations scale, and 6 or 7 items out of 7 for the heroic treatment scale.

[24] The following variables were examined in relation to activism: type of hospital affiliation, prestige of hospital affiliation, prestige of medical school, prestige of internship, prestige of residency, number of hospital beds/births, number of critical decisions, type of hospital control, social status of hospital patients, board certification of physician, physician status in hospital (full or part-time), religious affiliation, religiosity, religious affiliation and citizenship, social class origin, sex, professional age, respirator decision, narcotics decision. Only those variables where at least one correlation was .20 or above are shown in Table 7.14.

and the decision to resuscitate following cardiac arrest. The items were drawn from cases 2, 3 and 4. The proportions of very active physicians in the pediatric samples were also low. Seven percent of the residents were very active compared to 4 percent of the physicians.[25]

Again among the pediatric residents, but not among the physicians, religious affiliation, religious affiliation combined with citizenship, and religiosity were all strongly associated with activism. The proportions of pediatric residents belonging to Western religious faiths and having Western citizenship who had scores of 7–11 (the range was 7–21) on the pediatric resuscitation scale were very low (7 to 9 percent). By contrast, the proportions of Asian Protestants and Asian Catholics who had such scores were high (43 percent and 38 percent respectively). Fourteen percent of the Asian residents reporting Asian religious affiliations had such scores on this scale.

The respondents' rankings of the social characteristics of patients which influenced their decisions concerning treatment (social values) were also associated with activism (see Table 7.15).[26] For example, internists and medical residents who rated the patient's desire to die as an important influence upon their decision to treat a chronically ill patient were less likely to have high scores on the heroic treatment and resuscitation scales. Those who ranked the patient's chronological age as an important factor in their decisions to treat chronically ill patients were more likely to have high scores on the heroic treatment scale.

Among the pediatricians, concern with the impact of a damaged child upon his family was associated with less activism as was concern with the financial burden of the infant's condition to his family. Pediatricians who were concerned about the infant's potential usefulness to society or family were also likely to be less active. Three attitudinal variables — the infant's potential usefulness, concern with the impact of a damaged child upon his family and the fact that a particular pregnancy was "precious" to the mother — affected the behavior of the pediatric residents.

What is the relationship between activism, social values, and religious affiliation? Is religious affiliation associated with certain types of social values which are in turn related to activism?

Among the internists, religious affiliation (Jewish, Catholic, liberal Protestant) was negatively associated with the physician's evaluation of the im-

---

[25] "Very active" meant positive responses to 6 or 7 items out of 7 items. The following items were included: 30, 35, 36, 37, 42, 43, 44. See copies of questionnaires in Appendix 2. Low scores meant high activism.

[26] Table 7.15 shows Pearson's *r* correlation coefficients between respondents' ratings of the importance of social values and their scores on the activism scales. Respondents' ratings of social values are used here as scores to measure the extent to which they hold various attitudes.

portance of the patient's desire to die and positively associated with his evaluation of the importance of the patient's chronological age ($G = -.23$ and .24 respectively). Among the medical residents, these correlations were —.10 and .14 (Asian, Catholic, Jewish, liberal Protestant). The cultural background of medical residents of these faiths (Eastern citizenship, Western citizenship) was also correlated with these attitudes ($G = -.61$ and .29).

Among the pediatric residents, cultural background had more influence upon activism than religious background. Cultural background (Eastern citizenship, Western citizenship) was related to the physician's ranking of the importance of the fact that a particular pregnancy was "precious" upon his decisions ($G = .23$). It was not related to the resident's rankings of the child's impact upon his family or his potential usefulness. Since religious affiliation was not related to activism among the pediatricians, its relationship to social values is not relevant here.

Table 7.15

The Active Physician: Correlations Between Social Values and Activism Scale Scores[a]

A. Internal Medicine

| SOCIAL VALUES[b] | RESIDENTS | | PHYSICIANS | |
| | ACTIVISM SCALES | | | |
	RES.	TREAT	RES.	TREAT
Patient's desire to die	—.17	—.20	—.19	—.23
Patient's chronological age	.16	.20	.16	.21

B. Pediatrics

| SOCIAL VALUES[b] | RESIDENTS | PHYSICIANS |
	RESUSCITATION SCALE	
Impact of severely damaged child on his family	—.21	—.25
Infant's potential usefulness	—.16	—.22
Precious pregnancy	.20	—
Financial burden to family	—	—.17
Financial burden to state	—	—.15

[a] Pearson's *r* correlation coefficients less than .15 are not shown.

[b] Respondents' ratings of social characteristics of patients which influenced their decisions concerning treatment.

These findings suggest that the correlates of activism are not for the most part organizational variables but are deep-seated attitudes (of which a few examples have been examined here) concerning the value of life under different conditions. These attitudes probably precede medical training since they are not associated with the prestige of the respondents' hospital affiliations. Religious and cultural background (Western–non-Western) appears to play a role in shaping these attitudes. If these findings are correct, it suggests that socialization during medical training may be expected to have little effect on these attitudes since in all probability they are formed long before the individual begins his medical training and are thus likely to be resistant to change.

Conclusion

There is a continuing debate in the sociology of religion concerning the relationship between religious institutions and secular institutions in modern society. Some writers perceive the relationship as greatly attenuated. Others suggest that it is still important but that the traditional religious faiths have become increasingly secularized and as a result increasingly similar (Herberg 1967). This too has been questioned by recent data which suggest that there are important differences among Protestant denominations and between the latter and Catholicism (Glock and Stark 1965). Still other scholars (Luckmann 1967) argue that traditional religion is being replaced by private faiths.

The present study suggests that physicians affiliated with the major religious groups in America have somewhat different perceptions of the problems concerning the prolongation of life. It is interesting to note that their behavior remains distinctive in this area even when they are not very religious and are not guided by official church doctrines in these matters.

Consequently the role of religiosity appears to be less important than religious affiliation which seems to provide those who have been exposed to it (even if they no longer seriously practice it) a perspective on these issues that is remarkably consistent. Thus there is some indication that the activism of the Catholic is more ritualistic in its motivation (particularly since it is not sanctioned by Church doctrine with respect to adult patients) while that of the Jews appears to be more humanitarian. Liberal Protestants are less concerned than either of these groups about the preservation of life except when the individual expresses the desire to live. In this respect, identification with a religious group is much more significant than generational, social class or sex differences.

It had also been anticipated that members of Asian religions would be more fatalistic in their approach to these patients. Instead we find that these physicians are more likely than members of some Western faiths to say that they would resuscitate critically ill patients. Members of Asian religions as well as their fellow citizens who had adopted Western faiths were more likely than Westerners to be consistently active in the treatment of these patients as shown by the activism scales.

The present study suggests that the debate concerning an appropriate policy for the treatment of critically ill patients is made more difficult by the fact that physicians from various religious faiths perceive the issues differently. Since liberal Protestants appear to have an attitude toward the preservation of life different from that of the Catholics and the Jews and since these two groups in turn differ in the nature of their humanitarian concerns, it appears unlikely that controversies in this area will be speedily resolved.

Chapter 8: Departmental Dynamics and the Development of New Medical Technology

In previous chapters, we have discussed the allocation of medical care to patients under the conditions of normal medical practice. There are, however, a number of special medical situations where new medical technology is being developed and utilized in the treatment of patients. The best known examples of these situations are heart transplantation, kidney transplantation and cancer chemotherapy. Under these conditions, the allocation of medical resources is undoubtedly different in some ways from that to be found in general medical practice. These situations represent a variant of a more frequent but atypical situation in medical practice, that of medical experimentation. There, too, allocation of treatment is affected by the special goals of the research.

The development of new medical technology frequently necessitates heroic attempts to prolong the lives of unsalvageable patients. In this respect, these physicians are obliged to violate a norm which appears to be fairly general in the medical profession. If the result of these heroic efforts is a high mortality rate, other physicians may begin to impose negative sanctions upon the researchers. They may be forced to suspend their activities at least for a period of time (Swazey and Fox 1970). The organizational setting undoubtedly plays an important role in facilitating or inhibiting the physicians' adjustment to the strains involved in performing this type of research.

Doctor-patient relationships in these settings are different from those which occur in ordinary medical practice. In these situations, the relationship ceases to be that of a client seeking care from a disinterested professional. Instead, the professional often seeks the client because the latter is especially suitable for a particular medical experiment or clinical investigation. In other cases, clients may be forced to compete with one another for scarce innovational treatments. In these situations, the physician frequently relies more heavily on indicators of social status or social value in his selection of patients than he normally would (Simmons and Simmons 1971). Middle-class patients or those whose youth, prestige, or other social characteristics endow them with social value have an advantage in the selection process. Finally, under certain conditions, the doctor-patient relationship becomes much more intense than is normally the case with one or both parties becoming emotionally involved in the relationship (Fox 1959).

Medical researchers have seldom been studied from a sociological point of view. Fox (1959), in her study of a ward devoted to research on metabolic diseases and staffed by physicians from Harvard Medical School, concentrated upon the ways in which the researchers and the patients adjusted to the stress involved in studying or being studied in this fashion. The two parties coped with the situation by developing a type of doctor-patient relationship which was more similar to that which exists between two professionals than to the traditional doctor-patient relationship. Due to the fact that the subjects were few in number, stayed for considerable periods of time on the ward and often returned for lengthy subsequent visits, and tended to develop a high level of intellectual understanding and emotional involvement in the research process, the ideal of "informed voluntary consent" was truly observed in this setting.

Barber and his associates (1973) in a large questionnaire survey found some evidence of unethical behavior on the part of medical researchers which they attribute to inadequate socialization in medical school and to the overzealous pursuit of scientific recognition on the part of researchers who feel that they have been denied adequate recognition for their scientific work. Unlike Fox, they found close relationships between researchers and their patient-subjects to be relatively rare (Barber *et al.* 1973, pp. 112–113).

In the following pages, we will examine medical decision-making on two cancer chemotherapy wards in order to find out how organizational variables affect patient care in the context of this type of medical experimentation. The data which will be discussed in the following pages were collected by means of interviews with physicians and supporting medical personnel in two cancer chemotherapy wards. The research can best be described as exploratory. While most physicians in both settings consented to be interviewed,[1] cooperation varied depending upon the organizational

---

[1] On Ward I, nine senior physicians, three fellows, and two residents were inter-

characteristics of the wards, as will be discussed shortly. In dealing with such sensitive issues, it is difficult either to obtain entirely accurate information from respondents or to evaluate the reliability of the interview data and the extent to which they reflect actual behavior patterns in the setting.

Ethical Issues in Cancer Chemotherapy Research

In order to understand the ethical problems which arise in the course of cancer chemotherapy, it is necessary first to describe briefly the nature of the experimental procedures and their effects upon the patients. Ethical problems are likely to occur when patients in advanced stages of cancer are given a series of drug treatments which include high doses of exceedingly toxic drugs, alone or in combination, over a period of several days or weeks. The goal of the treatment is to bring about a remission in the disease process. Remissions when they occur are generally brief in duration although occasionally patients go into remission for a year or more. A number of drugs are tried in succession. If none of them works, the whole series may be repeated.

The immediate effects of the drugs upon the patients are generally negative. Nausea, vomiting, diarrhea, loss of hair, hematuria, and gastrointestinal upset are some of the debilitating symptoms which are likely to occur. Since patients become very susceptible to infection, it is sometimes necessary to isolate them in order to avoid infection. In this case, they are allowed to see family members and staff members only when they are wearing masks. The diagnostic procedures such as bone marrows which are necessary to evaluate their progress can be exceedingly painful. Psychological stress is not uncommon.

In response to increased concern in recent years for the subjects of medical experimentation,[2] a number of ethical codes have been developed. A primary difficulty with all such codes is that they are of necessity very general. It is not always clear how these general directives could be translated into medical practice. Sections of these codes which have the most

---

viewed as well as two nurses and a psychiatrist. One physician on Ward I refused to be interviewed. Papers written about the ward by an oncologist and another psychiatrist were also consulted. On Ward II, four senior physicians, 13 clinical associates, two nurses, and one social worker were interviewed. One physician was unintentionally not included in the study. Annual reports of the ward's activities were consulted. In the distributions presented in the text, the totals vary due to the fact that not all physicians responded to every question.

[2] Barber (1967, p. 96) reports that in addition to the Nuremberg Code which has been the model for many subsequent codes, codes have been written by the United Nations, the World Medical Association, the United States Public Health Service, the French National Academy of Medicine, and the American Medical Association.

relevance for experimentation with cancer chemotherapy are those concerning the patient's freedom to initiate the treatment process and to halt it while it is underway, the necessity of avoiding undue physical and mental suffering for the patient, and the stipulation that the risks to the patient should not outweigh the anticipated benefits to humanity if the medical problem is solved.

Voluntary consent by the patient to participation in a medical experiment is considered to be absolutely essential. In practice, it is an ideal which is difficult to realize particularly if the potential subjects are relatively uneducated and of lower social class status than the physician. The patient's freedom to bring the experiment to an end if he has reached the physical or mental state where continuation of the experiment seems unendurable to him is likely to be transgressed in practice. The physician is reluctant to terminate an experiment before it is finished since he thereby loses his total investment of time and money in the patient as a research subject. Since most experiments with cancer chemotherapy involve considerable discomfort for the patient, the point at which additional discomfort becomes "unnecessary" is extremely difficult to define in practice. Similarly, it is difficult to weigh potential risks to life against potential benefits to humanity in cases of patients who are terminally ill.

These issues were examined in two different settings. Ward I was associated with a prestigious university on the East Coast. Ward II was located in but administratively separate from a federal hospital in the same city. The two wards will be described separately. Comparisons between them will be made in a subsequent section.

Social Organization and Ethical Experimentation: Ward I

Ward I was a 22-bed research ward consisting of a combination of private rooms and a few four-bed rooms. The freshly painted white walls gave the area a clean but rather sterile appearance. The staff of the ward consisted of 10 senior researchers, three fellows (one of whom was directly in charge of the ward), and two residents. The occupants of the last two positions continually changed as residents rotated through the service for a few weeks at a time. In addition there were two or three medical students assigned to the ward for short periods. The senior researchers had their offices in a wing which was adjacent to the ward but separated from it by a short hallway.

The work was divided in such a way that the treatment and research roles were kept separate. Senior men did research; house staff were in charge of the day-to-day care of the patients. Research physicians took turns at monthly stints on the ward as attending physicians, countersigning the orders on the patients' charts. This is often described in the literature on medical experimentation as an ideal situation: the physician in charge of the research on a patient is not solely responsible for evaluating its benefits to the patient.

The senior members of the ward had developed a strong ideology which supported their activities. The most important aspect of the ideology consisted of a justification of the research role. In general, the senior men tended to justify what they were doing on the grounds that it was better for such patients to be treated than not to be treated. One of these physicians said:

> We are the only people who treat these patients. They are the outcasts of modern medicine.

The self-image of these physicians is suggested by the comment of one of them that he was the only physician in the city who was doing anything about leukemia.

The group's ideology also emphasized the amount of consensus which existed among the members. They saw themselves as a tightly-knit group who shared the same views toward the value of doing research on cancer patients. Much credit was given by members of the group to their director who had been on the service for many years. One of them said:

> We were selected by one man whose philosophy we probably had before we came here or we wouldn't be here. We are unanimous.

Many comments in the interviews referred to his influence and to their admiration for him as a physician. Along with this ideology went high morale among the senior men and a strong conviction that their ethical decisions were correct, as the following comment indicates:

> On Fridays at staff meetings we go over our morality which is quite high and which is controlled by each other.

The senior staff's ideology affected other members of the staff. The nursing staff appeared to be extremely committed to the goals of the ward. Some of the nurses had been working on the ward for long periods of time, a remarkable fact when one considers that their work involved daily contact with terminally ill patients undergoing extremely unpleasant courses of treatment. Members of the house staff who served for relatively short periods on the ward appeared to be rapidly socialized. A resident who was interviewed near the beginning of his rotation was somewhat critical of the activities of the ward but two weeks later the same resident was critical of the interviewer for raising questions about the functioning of the service.

The effects of this social system upon the quality of care which the patients received are difficult to evaluate precisely without a detailed examination of a series of patients including study of their records and interviews with physicians who had been associated with their course of treatment. This approach was not attempted during this study and there is some doubt as to whether it would have been possible to obtain sufficient cooperation in order to do so. Members of the senior staff tended to be defensive about their roles and to perceive the investigator as raising unnecessary issues. Persons occupying more peripheral roles in the setting such as medical students and psychiatrists were often more critical of the activities of the ward. Using their comments combined with an analysis of the kinds of controversies which were described by the ward's staff, it is possible to infer some of the effects of the ward's social structure upon patient care.

For example, it appeared that the technical separation of the research and treatment roles was not entirely effective. The disparity in status between researchers and practitioners was too great to permit a true separation of these roles. The practitioners who were the residents were transients on the ward, junior physicians with little experience handling these difficult types of cases, and numerically a minority (two as compared to ten). They were dependent upon the research staff for references to advance their future careers. This point was stressed by the physician who was in charge of the ward. On the one hand, he said that residents were encouraged to make their own decisions concerning patients. On the other hand, he also pointed out:

> In a university hospital everyone is very career-minded ... One is working for a chief of service and one does what his policy dictates. People who are not prepared to tow the line are out in private practice ... One's motives are dictated by one's career opportunities.

A psychiatrist who was attached to the ward brought out this theme even more sharply:

> The two residents are supposedly the responsible physicians but only theoretically ... Patients are not sure who their doctor is ... The residents are in the middle. They don't have complete autonomy. They are under more pressure in a sense because of this.

One type of conflict between researcher and practitioner which probably occurred fairly frequently was over whether or not a patient's treatment should be continued or whether he should be sent home to die. During the period when the field research was being conducted on the ward, several controversies of this kind arose. One patient, for example, had received the full series of drugs without going into remission. The research physician wanted the patient to stay on the ward and to receive the series of drugs a second time. The resident who was in charge of his case felt that the patient had experienced sufficient discomfort already, that it was unlikely that he would benefit from a repeat series of drugs, and that it would be desirable for him to go home to die where he could be with his family. Although the residents were low status members of the ward's social structure, their close involvement with the patients made it possible for them to manipulate the other members of the ward in order to obtain the kinds of decisions they wanted. For example, in presenting cases to the entire staff at the weekly conference, the resident could stress certain aspects of the case rather than others in order to win the group's approval of the course of action that he wanted rather than that wanted by the researcher who was associated with the case. A resident described this strategy very clearly:

> There is a tremendous amount of material on each patient. I obviously select certain things from it to emphasize. Today I stressed the social aspects of the case of Mr. Brown. I could have just glossed over these aspects of the case if I had wanted to. One of the staff wanted to use a very toxic drug on Mr. Brown. I don't want it used. I think most people would support me if they knew the case. Mr. Brown wants to go home. However, by myself, I can't say no. However, I used the rounds to get the group to say that they would rather let him go. So when this happened the staff member who wanted to continue the treatment had to agree.

Psychiatric observers claimed that the psychological problems of the patients were neglected. For example, the effects of being in isolation were at times very stressful for patients. One woman became hysterical under such conditions. The house staff were not prepared to handle the psychiatric aspects of their cases. As a result, they often abandoned patients by neglecting both their emotional and physical care. The nurses attempted to deal with the patient's psychological problems but this in turn meant that the patients discussed their problems less with the physicians and as a result obtained less information about their cases. The research staff were not interested in such problems and rarely attended a weekly psychiatric conference which was run by the ward psychiatrist. The staff's neglect of the psychiatric aspects of their cases was seen most clearly when they began to undertake a new type of operation, bone marrow transplants. When it was suggested to them that psychiatric screening of patients who were being selected for these operations would be desirable, the head of the program is reported to have said that he did not want any psychiatrists "messing around" with the project. The operation proved to be very traumatic for patients; some patients broke down emotionally. One patient proved to be a psychotic.

Members of the senior staff did not appear to recognize that there might be negative aspects to their organization's activities. One senior staff member commented:

Recently a medical student who had spent a quarter on the ward made a note on a patient's chart over at _____ Hospital. This was a 60-year-old female with lymphosarcoma. She said the woman was probably a candidate for chemotherapy but that it would be unfortunate to subject her to such a traumatic experience. She should be allowed to die. This comment took us by surprise. We wondered what sort of impression we were making on the medical students and the house staff. We've noticed that many medical students and house staff are very depressed. They think that what we are doing is wrong.

Social Organization and Ethical Experimentation: Ward II

Observations and interviews were also conducted on a second ward which was devoted to cancer chemotherapy research. This was a 45-bed ward composed of large rooms holding a dozen or more beds and a few private rooms. The walls were painted drab green and were in need of a fresh coat. The staff consisted of four senior men and 13 clinical associates, five who were spending their second year on the ward and eight who were spending their first year there. The clinical associates performed both experimental and treatment roles. Senior men were engaged primarily in research. All physicians except the director of the service had their offices inside the treatment complex.

Unlike the other group of researchers, this one lacked a strong ideology to support their activities. This was reflected in the attitude expressed by 12 out of 15 members of the department that there was no policy in the department regarding the treatment of cases. In Ward I only two out of 11 physicians expressed such an attitude. The absence of policy was seen as a result of the absence of strong leadership on the ward. The following comments illustrate this point of view:

This service has no policy-maker. If the head of a medical service feels one way or the other and makes his opinion heard and is looked up to, these questions become easier to deal with. You can defer your decision to the leader. There is nothing like that here. Each physician is pretty much encouraged to make his own decisions about his own patients.

X and Y are terrible leaders. Y has great difficulty dealing with patients or with colleagues. X is afraid of dying patients . . . There is a need for a philosophy but they don't provide it. I wanted to bring the new doctors together at the beginning of the year to prepare them a bit for what they were going to face. There isn't a philosophy from the top here. They are too mealy-mouthed.

Dr. X told us the first day that in the terminal situation we were to make our own decisions. Heroic measures were not expected if we felt them to be unnecessary. But we should work as hard as possible to save lives. Be active but don't overdo it. But this is very loosely stated so that it is interpreted differently by different people. It is a relatively non-specific thing. Dr. X is often excessively non-specific. He could have ended a controversy at rounds this morning simply by stating what should be done but he doesn't do that. Some things should be set down since the people who are making the decisions are not the ones who have the most experience. The most experienced person ought to set the policy.

The absence of an ideology to support their activities affected every aspect of the functioning of the ward. Morale was so low that it verged upon a state of demoralization. Ten out of 15 of the staff members reported that they were very or somewhat depressed when working with terminal patients. On Ward I, no physicians reported that they were very depressed. Four out of ten reported being somewhat depressed.

One source of the low morale on Ward II was a lack of conviction about the value of what they were doing. One of the younger physicians said:

> We test drugs. That's what we're here for. I think that certain drugs and certain protocols are not worth the morbidity to the patient. They cause so much discomfort, it's not worth it. I haven't decided whether I believe there is any future in this.

The combination of the lack of an ideology and their low morale affected patient care in a number of ways. There was a considerable amount of controversy concerning the appropriate treatment for particular patients. Fourteen out of 17 physicians on Ward II reported such controversies compared to eight out of 13 on Ward I. Only five out of 14 responded positively to a question concerning whether other physicians in the ward had influenced their thinking concerning the treatment of these patients. On Ward I, the comparable figure was nine out of 11. Some physicians reported that the director of the ward failed to criticize sloppy work on the part of the clinical associates. One physician said:

> Dr. X found that one of the men had not done an adequate write-up on one patient and had done no write-up on another patient. He should have given an ultimatum to that guy to do the write-ups but he didn't. He has no guts. He is wishy-washy.

Lack of leadership affected the performance of the nursing staff which was criticized by the physicians. In turn the nurses were critical of the physicians. They claimed on the one hand that the physicians avoided patients, and on the other, that some patients were overtreated. The social worker who was assigned to the ward corroborated the accusation of avoidance. He claimed that the patient charts showed that some physicians neglected their patients. At the same time, some of the doctors developed close relationships with certain patients.[3] The interviews suggested a tendency to identify with male patients who were approximately the same age as the physicians. Such patients became very dependent upon the physicians. Close relationships of this kind may have produced a lack of objectivity on the part of the physician with consequent effects on patient care.

It seems clear that the social organization of these two cancer chemotherapy wards affected the quality of patient care and the extent to which the patient's needs and rights were observed. In the following section, we will attempt to specify the effects of ward structure upon the ethical aspects of patient care in the two wards.

Social Organization and Ethical Codes

According to the Nuremberg Code for medical research involving human subjects, "the voluntary consent of the human subject is absolutely essential" (this and subsequent principles quoted in Barber 1967, pp. 96–97). A number of the problems involved in observing this principle are summarized in the following quotation from a physician who administered the day-to-day activities of Ward I. He was asked whether the patient's attitude influenced his decisions to continue their treatment:

> One case in point was the case of Mr. Jones who is an intelligent, well-educated attorney. He was here last summer. He knew a lot about the drugs and he asked that his life not be resuscitated or prolonged in a semi-coma. We respected his views. He didn't want to hang around indefinitely, if the medical possibilities had been exhausted. On the other hand, I think that Mr. Brown has only a hazy idea that he is not doing well and that he is in a very serious condition. I don't think he could grasp what is going on. I don't think he is capable of it. He doesn't understand his situation. He wants to go home. But the final decision has been dictated by medical policy and not by his personal feelings.

This quotation suggests that differences between social classes affect the extent to which informed consent actually takes place. It implies that scientific considerations rather than the attitude of the patient influence decisions to continue treatment in some cases. The same physician expressed general skepticism that patients could understand and benefit from the information which was given them:

> Patients who are going to have bone marrow transplants have the operation explained to them and they decide whether they want to go ahead. To me, this is ludicrous. Do they really understand what they are doing? I think that 99 percent of what they are told is lost.

---

[3] Only one senior physician was reported to have close relationships with his patients on Ward I.

A senior physician on Ward I doubted that even other physicians could really understand the value of their research. He commented:

> I can't even explain the value of a bone marrow transplant to physicians except after several hours of talk. If you asked me if other doctors at this hospital have difficulty understanding what we do, the answer is yes. We have serious conflicts with them.

The psychiatrist attached to Ward I doubted whether the patients were actually told what alternative treatments were available to them. He said:

> Very few people have refused treatment on that ward. This is probably because the alternatives are not presented to them. They are told that you will be killing yourself if you don't take these drugs, but this may not be true.

On the other hand, a member of the senior staff presented a very different picture of this process:

> The decision to prolong life is a two-way decision. The patient has to consent. It is very rare to treat a patient who is incapable of making the decision. Occasionally they are mentally confused and a member of the family makes the decision.

A case on Ward II illustrated another type of problem which is involved in obtaining the patient's consent. In this case, the patient stated an opinion which conformed to cultural expectations of her social role but which she evidently did not really believe. The patient was a housewife with three children who was carrying a fourth child when the diagnosis of leukemia was made. The physicians faced the dilemma of deciding whether to abort and treat her or to wait until the baby was born and treat her afterward. The patient expressed the desire to have the child but evidently suffered from a conflict between her desire for chemotherapy and her belief that abortion was immoral. At one point when she was five months pregnant she developed abdominal pains while on the ward. She interpreted these pains to the physician in charge as labor pains and expressed satisfaction that she would have the child soon and then be able to begin chemotherapy. Absence of psychiatric assessment of her case probably prevented the physicians from discovering her true feelings toward the child and toward treatment.

There was relatively little discussion of informed consent on Ward II. No direct questions were asked on this topic on the interview schedule but questions about prolongation of life for experimental purposes and the patient's attitude toward treatment which elicited such discussion on the other ward did not do so on this ward.

Item 9 of the Nuremberg Code states that "During the course of an experiment, the human subject should be at liberty to bring the experiment to an end if he has reached the physical or mental state where continuation of the experiment seems to him impossible." The case of Mr. Brown on Ward I which has been referred to earlier was perhaps the most clear-cut example of this situation during the period when observations were being made on that ward although there were other similar cases. Mr. Brown had received the full cycle of drugs without going into remission and some of the physicians wished to begin the treatment again. The physician who was in charge of the ward commented:

> We really face the question of whether we should go ahead when there is very little hope of remission. However, we intend to carry on. The alternative is that he goes home, gets pneumonia, bleeds and dies.

One of the medical students said:

> I sense that Mr. Brown wants to go home. They want to give him an extremely toxic agent. That will make him miserable and the chances of curing him are very poor.

The physician's ambivalence toward this principle was clearly stated by an informant who had formerly served as a clinical associate on Ward II:

> I think that you have to be more stringent about keeping people alive in that situation because your data depend on how long the patient lives.

There did not appear to be specific controversies of this kind on Ward II, although it was evident that some physicians felt that patients were overtreated. Physicians on both wards were asked the following question: "It has been claimed that lives of patients upon whom new drugs are being tested are sometimes prolonged until the experiment is finished." Two out of 11 physicians on Ward I replied affirmatively to this question compared to 11 out of 14 on Ward II. These questions evoked a great deal of resistance on Ward I but not on Ward II, perhaps due to the absence of an ideology or policy concerning these matters on that ward.

There were also allusions to another practice which reflects overtreatment, that of trying drugs "just to see what will happen." This type of approach was criticized by several physicians on Ward I on the grounds that its scientific value was nil. Another set of experiments which had been conducted on Ward II involved resuscitation of every patient on the ward regardless of his case in order to study the effects of resuscitation upon these kinds of patients. If the resuscitation succeeded in reviving the patient, he experienced considerable discomfort while the gain in useful life was minimal.

However, when asked how much the patient's attitude affected their decisions to continue treatment, the majority of physicians on both wards said that it did (seven out of 11 on Ward I; nine out of 14 on Ward II). But they also indicated that they were more responsive to the patient who wanted to be treated than to the patient who did not want to be treated. The family's attitude toward these matters had no influence whatsoever on Ward I (none of the physicians reported that they were influenced by the family's attitude) while half the physicians on Ward II said that they were influenced by the family's attitude. The physician who was in charge of Ward I said:

> Most families don't understand. They're not in a position to assess what is going on. In general the family doesn't influence me here.

A senior physician on Ward II said:

> You can't let the family influence you. But it is necessary to handle them diplomatically, so they will go along with your decisions. I steer them to my way of thinking. They don't want to make the decisions themselves.

The Nuremberg Code also states that "the experiment should be so constructed as to avoid all unnecessary physical and mental suffering and injury." As far as mental suffering is concerned, it appeared that the physicians on both wards tended to deny or ignore the psychiatric aspects of these cases. Avoidance of physical suffering was complicated by the fact that narcotics interfere with the effects of chemotherapy. As a result the physicians on Ward I tended to use placebos in place of narcotics to alleviate pain. The senior physicians denied that the patients experienced severe pain although the house staff reported that they did. Narcotics were apparently used more frequently on Ward II. However, a former member of that ward commented:

> You have to hurt people to do the research. Knowing what the therapy is like, I wouldn't choose to have it . . . You couldn't plan a death more horrible than intensive chemotherapy.

Finally, the Nuremberg Code states that "the degree of risk to be taken should never exceed that determined by the humanitarian importance of the problem to be solved by the experiment." This issue also becomes ambiguous in this type of setting. A young physician on Ward II described such ambiguities in a case which he was handling at the time:

> Mrs. Smith is 76. Recently she had a temperature of 107 degrees and she went into shock. She was given antibiotics and she came through shock. This was remarkable . . . The question now is what to treat her with. There are two ways of thinking about this. Is this a good time to treat her? She is so badly off that we might just make things worse by treating her. I used to think we shouldn't treat people in this situation but I have changed my mind. The chances of success are low but the outcome is so certain that she is going to die that I don't think treatment will really make her worse. If she gets a remission, then her white count will go up and her normal body responses to infection will be increased. Otherwise she will just get infection or maybe bleed to death. The other possibility is not to treat her and just transfuse her. But you can't do that for long because the bleeding will continue. You would

just be putting the blood in one place and it will come out at another. Her ultimate chances of survival are zero. But you can try and see what happens with various drugs. However, you can also argue that you are prolonging her misery if you get a remission because she will relapse very soon after. I can't answer that question.

In conclusion, additional insight into the nature of this experimental situation can be obtained from the fact that informants commented that they would treat patients differently if they were in private practice. The Nuremberg Code and others like it imply that patients should not be treated differently when they are experimental subjects than when they are private patients.

Ethical Treatment of Unsalvageable Patients

The data which have been presented in this chapter are based on field studies so that it is impossible to generalize the findings to other settings. Since studies have been done in similar settings, it is appropriate to compare this study with others and to attempt to develop a model of the factors that affect the behavior of physicians in such settings.

It is necessary to consider not only situations in which experimentation on human beings is taking place but all situations in which heroic attempts are being made to prolong the lives of unsalvageable patients. This type of situation is contrary to the norms of the medical profession as revealed by the present study. The unsalvageable patient is typically not treated heroically. Attempts to treat him are exceedingly stressful for both patient and physician. As a result, physicians who decide to treat such patients actively must develop a set of norms and a special organizational structure to protect themselves from demoralization and to protect the patients from exploitation. From this point of view, the problems of artificial kidney units where experimentation is not generally conducted are similar to those of cancer chemotherapy units, to the kind of situation described by Fox (1959), and to those in which an innovative operation such as a heart or kidney transplant is used to treat the patient. On the other hand, a large category of medical experiments, those which are conducted upon salvageable patients, is excluded from consideration.

What are the factors that affect the ethical treatment of unsalvageable patients undergoing experimental or heroic treatments? Fox found that the physicians on the ward which she studied typically treated their patients like close friends and almost like colleagues in some respects. Since the physicians needed to obtain the cooperation of these patients over periods of several years, they explained many of the scientific aspects of their illness to them in order to motivate them to continue to participate in the activities of the ward.

On Ward I, the possibilities for such involvements were limited because of the transience of the house staff and the sharp separation between the roles of researcher and practitioner. In addition, the researchers' strong ideology provided them with all the emotional support which they needed for their work. In fact, on Ward I there was a tendency to dehumanize the patients and to think of them as being incapable of making decisions.[4]

The demoralized junior physicians on Ward II also became friendly with their patients occasionally but for different reasons. The absence of a strong ideology to justify their work meant that colleague relationships were strained and that it was very difficult for them to maintain their own motivation to continue their work. Under these circumstances, they sometimes sought emotional satisfaction through friendships with patients.

Kuty (1973) who made field observations in four artificial kidney units in France and Belgium concluded that the patients' rights were more adequately protected in units which were democratically organized as compared to those which were hierarchically organized. He advocates a situation somewhat like the one Fox described, where the physicians treat the patients almost like colleagues. He suggests that the physician in these circumstances becomes somewhat deprofessionalized while the client becomes somewhat professionalized (Kuty 1973, p. 446). Under these conditions, the patient is aware of what is happening to him and can participate in the decision-making process.

However, this type of doctor-patient relationship is ineffective if the physicians are demoralized and deprofessionalized as a result of inadequate leadership. It would appear that both strong leadership, including a clearly defined set of norms and values and effective social control, is needed as well as the willingness to treat the patient as a kind of collaborator rather than as an object.

As we discussed above, ethical codes generally specify desirable consequences of physician behavior. However it appears that such codes are of limited usefulness. It is more important to specify the organizational variables which are conducive to ethical behavior. It appears that where medical experimentation and life-prolonging technologies in general are being used, the traditional relationships between physicians and between physician and patient are inappropriate. On the one hand, a more cohesive set of relationships among the physicians involved in such units including strong leadership is necessary.[5] On the other hand, a less hierarchical, less authoritarian

---

[4] The one physician on Ward I who did form close relationships with his patients was involved in developing techniques for bone marrow transplant surgery. The consequences of experimental surgery and of experimental treatments for relationships between physicians and patients will be discussed shortly.

[5] Barber *et al.* (1973) suggest that in some cases the absence of strong leadership by senior men in a research unit was associated with unethical behavior by their junior colleagues.

relationship between doctor and patient in which information can be freely exchanged is required. These conditions are most likely to occur when the social value of the patient to the physician and the social visibility of the unit are both high. In the absence of these two conditions, considerably greater effort and self-discipline on the part of the physician is required to create the appropriate organizational environment for ethical treatment of unsalvageable patients.

Fox and Swazey's studies of heart surgeons suggest that the patient upon whom experimental surgery is performed is the one whose rights are most likely to be protected for several reasons. First, the social value of the patient to the surgeon is very high due to three factors: (a) the number of patients who can be treated by each physician in this fashion is relatively small; (b) important results can be obtained from a single patient (by contrast, most forms of treatment and especially drug tests require trials on extensive series of patients); (c) the amount of time invested in each patient by the physician is high.[6] Second, the social visibility of the unit is likely to be high. Other physicians and the public are likely to be watching its activities and monitoring the results. If the mortality rate is too high, other physicians will exert social control, thus bringing the work at least temporarily to an end (Swazey and Fox 1970, Fox and Swazey 1974, Chapter 6).

The variables which tend to protect the surgical patient from exploitation by his physician are less likely to occur when the patient is the subject of medical research or treatment. The social value of each patient to the investigator is likely to be low because he deals with many patients on a short-term basis and the results obtained from each one are significant only as part of a series of trials. The social visibility of such units is apt to be low, since the research is not sufficiently dramatic or innovative to attract the attention of other physicians or of the public. It is not surprising that four out of the six case studies of unethical experiments which Barber and his associates (1973, Chapter 8) present are experiments involving drug tests.

On the other hand, when ethical standards are high in experimental units involving medical treatment, such as in the setting described by Fox (1959), the two variables which we have specified are likely to be positive. On Fox's Metabolic Ward, the social value of the patient to the investigators was high since they dealt with few patients, could obtain results from a single patient, and invested extensive amounts of time in each patient. Since the researchers were associated with a very prestigious medical school, the social visibility of the unit was probably higher than it would have been had it been connected with a less prestigious medical school.

---

[6] See Fox and Swazey 1974, Chapter 4, for case studies of kidney and heart transplant surgery teams which substantiate these observations.

Conclusion

As we have suggested, the use of any kind of treatment to prolong the life of an unsalvageable patient is stressful for patient and physician alike, whether experimental or not (Simmons and Simmons 1970 and 1971). The high suicide rates among patients in artificial kidney units is one indication of this (Abram *et al.* 1971). Under such conditions, the emotional well-being of a patient requires that he be more fully informed about the hazards and potentialities of his treatment than would be necessary under normal conditions.

On the other hand, the physician tends to reject these difficult patients. In order to handle them, he needs to be part of a cohesive group of physicians which provides both a set of norms to guide the behavior of its members and exercises social control when deviations occur.

In addition to the organizational variables which we have discussed, stronger external controls are needed, probably in the form of modifications of the already existing peer review mechanism, local committees of physicians which currently review medical research before it is undertaken (Barber *et al.* 1973, Chapter 9). Making these committees responsible to a central organization, as Pappworth (1968) proposes, would have the effect of making all of these groups conform to minimum standards. In addition, as Barber *et al.* suggest, the inclusion of more non-medical members and the institutionalization of reviews of research in progress would provide important additional checks on the ethical behavior of researchers. Extension of the activities of these peer-review committees to cover all those who apply life-prolonging technologies to unsalvageable patients would be advisable.

Chapter 9: Conclusion

Summary of Findings Concerning the Treatment of Critically Ill Patients

Evidence from the present study suggests that physicians respond to the chronically ill or terminally ill patient not simply in terms of physiological definitions of illness but also in terms of the extent to which the patient is capable of interacting with others.[1] The treatable patient is one who can interact or who has the potential to interact in a meaningful way with others in his environment. The physically damaged salvageable patient whose life can be maintained for a considerable period of time is more likely to be actively treated than the severely brain-damaged patient or the patient who is in the last stages of terminal illness. The brain-damaged infant is also defined as untreatable by many physicians since he lacks the potential to establish social relationships with others. The unsalvageable infant is less likely to be actively treated than the salvageable infant, even if the latter is physically or mentally damaged.

Consistent with the interpretation that physicians are using a social definition of life are the findings from this study which show that the family's attitude toward the treatment of the brain-damaged child is an important influence upon the physician's decision to treat the child. If the family does

---

[1] The findings from the study are generalizable (a) to internists and pediatricians practicing in hospitals which have residencies in these specialties; (b) to all neurosurgeons and pediatric heart surgeons practicing in the United States.

199

not define such an infant or child as socially dead, it is more likely to be treated. By contrast, the adult patient's attitude rather than his family's attitude affects the doctor's decision to treat or not to treat the terminally ill patient. However, the surveys indicate that consent is only one factor in the physician's decision to treat. He sometimes withdraws treatment when the patient is incapable of giving consent and gives treatment when the patient or his agent have expressed a desire that treatment be discontinued.

Although the data are not entirely consistent or conclusive on this point, it appears that social capacity rather than social value is the more important factor in the physician's decision to treat these patients. In other words, the patient's capacity or potential capacity to engage in social interaction is a more important factor in the decision to treat him than his social status or prestige.

While some physicians are reluctant to withdraw all treatment from dying patients even when the patient is incapable of benefiting from the treatment (the extreme example of this is the case of the anencephalic infant), the number of physicians who consistently treat different types of patients actively, regardless of their social potential, is small.

Certain types of problems which the physician encounters in the treatment of the dying and the dead occur so frequently and are so visible to the medical profession and even to the general public that norms have emerged which permit the physician in effect to hasten deaths in these situations. Two examples of this are the prescription of narcotics to terminal patients in pain and the termination of respirator treatment for the patient who has suffered irreversible brain death.

The data suggest that while negative euthanasia with respect to certain types of cases — the severely brain-damaged patient and the severely physically damaged terminal patient — is widespread, positive euthanasia is relatively rare. In fact, there appears to be a very strongly held norm in the medical profession against direct killing, even when the individual has no capacity whatsoever to develop social relationships. Only a handful of pediatricians said that they would be likely to kill an anencephalic infant. On the other hand, close to half of the internists said that they would be willing to increase the dosage of narcotics for a terminally ill cancer patient to the point where it would probably lead to respiratory arrest. In this situation, the physician interprets his behavior as an attempt to alleviate pain rather than as an act which is intended to kill the patient.

There appears to be a puzzling inconsistency between the physician's attitudes toward the treatment of critically ill patients and his responses to the patient who has just died. Although resuscitation procedures are not recommended for terminal patients, a substantial proportion of respondents indicated that they would resuscitate patients who had died of terminal illness.

The internist is less likely to say that he would treat some types of critically ill patients actively than to say that he would resuscitate them after they have died. Actual behavior in the two areas may be more similar than are attitudes concerning the two areas since examination of hospital records indicates that resuscitation occurs less frequently than the attitude data suggest. In other words, physicians' attitudes but not necessarily behavior toward the patient who has died are closer to the traditional norm that life must be preserved as long as possible.

An analogous phenomenon was observed among pediatric surgeons. An analysis of records of mongoloid children with heart defects who were evaluated for surgery in a hospital where the pediatric service was very much in favor of treating mentally retarded children, indicated that the proportion of mongoloid children who received cardiac surgery was lower than the questionnaire results would suggest.

In general, the findings concerning the attitudes and behavior of physicians towards these types of patients were remarkably consistent in the various samples. The consistency of the findings using examples of patients from four different specialties and at both ends of the life cycle is an important element in their credibility.

While there is considerable consistency among the attitudes of these physicians concerning priorities for the treatment of critically ill patients, how much consensus is there among them concerning the allocation of treatments to specific patients? The highest levels of consensus appeared in the surgical samples, probably as a consequence of the small size of these specialties. In both these samples over 95 percent of the surgeons indicated that they would usually or sometimes operate upon salvageable patients with physical damage. Over 75 percent in both samples would usually or sometimes operate upon salvageable patients with mental damage. Among the neurosurgeons, over 75 percent said that they would usually or sometimes operate upon an unsalvageable patient with physical damage (age 40). However, only 50 percent made similar replies to the question concerning the unsalvageable patient with mental damage.

Among the internists, the highest level of consensus also occurred in the case of the salvageable patient with physical damage. Over two-thirds of both residents and physicians said that they would or might resuscitate this patient and about 90 percent said that they would treat him (defined as scores in the lowest third of the distribution). Between one-half and two-thirds of these physicians would treat and resuscitate the salvageable patient with moderate mental damage. With respect to three other patients, the salvageable patient with severe mental damage, the unsalvageable patient with moderate physical damage, and the unsalvageable patient with severe physical damage, the consensus was highest concerning whether or not these patients should be resuscitated — between half and three-quarters of both residents and physicians agreed on this point. There was much less consensus concerning the treatment of these patients. Approximately one-third of the residents and physicians agreed that these patients should be treated and another third agreed that they should receive minimal treatment (defined as scores in the highest third of the distribution).

Among the pediatricians, there was considerable agreement concerning the treatment of the salvageable infant with physical damage and the salvageable mongoloid child. Over two-thirds of both the residents and physicians agreed that these children should be treated (scores in the lowest third of the distribution). Similar proportions of both samples agreed that the mongoloid child should not be resuscitated, but both samples were almost equally divided on the question of resuscitating the physically damaged (myelomeningocele) salvageable infant. Over 90 percent of the residents and physicians agreed that the anencephalic infant (unsalvageable, mentally damaged) should not be resuscitated. While over two-thirds of the physicians agreed that this child should receive minimal treatment, only 61 percent of the residents agreed on this point. There was least agreement about the unsalvageable, physically damaged child. Between one-half and two-thirds of the physicians and residents agreed that this child should not be resuscitated. Almost three-quarters of the residents were willing to treat it but only one-half of the physicians were of this opinion.

To summarize, the highest levels of consensus were found among the surgeons, followed by the pediatricians. The highest levels of disagreement occurred among the internists' decisions about whether or not to treat severely damaged salvageable and unsalvageable patients. In general, it appeared that there was less consensus about the treatment and resuscitation of unsalvageable patients than salvageable patients. The treatment of severely damaged patients was also controversial, perhaps because the social potential of these patients was ambiguous to many physicians.

The findings concerning the characteristics which differentiate physicians who appear to have traditional attitudes toward treatment from those whose attitudes are more permissive were less consistent. However, it seems clear that house staff physicians working in prestigious hospital settings are more active in their treatment of critically ill patients than older physicians. While they also tend to be more active than their counterparts in other types of hospials, they are less concerned with the social aspects of the treatment of their patients in some cases and more concerned in others. The emphasis upon high standards of treatment in prestigious hopsitals leads to the aggressive treatment of some types of patients who are unlikely to be able to resume their social roles. On the other hand, these residents were more responsive to the wishes of their patients concerning treatment than were residents in less prestigious hospitals.

There was also some evidence that the norms concerning the treatment of critically ill patients which are followed by residents and physicians in these hospitals are different. Physicians are less likely than residents to be active in their treatment of critically ill patients in prestigious hospitals but are as active as residents in other hospitals. The existence of two distinct hospital subcultures, one consisting of house staff and attending physicians and the other consisting of part-time physicians, was inferred.

Among the medical and pediatric residents, hospital setting was the most important influence upon decisions to treat patients (in prestigious settings, more aggressive treatments were used), while religious affiliation had the most influence upon decisions which affect the patient when he has died or is close to death, such as resuscitation. Among the physicians in these specialties, religious affiliation was the major factor both in decisions to resuscitate and to a lesser extent in decisions to treat. In some cases, hospital prestige was negatively correlated with these types of decisions.

Differences in the behavior of members of the three major religious faiths (Catholicism, Judaism, and Protestantism) seem to reflect their status as members of ethnic groups rather than the official policies of the religious organizations concerned. Catholics and Jews seem to be most concerned with the preservation of life and liberal Protestants least. The data indicate that religious norms concerning euthanasia have virtually no influence upon physicians' decisions concerning critically ill patients. Even very religious physicians are relatively unaffected by the positions which representatives of their religious faiths have taken on these issues.

Religious affiliation also appeared to be the factor most consistently associated with a general tendency to treat actively regardless of the characteristics of the patient. The findings suggest that the correlates of activism are not for the most part organizational variables but are deepseated attitudes concerning the value of life under different conditions. Religious and cultural (Western–non-Western) background appears to play a role in shaping these attitudes. Since physicians from different religious faiths perceive these issues in various ways, it appears unlikely that controversies regarding appropriate policies for the treatment of critically ill patients will be speedily resolved.

Social Control Over Medical Care for the Critically Ill Patient: Some Recommendations

I have stressed that this study, unlike other treatments of the subject, has been concerned not with what physicians *should* do for the critically ill patient but with his *actual* behavior. What are the implications of these findings for those groups in our society who are concerned with formulating policy in this area and with developing new ethical imperatives for medical practice?

The findings from this study of the treatment which doctors say they give to critically ill patients suggest that the system whereby this type of behavior is controlled by peers, clients, and other social institutions such as the law, is in need of reformulation. The problem arises because there is clearly a disparity between official medical policy concerning the treatment of these patients and the actual behavior of physicians. Officially, treatment is meant to be continued as long as life, defined in physiological terms, can be preserved. In fact, as we have seen, treatment is generally withdrawn when the quality of life as defined in social terms has deteriorated or disappeared irrevocably.

In a sense, social control over these kinds of decisions is maintained by stressing the preservation of life at all costs, rather than by specifying conditions under which the norm may be relaxed. This suggests that deviance is widespread and that it is considered a threat to existing norms. The system responds to this danger by overstressing the importance of treating, even when the patient cannot benefit from treatment, in order to avoid the possibility that individuals who might benefit from treatment will not be treated. Following Scheff's analysis (1963) of decision rules in medical diagnosis, the system is arranged in such a way that physicians will avoid making Type One errors (not treating a patient who could have benefited from treatment) even at the risk of making a certain number of Type Two errors (treating patients who could not benefit from treatment).

Since both the attitudes and the actual behavior of physicians indicate that they avoid treating patients who could not benefit from treatment, it is possible that the likelihood of making Type Two errors (treating patients who could not benefit from treatment) has increased to such an extent that informal norms have developed to cope with the situation. Informally, social criteria for defining the treatable patient have replaced the official physiological criteria but the new criteria are not universally accepted.

Considerable stress is being placed upon this social control system by the disparity between the formal and informal norms and by the fact that the number of patients for whom application of the formal norms would be undesirable is steadily increasing due to improvements in medical technology. At the same time, in a number of other areas such as abortion and genetic engineering, the same dilemma of choosing between social and physiological definitions of life is being resolved in favor of the former.

This suggests that an attempt should be made to alter the formal norms in this area. Since the present study shows that these decisions are made on the basis of criteria which are specific to individual patients, this could be done by developing ethical guidelines for the withdrawal of treatment with respect to certain specifically defined conditions. In fact, such a set of guidelines has already been formulated to deal with one pressing problem in the treatment of the critically ill patient: the problem of the irreversibly comatose patient whose respiratory functions are being maintained mechanically. As the data presented in the book indicate, this set of guidelines has already been widely although not universally accepted by physicians in four major medical specialties.

Since there appear to be certain cases in each medical specialty which repeatedly cause controversy, some attempt ought to be made to specify the medical and social conditions under which treatment would be desirable. For example, it should be possible to define guidelines for withdrawing all life-saving or death-prolonging treatment from the patient whose capacity for meaningful social interaction has been irreversibly impaired by a stroke. In such cases only the use of treatment which alleviates suffering is appropriate, if the treatable patient is being defined in social as well as physical terms.

Similarly the case of the anencephalic infant would appear to be one where specific guidelines could resolve the inconsistencies which now exist between the treatment of these infants and those whose conditions meet the criteria of irreversible brain death. Treatment can be discontinued in the latter case as specified in existing ethical guidelines. There is no reason to continue it in the former case.

Another example is the case of the infant with a myelomeningocele, a condition which if severe produces paraplegia, lack of bladder and urinary control, and brain damage in newborn infants. A recognized medical authority on this type of ailment (Lorber 1971) has recently stated the criteria for not treating certain children with this ailment. Unfortunately, such children can live untreated for several months, enduring considerable pain and suffering. J. M. Freeman (1972) has recently suggested that this is one instance where withholding treatment should not be considered to be ethically superior to terminating life. In other words, it would be more ethical to kill such a child than to permit it to linger in the hospital for weeks or months untreated, waiting to die. In this type of case, also, specific guidelines for the withdrawal of treatment and even for the termination of life would appear to be highly desirable.

Many difficult medical problems which physicians now face will obviously not be amenable to this approach. However, with improvements in medical knowledge it will no doubt be possible to specify such guidelines for increasing numbers of medical conditions.

What is meant here by ethical guidelines is very different from the ethical codes which have been developed particularly in the area of medical experimentation, but also for general medical practice. These codes are stated in such general terms that they provide no useful guidance in dealing with the highly differentiated situations which physicians face. Instead, ethical guidelines concerning the appropriate levels of treatment for specific conditions or diseases are needed.

The decision to withdraw treatment in accord with such guidelines should be subject to review by the physician's colleagues. Peer review is already used to monitor ethical aspects of medical behavior in the area of medical experimentation on human beings. Many hospitals already have committees which monitor medical performance with respect to operative procedures and deaths. The individualistic character of medical practice has made any sort of regulation of medical practice extremely difficult. However, now that it has become evident that the rule that life should be preserved in every instance is unworkable, some sort of regulation to resolve the most difficult cases is a necessity.

Such guidelines would probably be of greatest value for the young physician. The older physician has discovered the range of acceptable behaviors with respect to difficult cases but also is less likely to have to make life-saving or death-prolonging decisions. The younger physician faced with such decisions is usually given generalities in place of guidance. Programs which attempt to teach medical ethics are probably of limited usefulness in resolving the dilemmas which young physicians face since the kind of philosophical approach that is often used tends to highlight these ambiguities in such difficult cases rather than to develop a framework within which they could be resolved. Discussions of the quality of life are not useful unless it can be operationally defined.

Current Medical Practice on Euthanasia and Its Social Implications

The implications of this study and of new developments in related areas are that our culture is in the process of changing its definition of human life. We are moving away from a definition of life in purely physiological terms toward a social definition. Increasingly a life is being defined as human on the basis of its capacity for social interaction. Indications of this fundamental shift in cultural values can be seen not only in the medical area but also in recent legal decisions and in changes in popular attitudes as measured by public opinion polls.

When a physician chooses to challenge the right of a patient or his agent to refuse treatment, the issue may be decided by the courts.[2] Until recently, the law has upheld the position that life should be preserved under all circumstances. In general, competent adults have not been permitted to refuse procedures which save life or prolong the process of dying. In such cases, the judge declares the patient "incompetent" so that his wishes can be overridden by a court-appointed guardian. Families have also not been permitted to refuse life-saving or dying-prolonging procedures for their incompetent rela-

---

[2] I am grateful to Robert M. Veatch for suggesting materials in this area and for his memo on this issue (Veatch and Sollitto 1973).

tives. However, there appear to be signs of a trend toward judicial refusals of physicians' requests to override a patient's rejection of death-prolonging medical treatment (Cantor 1973). In some recent cases competent adults without dependents have been permitted to refuse treatment (Holman 1972, Hendin 1973). In one of these cases, the judge permitted a woman who was mentally competent but unable to speak to refuse further leg amputations (Hendin 1973, pp. 67–69). While families have not generally been permitted to refuse treatment for incompetent relatives, a recent case of an elderly woman with hemolytic anemia set a precedent in that her daughter was permitted to refuse treatment for her which was prolonging her life (Dilemma in Dying 1971).

The legal principles underlying these decisions have been discussed by Cantor (1973). On the one hand, the law is concerned with upholding society's interest in the preservation of life. This principle underlies the law's unwillingness to permit the patient to refuse life-saving or death-prolonging techniques. He argues that there is another principle that is equally important in Western law which might be considered in these cases. The principle is that of respect for individual self-determination and for bodily integrity as dictated by constitutional rights of personal privilege. On this ground he argues that the right of the competent individual to refuse treatment must be upheld and that the law must recognize that refusals of treatment do not pose a threat to social well-being. Thus the government does not have a valid interest in compelling the individual to accept medical treatment. He also considers that the individual's right to refuse treatment should be upheld regardless of whether the patient has dependents. The law has no right to intervene in order to protect the survivor's emotional or economic interests. In his view, respecting the patient's right to decline treatment reflects sensitivity toward personal freedom, *not* lack of respect for the sanctity of life. To the extent that recent court decisions have tended to uphold the individual's right to decline treatment, it is possible that Cantor's views reflect a position toward which the law is gradually moving.

Information about popular attitudes toward the definition of life is most readily available in the area of abortion. Judging from public opinion surveys, abortion of potentially deformed children appears to be well accepted by the general public (Blake 1971, p. 540). In 1969, 75 percent of a national sample approved of abortion if it was known that the child would be deformed. There is much less public support for abortion when the fetus is rejected by its mother for discretionary (selfish) reasons, but support for this point of view is rapidly growing. Twenty-one percent of a national sample would accept abortion in cases where the parents did not want an additional child, a figure which is 12 percent higher than that obtained in a similar poll taken in 1965. These data also suggest that popular attitudes are moving toward a social interpretation of life. Similarly, juries have tended not to recommend punishment in cases of so-called "mercy-killing" (Sanders 1969).

There appear to be certain important differences between the doctor's perspective and that of the layman. It seems that the physician makes a distinction among chronically ill patients which is not always obvious to the layman. The physician differentiates between those patients who can be maintained over a considerable period of time and those patients whose condition is clearly terminal. When there is severe physical discomfort or irreversible mental damage the layman is likely to view salvageable patients in the same light as unsalvageable patients.

It is probably in this area that some of the most serious conflicts between physicians and patients or patients' families arise. Recent court cases confirm this impression. For example, the dispute between a New York City hospital and the wife of an irreversibly brain-damaged man over the insertion of a new battery in the pacemaker which was maintaining his cardiac function can be seen in this light (Crafton 1972). The physicians did not perceive this man's condition as terminal. Therefore, they considered that it was necessary to continue treatment. The wife did not see the problem in these terms but felt that her husband's level of functioning did not justify the use of such a surgical procedure. The court held that the physicians were correct and appointed a guardian for the patient. Another case, with a different outcome — that of an elderly woman suffering from hemolytic anemia which was resolved by a court order permitting the patient's daughter to refuse treatment for her — also represented a situation which doctor and layman interpreted differently (Dilemma in Dying 1971). The physician sees such a patient as one whose condition can be maintained in spite of acute physical discomfort. The layman tends to feel that the level of discomfort is too high to justify the additional weeks or months of life.

According to the survey, the patient with severe physical damage whose condition can be maintained for a considerable period of time is likely to be actively treated against his wishes or those of his agent. Patients in the other three categories (i.e., the salvageable patient with severe mental damage, the unsalvageable patient with physical damage only, and the unsalvageable patient with mental damage) are less likely to be actively treated against their wishes or those of their agents. Sixty-seven percent of the physicians in internal medicine indicated that they would treat very actively a severely debilitated, semi-comatose but salvageable patient suffering from chronic pulmonary fibrosis whose wife was described as being reluctant to authorize an essential life-saving procedure (a tracheostomy). However, only 16 percent of the internists indicated that they would treat very actively a severely brain-damaged patient who could not communicate meaningfully with others and whose family had indicated that they were unwilling to care for her at home after discharge from the hospital. The patient who wants active treatment is likely to receive it but withdrawal of treatment by the physician depends less upon the consent of the patient or his agent than on the physician's assessment of the patient's prognosis and type of damage.

While the survey suggests that the terminal patient who indicates that he does not want vigorous treatment will not receive such treatment, not all patients are aware of their rights to refuse treatment. Numerous studies show that certain types of patients, particularly those whose ethnic and educational backgrounds are different from those of their physicians, find it difficult to communicate with physicians and presumably to engage in the delicate type of negotiations required in order to obtain withdrawal of medical treatment.

It is important that the element of individuality in these decisions, the right of the patient or his family to select more or less treatment depending on their needs and preferences, be strengthened, since the element of individual choice is what makes such decisions the antithesis of the mass killings of the physically and mentally damaged which occurred in Nazi Germany. Legislation to strengthen the rights of patients or their families to refuse treatment may help to resolve some of the difficulties which now exist in this area. Legislation which would permit physicians to cease treatment of certain types of cases has been proposed in several states (Veatch 1972). There are a number of problems in developing suitable legislation. Some of the legislation which has been proposed is too general such as the Florida Death with Dignity Bill of 1970 which would guarantee that life would not be prolonged beyond the point of "meaningful existence." Another proposed bill, the West Virginia Bill of 1972 is too specific, since the right to refuse treatment is limited to "artificial, extraordinary, extreme or radical medical or surgical means or procedures." Still another bill, the Idaho Euthanasia Act,[3] which was modeled after legislation which has been introduced in the British parliament would legalize active hastening of death when requested by the patient. This feature is more controversial than the right to refuse treatment and is opposed by those who fear that it would weaken the prohibition against killing and hence respect for the sanctity of life. Veatch (1972) contends that there is no real need for such a bill. Instead he argues that what is needed is legislation which would strengthen the right of the patient to refuse treatment, including a clear statement of law that refusal of treatment itself is not to be taken as grounds for mental incompetence. He also sees a need to modify the law to permit refusals of treatment by relatives when the patient is incompetent.

There are of course limitations to what can be accomplished by legislation.

---

[3] Similar positive euthanasia proposals were introduced in Montana and Oregon in 1973. At least sixteen bills of various types have been introduced in state legislatures but to date none has passed.

While it is easy to impose sanctions upon the physician who hastens death or withdraws treatment without the permission of his patient or the patient's guardians, it is more difficult to impose sanctions upon a physician who refuses to hasten death or withdraw treatment.[4] The Idaho Bill permits physicians who are reluctant to hasten death to withdraw from the case but circumstances might often make it difficult for a patient to change doctors in such a situation. For example, other physicians might be unwilling to cooperate.[5]

While legislation may provide valuable support for the patient or his relatives in these situations, other changes will also be necessary. If they are to exercise their rights in a meaningful fashion, patients and families alike will have to educate themselves in advance about the complexities of medical technology and the problems which it can create for medical care. By the time they are actually faced with such decisions, they should know what sort of alternatives they prefer.[6]

Additional support for the patient has recently been provided by the American Hospital Association which has published as a statement of its national policy a "bill of rights" for patients. Among these rights, the bill includes that of refusing treatment "to the extent permitted by law." Some hospitals are introducing ombudsmen who concern themselves with the problems which patients face in obtaining appropriate medical care. These people

---

[4] While sanctions have not been imposed, a court decision against the use of life-saving treatment was rendered after the death of a Jehovah's Witness who had refused blood transfusions but received them as a result of a decision by a court-appointed guardian (Holman 1972).

[5] The law could also deal with the problem of patients whose respiratory function is being supported by a respirator after spontaneous brain function has ceased by establishing statutory definitions of death which would define as dead patients who have experienced brain death. A movement is under way to enact legislation which would define acceptable criteria for declaring a patient to be dead. One such statute has been enacted in Kansas; other states have passed or are considering such legislation. Although this type of legal approach is controversial, proponents of a model statute of this sort argue that such a statute is necessary because it will "dispel public confusion and disquiet and protect both physicians and patients" (Capron and Kass 1972).

[6] Letters, sometimes called "living wills," can be used to indicate preferences concerning treatment in advance of illness. Such documents executed before the illness occurs must necessarily be vague and as a result may not be useful when illness actually occurs. The physician is under no obligation to follow such documents. Whether or not he does is probably a function of the type of doctor-patient relationship which has been established before the illness occurs. Since the family doctor appears to be becoming a rarity, the optimal conditions for the observance of the patient's wishes as expressed through such letters are unlikely to occur. However, if the patient is incompetent, such letters may assist relatives to confirm their impressions of his attitudes concerning treatment. For further discussion of such letters, see Veatch 1972.

could be especially useful in assisting lower-class patients and in informing them of their rights with respect to these issues. It appears that ombudsmen are most effective when they belong to a separate organization rather than to the hospital's administrative staff.[7]

It is possible that growing public concern with these issues reflects an increasing desire by individuals to control their own lives (and deaths) and increasing unwillingness to accept unquestioningly the physician's judgment in these matters. Physicians in the future may find it necessary to treat the chronically ill patient less as a dependent for whom decisions have to be made and more as an equal. Concern with these issues can already be found in the literature (Freidson 1970, pp. 352, 355–56, Reeder 1972).

Finally, the traditional sociological perspective on these issues also requires some modification. The Parsonian model of the physician's role gives the physician complete authority over the definition of illness and the decision to treat it. Lay evaluation and control over the physician's behavior are considered to be minimal, except in cases where the physician may treat complaints that he considers to have no medical basis in order to expand his practice (Freidson 1970, p. 107).

In a sense, the Parsonian model reflects the nature of medical practice during approximately the first half of the twentieth century. The physician did not have the kind of authority which the sociological model of a medical professional now attributes to him 150 years ago when his capacity to treat acute illness, much less chronic illness, was more limited than it is now. The professional role of the physician as described by the current sociological model seems to have emerged in the second decade of this century and appears now to be undergoing significant alterations.

According to Daniel Bell (1966), these kinds of changes are to be anticipated as part of the post-industrial society. He suggests that in the post-industrial society professionals will increasingly be challenged by their clients who will be concerned to defend their rights:

> If the struggle between capitalist and worker, in the locus of the factory, was the hallmark of industrial society, the clash between the professional and the populace, in the organization and in the community, is the hallmark of conflict in the post-industrial society. [p. 167]

The steady decline in the proportion of acute illness and concomitant increase in the proportion of chronic illness means that the results of medical treatment are no longer unequivocally desirable. While the patient can be given extra months or years of life, the cost in terms of suffering and in the reduction of his life space may mean that the patient himself will define the

---

[7] I am grateful to Rick Cortez for documentation on the role of the ombudsman.

results as undesirable. As the results which the physician can offer become more ambiguous in terms of their social value to the patient, one can expect that the physician's authority will increasingly be questioned.

Appendix 1: Charts

CHART A.1. NEUROSURGERY — SUMMARY OF RESEARCH DESIGN

(1) *Type of Condition: Cerebral hematoma (salvageable)*

    Op. 1a — Severe brain damage   Op. 1b — Physical damage

(2) *Type of Condition: Broken neck with quadriplegia — Severe Physical Damage in Adult*

    Op. 2a — Family attitude high   Op. 2b — Family attitude neutral

(3) *Type of Condition: Myelomeningocele—Severe Physical Damage in Newborn (salvageable)*

    Op. 5a — Low social status   Op. 5b — High social status

(4) *Type of Condition: Mongoloid hydrocephalic — Brain Damage in Newborn (salvageable)*

    Op. 6a — Family attitude low   Op. 6b — Family attitude high

(5) *Type of Condition: Solitary metastatic brain tumor — Terminal Illness in Adult*

    Op. 3 a.i. — 40-yr-old patient   Op. 3 a.ii — 40-yr-old patient
              Mild physical   Severe mental
              impairment   impairment

    Op. 3 b.i — 65-yr-old patient   Op. 3 b.ii — 65-yr-old patient
              Mild physical   Severe mental
              impairment   impairment

(6) *Type of Condition: Metastatic tumor with paraplegia — Terminal Illness in Adult*

    Op. 4 — Severe physical impairment

CHART A.2. INTERNAL MEDICINE: SUMMARY OF RESEARCH DESIGN

Case #	Salvage-able	Intellectual or Physical Disability	Disease	Physician Error	Patient Age	Family Finances	Family Attitude	Patient Attitude	Social Status	Sex
1 A	No	Phys.	Cancer	none	45	Hi	Pos.	Unknown	Hi	Male
B	No	Phys.	Cancer	none	45	Lo	Pos.	Unknown	Hi	Male
C	No	Phys.	Cancer	none	45	Lo	Pos.	Unknown	Lo	Male
5 A	No	Phys.	Cancer	none	30	—	None	Neg.	—	Male
B	No	Phys.	Multiple Sclerosis	none	30	—	None	Neg.	—	Male
C	No	Phys.	Cancer	none	30	—	None	Pos.	—	Male
2 A	Yes	Moderate Intellec.	Stroke	none	65	—	Neg.	Unknown	Lo	Female
B	Yes	Severe Intellec.	Cerebral atrophy	none	65	—	Neg.	Unknown	Lo	Female
C	Yes	Moderate Intellec.	Stroke	none	65	—	Pos.	Unknown	Lo	Female
6 A	Yes	Phys.	Pulmonary disease	none	35	—	Neg.	Unknown	Non-deviant	Male
B	Yes	Phys.	Pulmonary disease	none	35	—	Neg.	Unknown	Deviant	Male
C	Yes	Phys.	Pulmonary disease	none	65	—	Neg.	Unknown	Non-deviant	Male
3 A	No	—	Cardiac arrest	yes	67	—	—	—	—	Female
B	No	—	Cardiac arrest	no	67	—	—	—	—	Female
C	No	—	Cardiac arrest	yes	47	—	—	—	—	Female

4 A	Uncertain	Phys.	Myocardial infarc.;	none	47	Hi	—	Pos.	Hi	Male
B	Uncertain	Phys.	jaundice;	none	47	Lo	—	—	Lo	Male
C	Uncertain	Phys.	hist. of cancer	none	47	Hi	—	Neg.	Hi	Male
7 A	Uncertain	Phys.	Dyspnea;	none	45	—	Pos.	—	—	Male
B	Uncertain	Phys.	hypotension;	none	75	—	Pos.	—	—	Male
C	Uncertain	Phys.	possib. of cancer	none	75	—	Neg.	—	—	Male

CHART A.3. PEDIATRICS — SUMMARY OF RESEARCH DESIGN

(1) *Type of Condition: Congenital anomaly — Anencephaly; hypoplastic left ventricle (unsalvageable)*

A: Severe brain damage

Family attitude: high (would encourage physician to get rid of the child)

B: No brain damage

Family attitude: Low (would not encourage doctor to be active)

(2) *Type of Condition: Congenital anomaly — Myelomeningocele (salvageable)*

A: Severe physical damage; some possibility of brain damage but this is less likely since the child does not have hydrocephalus at birth.

Social status: high

B: Same.

Social status: low

(3) *Type of Condition: Congenital anomaly — Mongolism (salvageable)*

A: Mental retardation plus hyaline membrane disease or pneumonia

Family attitude: low

Social status: high

B: Same.

Family attitude: high (precious pregnancy)

Social status: low

(4) *Type of Condition: Birth defect — Brain damage (salvageable)*

A: Premature separation of placenta followed by seizures, spasticity and hypertonia

Family attitude: high (precious pregnancy)

Social status: high

B: Same

Family attitude: low

Social status: low

(5) *Error*

A: Physician error

B: Mechanical error

CHART A.4. PEDIATRIC HEART SURGERY — SUMMARY OF RESEARCH DESIGN

(1) *Type of Condition: Moderate heart defect combined with mongolism*
Op. 1a: Family attitude high   Op. 1b: Family attitude low

(2) *Type of Condition: Severe heart defect combined with mongolism*

Op. 2a: Family attitude high   Op. 2b: Family attitude low

(3) *Type of Condition: Severe heart defect combined with severe mental retardation (Op. 3)*

(4) *Type of Condition: Moderate heart defect combined with severe but treatable urogenital anomaly*

Op. 4a: Social status high   Op. 4b: Social status low
      Family attitude high   Family attitude neutral

(5) *Type of Condition: Severe heart defect combined with severe but treatable urogenital anomaly*

Op. 5a: Social status high   Op. 5b: Social status low
      Family attitude high   Family attitude neutral

(6) *Type of Condition: Mild heart defect combined with multiple physical defects*

Op. 6a: No developmental   Op. 6b: Developmental retardation
      retardation

Appendix 2: Questionnaires

1. **Critical Decisions in Neurosurgery**

2. **Critical Decisions in Medical Practice, Versions A, B, and C**

3. **Treatment of Congenital Anomalies and Severe Birth Defects in Newborns, Versions A and B**

4. **Critical Decisions in Pediatric Cardiac Surgery**

1: Critical Decisions in Neurosurgery

Instructions-- Either pen or pencil may be used to complete the questionnaire. Please disregard the numbers which appear in the text of the questions. They are for the use of IBM tabulating machine operators.

The object of this survey is to determine your attitudes toward performing operations which can only partially correct extremely debilitating conditions or which involve risk of worsening the patient's physical or social condition or that of his family. In responding to these questions please keep in mind similar cases which you have treated *in the hospital in which you perform the majority of your operations.*

Operation 1: (a) A 40 year old right-handed married lawyer with a past history of mild hypertension has suffered a large, intracerebral, left, deep frontal hematoma. He has severe aphasia, moderate right hemiparesis, and mild nuchal rigidity. He is drowsy but is able to say his name in a garbled manner. BP is 190/100. Arteriogram shows 1 cm. shift of anterior cerebral artery to right and no evidence of tumor, aneurysm, or A-V malformation. During the first 12 hours of observation, his level of consciousness has steadily declined. Needle evacuation of the hematoma has been attempted but only a negligible quantity of liquified blood could be aspirated. Although trans-cortical incision with direct surgical evacuation of the hematoma might prove fatal, he might also die if the hematoma is not evacuated. Assuming that he survives surgical evacuation, it is very likely that he may have severe residual intellectual and neurological impairment. Under these circumstances, would you operate? *(Check one of the following).*

5. ☐ 1. Would *usually* perform.
   ☐ 2. Would *sometimes* perform.
   ☐ 3. Would *rarely* perform.

(b) In this same patient, the hematoma has occurred in the nondominant right parietal-occipital area and the residual deficit has left him with a visual field-cut and left hemiparesis but no significant intellectual or speech impairment. In this instance, again, needle evacuation of the hematoma was ineffective and it appears that the patient may die if surgical evacuation is not performed. What would be your likely course of action with respect to surgical evacuation of the hematoma? *(Check one of the following).*

6. ☐ 1. Would *usually* perform.
   ☐ 2. Would *sometimes* perform.
   ☐ 3. Would *rarely* perform.

Operation 2: A 20 year old college student has a fracture dislocation at C.5-6 which is now in good position 24 hours after reduction in tongs. He has shown no motor or sensory function below the C.5 level from the time of admission and there is no manometric block on L.P. *Irrespective* of your plans regarding possible anterior or posterior cervical fusion, would you do a *cervical decompressive laminectomy* under either of the following circumstances?

221

(a)   The family is financially comfortable and is anxious that everything possible be done for their son. *(Check one of the following)*.

    7. ☐ 1. Would *usually* perform.

          ☐ 2. Would *sometimes* perform.

          ☐ 3. Would *rarely* perform.

(b)   The same family is applying no pressure upon you for action. *(Check one of the following)*.

    8. ☐ 1. Would *usually* perform.

          ☐ 2. Would *sometimes* perform.

          ☐ 3. Would *rarely* perform.

Operation 3: (a)   A 40 year old man presents with a solitary metastatic brain tumor. The primary cancer is inoperable bronchogenic. The patient is still in good general physical condition. He has a wife and three teenage sons. Would you remove the tumor under either of the following conditions? Headache is not a problem in either case.

(i)   The tumor is in the non-dominant right frontal lobe. *(Check one of the following)*.

    9. ☐ 1. Would *usually* perform.

          ☐ 2. Would *sometimes* perform.

          ☐ 3. Would *rarely* perform.

(ii)   The tumor is adjacent to the speech area in the left temporo parietal area. *(Check one of the following)*.

    10. ☐ 1. Would *usually* perform.

           ☐ 2. Would *sometimes* perform.

           ☐ 3. Would *rarely* perform.

(b)   The same patient is 65 years old. Would you remove the tumor under either of the following conditions? Headache is not a problem in either case.

(i)   The tumor is in the non-dominant right frontal lobe. *(Check one of the following)*.

    11. ☐ 1. Would *usually* perform.

           ☐ 2. Would *sometimes* perform.

           ☐ 3. Would *rarely* perform.

(ii)   The tumor is adjacent to the speech area in the left temporo parietal area. *(Check one of the following)*.

    12. ☐ 1. Would *usually* perform.

           ☐ 2. Would *sometimes* perform.

           ☐ 3. Would *rarely* perform.

Operation 4:   To remove a tumor which is metastatic from the kidney to the thoracic epidural space and which has produced paraplegia within the last 24 hours. He has also suffered complete loss of bladder function in the last 24 hours. Pain is not a problem. The patient is a 45 year old married man. Would you remove the tumor? *(Check one of the following)*.

    13. ☐ 1. Would *usually* perform.

☐ 2. Would *sometimes* perform.

☐ 3. Would *rarely* perform.

Operation 5:   To correct high lumbar myelomeningocele which is leaking CSF in a newborn. There is no evidence of hydrocephalus or of Arnold-Chiari malformation. He has no nerve function in his legs and no bladder or rectal sphincter control. Would you correct this condition under either of the following conditions?

   (a)   This is the first child of 20 year old parents neither of whom have completed high school. *(Check one of the following).*

       14.   ☐ 1. Would *usually* perform.

              ☐ 2. Would *sometimes* perform.

              ☐ 3. Would *rarely* perform.

   (b)   The parents of the infant are well educated and financially comfortable. *(Check one of the following).*

       15.   ☐ 1. Would *usually* perform.

              ☐ 2. Would *sometimes* perform.

              ☐ 3. Would *rarely* perform.

Operation 6:   To shunt a rapidly progressive hydrocephalic with a cortex of 2 cms. The infant also has the characteristics of a mongoloid. Would you correct this condition under either of the following conditions?

   (a)   The parents of the infant have three other healthy children. They do not want the child and plan to institutionalize him. *(Check one of the following).*

       16.   ☐ 1. Would *usually* perform.

              ☐ 2. Would *sometimes* perform.

              ☐ 3. Would *rarely* perform.

   (b)   The parents of the infant want him and plan to care for him at home. *(Check one of the following).*

       17.   ☐ 1. Would *usually* perform.

              ☐ 2. Would *sometimes* perform.

              ☐ 3. Would *rarely* perform.

Question 1:   Which of the following best describes the attitude of the majority of your neurosurgical colleagues in the department of surgery *in the hospital where you perform the majority of your operations?*

   (a)   Toward operations to correct severe myelomeningocele in a newborn. *(Check one of the following).*

       18.   ☐ 1. They are in favor of performing such operations in most cases.

              ☐ 2. They are *not* in favor of performing such operations in most cases.

              ☐ 3. There is no consensus among them about such operations.

   (b)   Toward operations to remove a solitary metastatic brain tumor. *(Check one of the following).*

       19.   ☐ 1. They are in favor of performing such operations in most cases.

              ☐ 2. They are *not* in favor of performing such operations in most cases.

              ☐ 3. There is no consensus among them about such operations.

Question 2: (a)   Assuming that the patient is a 45 year old man with a concerned family, please rank the following conditions in terms of the likelihood that you would operate. Place a 1 next to the condition in which you would be most likely to operate, a 4 next to the condition in which you would be least likely to operate, and 2 or 3 next to the conditions in which you would be moderately likely to operate.

    20. _____ a. Intracerebral hematoma.

    21. _____ b. Neck fracture with quadriplegia.

    22. _____ c. Solitary metastatic brain tumor.

    23. _____ d. Tumor metastatic to spine.

(b)   *Approximately* how many cases of the following conditions do you see in an average year?

    24. _____ a. Hydrocephalus.

    25. _____ b. Intracerebral hematoma.

    26. _____ c. Myelomeningocele.

    27. _____ d. Neck fracture with quadriplegia.

    28. _____ e. Solitary metastatic brain tumor.

    29. _____ f. Tumor metastatic to spine.

Question 3: (a)   A 25 year old man with head trauma is in deep coma on a respirator. There is no evidence of intracranial hematoma. He has had two flat EEG's over a 2-day period and is unresponsive to painful stimuli. Brain stem reflexes are absent. Cardiac activity is present but there is no spontaneous respiratory activity. Which of the following would you be likely to do? *(Check one of the following).*

    30. ☐ 1. Leave respirator running until spontaneous cardiac activity ceases.

    ☐ 2. Turn off respirator without consulting colleagues or family.

    ☐ 3. Turn off respirator after consulting colleagues and finding a consensus of their opinion in favor of doing so.

    ☐ 4. Turn off respirator after consulting family and finding that they will accept this decision.

    ☐ 5. Turn off respirator after consulting both colleagues and family and finding both groups in favor of it.

(b)   In the past year, how many patients have you treated on respirators in whom there was a question of brain death?

    31. _____

Question 4: (a)   When you are uncertain about whether to operate upon a patient with an extremely debilitating condition, how much do the following *professional considerations* influence your decision? Please place a 1 next to the factor which influences you most, a 6 next to the factor which influences you least, and a 2,3,4 and 5 next to the factors which have intermediate degrees of influence upon your decision.

    32. _____ a. Your previous success in treating a similar and equally difficult case.

    33. _____ b. The advice of residents and interns.

34. _____ c. The advice of senior physicians.

35. _____ d. Legal consequences which might ensue if medically indicated therapy were omitted

36. _____ e. Scientific studies showing the success rate of a particular type of treatment.

37. _____ f. Opportunity to learn, practice or teach new techniques.

Question 4: (b) When you are uncertain about whether to operate upon such a patient, how much do the following *characteristics of the patient* influence your decision? Please place a 1 next to the factor which influences you most, a 7 next to the factor which influences you least, and a 2,3,4,5 and 6 next to the factors which have intermediate degrees of influence upon your decision.

38. _____ a. The patient's chronological age.

39. _____ b. The patient's physiological age.

40. _____ c. The patient's desire to die.

41. _____ d. The family's concern for the patient.

42. _____ e. The financial burden of his illness to his family.

43. _____ f. The financial burden to society, i.e. insurance and welfare.

44. _____ g. The patient's potential usefulness to society or family if he recovers.

Question 5: (a) *Approximately* how many operations of all types (excluding diagnostic procedures) do you perform per year?

45. _____

(b) In what type of hospital do you perform the *majority* of these operations? *(Check one of the following).*

46. ☐ 1. A teaching hospital which is the major unit in a medical school's teaching program.

☐ 2. A teaching hospital which is used to a limited extent in a medical school's teaching program.

☐ 3. A teaching hospital which is used for graduate training only in a medical school's teaching program.

☐ 4. A teaching hospital with no medical school affiliation.

☐ 5. A hospital with no teaching program.

Question 6: (a) In what year did you receive your M.D.?

47. _____

(b) In what hospital (s) did you do your neurosurgical residency? *(Please give name and city where hospital is located for each hospital).*

48. _____

(c) What is your status now?

49. ☐ 1. Full-time neurosurgeon on hospital staff.

☐ 2. Part-time neurosurgeon on hospital staff (private practice).

Question 7: Are you board certified in neurosurgery?

50. ☐ 1. Yes

☐ 2. No

Question 8: (a) What is your marital status? *(Check one of the following).*

51. ☐ 1. Single.

☐ 2. Married.

☐ 3. Divorced or separated.

☐ 4. Widowed.

Question 8: (b)   How many children do you have?

        52. _____

Question 9: (a)   In what religious faith were you raised? *(Check one of the following).*

        53. ☐ 1. Catholic ·

             ☐ 2. Jewish.

             ☐ 3. Protestant *(Please specify denomination, e.g. Congregationalist).*

             _____

             ☐ 4. Other *(Please specify religion, e.g. Buddhist).*

             _____

             ☐ 5. None.

        (b)   If you have changed your religion, please indicate your new faith.

        _____

        (c)   How important is your religion to you now? *(Check one of the following).*

        54. ☐ 1. Extremely important.

             ☐ 2. Fairly important.

             ☐ 3. Fairly unimportant.

             ☐ 4. Not at all important.

Question 10:   What is your father's occupation? (If he is retired or deceased, please indicate his occupation before his retirement or decease).

        55. _____

PLEASE MAIL THE POSTCARD WHICH IS ENCLOSED WITH THE QUESTIONNAIRE. THIS WILL INDICATE THAT YOU HAVE RETURNED IT WITHOUT REVEALING YOUR IDENTITY ON THE QUESTIONNAIRE IN ANY WAY. THESE POSTCARDS WILL BE USED TO COMPILE A MAILING LIST OF PHYSICIANS TO WHOM COPIES OF THE FINDINGS FROM THIS STUDY WILL BE SENT.

IF YOU HAVE ANY COMMENTS ON THESE QUESTIONS OR A PERSONAL PHILOSOPHY CONCERNING THESE ISSUES, PLEASE WRITE THEM BELOW. THANK YOU VERY MUCH FOR YOUR COOPERATION.

2: Critical Decisions in Medical Practice: A

Instructions-- Either pen or pencil may be used to complete the questionnaire. Please disregard the numbers which appear in the text of the questions. They are for the use of IBM tabulating machine operators.

The following cases are designed to simulate the decision-making process which the physician faces in dealing with patients suffering from chronic diseases. In responding to these questions, please keep in mind similar cases which you have treated in the hospital named in the covering letter.

A (1) A 45 year old lawyer with a history of mild hypertension and biopsy-proven carcinoma of the upper esophagus develops a severe esophageal obstruction. He is not able to swallow liquids and has considerable local discomfort requiring morphine on admission to the hospital. Chest x-rays reveal an enlarged cardiac silhouette and it is suspected that he may have pericardial effusion. His wife and three teenage sons are deeply concerned and ask you to spare no expense in treating him. Which of the following would you be likely to perform? *(Check yes, maybe, or no for each item).*

Yes	Maybe	No		
☐	☐	☐	10.	Intravenous fluids for dehydration.
☐	☐	☐	11.	Heart scan for diagnosis.
☐	☐	☐	12.	Pericardiocentesis for cardiac tamponade.
☐	☐	☐	13.	Thoracotomy and pericardial window for recurrent tamponade due to spread of cancer.
☐	☐	☐	14.	Colon bypass for palliation if liver biopsy contains tumor and life expectancy is one month.
☐	☐	☐	15.	Feeding gastrostomy if liver biopsy contains tumor and life expectancy is 9 months.
☐	☐	☐	16.	If life expectancy is one month and respiratory insufficiency due to pneumonia became severe, would you use endotrachial tube and respirator?
☐	☐	☐	17.	If respiratory distress lasted 2 days, would you perform tracheostomy?
☐	☐	☐	18.	If cardiac arrest occurred, would you begin resuscitation?
☐	☐	☐	19.	If resuscitation was unsuccessful after 15 minutes, would you continue?

A (2) A 65 year old woman had a severe stroke one year ago. As a result, she cannot walk, eats with difficulty and has mild difficulty expressing herself. She is admitted to the ward service dehydrated and septic. Her family is unwilling to care for her at home if discharged from the hospital following treatment. Which of the following would you be likely to perform? *(Check yes, maybe, or no for each of the following).*

Yes	Maybe	No		
☐	☐	☐	20.	Intravenous feeding for dehydration.
☐	☐	☐	21.	Lumbar puncture for stiff neck and fever.

227

☐ ☐ ☐ 22. Urine culture for pyuria.

☐ ☐ ☐ 23. Six blood cultures for fever and murmur.

☐ ☐ ☐ 24. Appendectomy for incidental suspected appendicitis.

☐ ☐ ☐ 25. Small bowel resection for suspected infarcted bowel.

☐ ☐ ☐ 26. If respiratory insufficiency due to pneumonia became severe, would you use endotrachial tube and respirator?

☐ ☐ ☐ 27. If respiratory distress lasted 2 days, would you perform tracheostomy?

☐ ☐ ☐ 28. If cardiac arrest occurred, would you begin resuscitation?

☐ ☐ ☐ 29. If resuscitation was unsuccessful after 15 minutes, would you continue?

A (3) A 67 year old retired social worker is admitted to your service. She has previously been in excellent health except for shortness of breath. You obtain blood gases and treat the patient for pulmonary edema. After giving a second large dose of morphine, the patient's heart suddenly stops. Blood gas report is then called to the ward, indicating that PCO_2 before repeated morphine was 87 mm Hg. After three minutes, you insert endotracheal tube and restore respirations and a normal sinus rhythm. Which of the following would you be likely to perform? *(Check yes, maybe, or no for each item)*.

Yes   Maybe   No

☐ ☐ ☐ 30. Monitor EKG constantly.

☐ ☐ ☐ 31. Order special nurses on 24-hour duty or place in an intensive care unit.

☐ ☐ ☐ 32. Measure arterial blood gases.

☐ ☐ ☐ 33. Respirations become labored, would you begin artificial ventilation?

☐ ☐ ☐ 34. Two days later respirations remain depressed, would you perform a tracheostomy?

☐ ☐ ☐ 35. Acute renal shutdown with uremia develops; her heart functions but she is in coma; would you perform peritoneal dialysis when urea nitrogen reached indicated level?

☐ ☐ ☐ 36. One month later she opens eyes, follows objects, cannot speak or use extremities. Pneumonia recurs; would you give antibiotics ?

☐ ☐ ☐ 37. Breathing is labored again, would you use respirator?

☐ ☐ ☐ 38. Two EEG's are flat in a 24-hour period, heart is still beating; brother *reluctantly* agrees to consider donation if she *"dies"*; kidneys are needed by young patient with excellent match. Would you pronounce dead or call the death committee?

☐ ☐ ☐ 39. Two EEG's are flat in a 24-hour period; heart is still beating; brother agrees *willingly* to donation. Would you pronounce dead or call the death committee?

A (4) A 47 year old married banker with recent pneumonectomy for lung cancer is brought to the hospital by his wife and daughter because he has become jaundiced. On the night of admission to the hospital he talks about his plans for the future. Later that evening he has a myocardial infarction and a few PVC's. Which of the following would you be likely to perform? *(Check yes, maybe, or no for each item).*

Yes	Maybe	No	
☐	☐	☐	40. Would you order 24-hour special nurses or place in intensive care unit?
☐	☐	☐	41. Respirations become labored; would you use endotrachial tube and respirator?
☐	☐	☐	42. Two days later, respirations are still poor; would you perform tracheostomy?
☐	☐	☐	43. Ventricular tachycardia occurs. Would you use IV xylocaine if you had to sit by bed all night?
☐	☐	☐	44. Would you use constant IV xylocaine if nurses monitored all night?
☐	☐	☐	45. He survives MI but has acute tubular necrosis. Would you perform peritoneal dialysis when urea nitrogen reached indicated level?
☐	☐	☐	46. Would you use antibiotics for pneumonia?
☐	☐	☐	47. He suddenly arrests; would you begin resuscitation?
☐	☐	☐	48. After 20 minutes, no stable rhythm is obtained; would you continue to resuscitate?
☐	☐	☐	49. If chest cardiac massage did not produce an effective pulse, would you open the chest?

A (5) A 30 year old bachelor has been suffering from melanoma of the leg that has metastasized to the spinal cord and he becomes paraplegic. You have been treating him for several months on an out-patient basis. He then develops a severe urinary tract infection. He is admitted to the hospital, alert but septic and in severe distress. He requests that he not be treated vigorously. Which of the following would you be likely to perform? *(Check yes, maybe, or no for each of the following).*

Yes	Maybe	No	
☐	☐	☐	50. Intravenous fluids for dehydration.
☐	☐	☐	51. Antibiotics.
☐	☐	☐	52. Lumbar puncture because he has stiff neck and fever.
☐	☐	☐	53. Urethral catheter for urinary retention.
☐	☐	☐	54. Suprapubic tube if catheter can't be inserted.
☐	☐	☐	55. Appendectomy for incidental appendicitis.
☐	☐	☐	56. Upper G.I. series for acute upper G.I. bleeding.
☐	☐	☐	57. Esophagoscopy and gastroscopy for acute upper G.I. bleeding.
☐	☐	☐	58. If cardiac arrest occurred, would you begin resuscitation?
☐	☐	☐	59. If resuscitation was unsuccessful after 15 minutes, would you continue?

A (6) A 35 year old man is brought to the hospital by his wife. He has a history of severe chronic pulmonary fibrosis and for three years has been unable to climb stairs or walk more than 10 feet due to shortness of breath. He is found to have pneumococcal pneumonia, but during his first hospital day he becomes cyanotic and semicomatose. If a tracheostomy is performed, he will probably survive without further impairment of lung function. His wife is reluctant to authorize this procedure. Which of the following would you be likely to perform? *(Check yes, maybe, or no for each of the following).*

Yes   Maybe   No

☐ ☐ ☐ 60. Would you attempt to persuade his wife to authorize tracheostomy?
☐ ☐ ☐ 61. Intravenous feeding for dehydration.
☐ ☐ ☐ 62. Antibiotics.
☐ ☐ ☐ 63. Arterial puncture for blood gas analysis.
☐ ☐ ☐ 64. Urine culture for pyuria.
☐ ☐ ☐ 65. Urethral catheter for urinary obstruction.
☐ ☐ ☐ 66. Appendectomy for incidental suspected appendicitis.
☐ ☐ ☐ 67. Small bowel resection for suspected infarcted bowel.
☐ ☐ ☐ 68. If cardiac arrest occurred, would you begin resuscitation?
☐ ☐ ☐ 69. If resuscitation was unsuccessful after 15 minutes, would you continue?

A (7) A 45 year old man is brought to the hospital by his concerned family. Chest x-ray reveals a mass in the right hilum which is thought by the radiologist to represent lung cancer. He admits to smoking and hemoptysis. His family expresses concern for his welfare and asks you to do all you can for him. While you are talking to the family, the nurse tells you that he has become dyspneic while getting into bed and has developed hypotension. Which of the following would you be likely to perform? *(Check yes, maybe, or no for each item).*

Yes   Maybe   No

☐ ☐ ☐ 70. Do EKG.
☐ ☐ ☐ 71. Lung scan for suspected pulmonary emboli.
☐ ☐ ☐ 72. Pulmonary arteriogram for suspected emboli.
☐ ☐ ☐ 73. Heparin therapy for proven pulmonary emboli.
☐ ☐ ☐ 74. A proven massive embolus occurs and he has approximately a 20% chance of living only if he has embolectomy. Would you ask surgeon to operate?
☐ ☐ ☐ 75. He survives embolus only to have a myocardial infarction and develops shock requiring your constant monitoring of an intravenous infusion of Levophed. Would you stay by bed all night?
☐ ☐ ☐ 76. After he has recovered from MI and if respiratory insufficiency due to pneumonia became severe, would you use endotrachial tube and respirator?
☐ ☐ ☐ 77. If respiratory distress lasted 2 days, would you perform tracheostomy?
☐ ☐ ☐ 78. If cardiac arrest occurred, would you begin resuscitation?

☐ ☐ ☐ 79. If resuscitation was unsuccessful after 15 minutes, would you continue?

8 (a) In the hospital named in the covering letter, what is the average number of patients which you treat per month?

10. _____

(b) On the average, how many of these patients require decisions of the type described above?

11. _____

(c) Do you generally refer these patients or do you treat them yourself?

_____ I generally refer these patients.

_____ I generally treat them myself.

9 (a) A 25 year old man with head trauma is in deep coma on a respirator. There is no evidence of intracranial hematoma. He has had two flat EEG's over a 2-day period and is unresponsive to painful stimuli. Brain stem reflexes are absent. Cardiac activity is present but there is no spontaneous respiratory activity. Which of the following would you be likely to perform? *(Check one of the following).*

12. _____ 1. Leave respirator running until spontaneous cardiac activity ceases.

_____ 2. Turn off respirator without consulting colleagues or family.

_____ 3. Turn off respirator after consulting colleagues and finding a consensus of their opinion in favor of doing so.

_____ 4. Turn off respirator after consulting family and finding that they will accept this decision.

_____ 5. Turn off respirator after consulting both colleagues and family and finding both groups in favor of it.

(b) In the past year, how many patients have you treated on the respirator in whom there was a question of brain death?

13. _____

10. A 45 year old, 140 pound man in the last stages of terminal cancer has been receiving 40 mg. of morphine p.r.n. Later 40 mg. of morphine no longer gives him relief from pain. Which of the following would you be likely to prescribe? *(Check one of the following).*

14. _____ 1. No increase in dosage.

_____ 2. Increased dosage but not to the extent that there is danger of producing respiratory arrest.

_____ 3. Increased dosage to the point where pain is relieved even if it might risk respiratory arrest.

_____ 4. If dosage described in (3) was not effective, increased dosage to the point where pain is relieved even if it will probably lead to respiratory arrest.

11. (a) Assuming that the patient is a 45 year old man with a concerned family, please rank the following illnesses in terms of how actively you would treat them. Place a 1 next to the illness which you would treat *most* actively, an 8 next to the illness you would treat *least* actively, and 2, 3, 4, 5, 6, and 7 next to the illnesses to which you would give intermediate degrees of attention.

15. _____ a. Chronic pulmonary disease.

_____ b. Chronic uremia.

_____ c. Meningitis.

_____ d. Metastatic carcinoma to the brain.

_____ e. Metastatic carcinoma to the spine.

_____ f. Multiple strokes.

_____ g. Myocardial infarction.

_____ h. Pneumonia.

(b) *Approximately* how many cases of these illnesses do you treat in an average year in the hospital named in the covering letter?

16. _____ a. Chronic pulmonary disease.

17. _____ b. Chronic uremia.

18. _____ c. Meningitis.

_____ d. Metastatic carcinoma to the brain.

_____ e. Metastatic carcinoma to the spine.

_____ f. Multiple strokes.

_____ g. Myocardial infarction.

_____ h. Pneumonia.

12.(a) When you are uncertain about how actively to treat a patient with debilitating chronic disease, how much do the following *professional considerations* influence your decision? Please place a 1 next to the factor which influences you most, a 6 next to the factor which influences you least, and a 2,3,4, and 5 next to the factors which have intermediate degrees of influence upon your decision.

19. _____ a. Your previous success in treating a similar and equally difficult case.

20. _____ b. The advice of residents and interns.

21. _____ c. The advice of senior physicians.

22. _____ d. Legal consequences which might ensue if medically indicated therapy were omitted.

23. _____ e. Scientific studies showing the success rate of a particular type of treatment.

24. _____ f. Opportunity to learn, practice or teach new techniques.

(b) When you are uncertain about how actively to treat such a patient, how much do the following *characteristics of the patient* influence your decision? Please place a 1 next to the factor which influences you most, a 7 next to the factor which influences you least, and a 2,3,4,5, and 6 next to the factors which have intermediate degrees of influence upon your decision.

25. _____ a. The patient's chronological age.

26. _____ b. The patient's physiological age.

27. _____ c. The patient's desire to die.

28. _____ d. The family's concern for the patient.

29. _____ e. The financial burden of his illness to his family.

30. _____ f. The financial burden to society (i.e. insurance and welfare).

31. _____ g. The patient's potential usefulness to society or family if he recovers.

13. How would you rate the quality of intensive nursing care on the medical service of the hospital named in the covering letter? (*Check one of the following.*)

    32. _____ 1. Very good.
           _____ 2. Good.
           _____ 3. Fair.
           _____ 4. Poor.
           _____ 5. Very poor.

14.(a) What is the name of the medical school from which you obtained your M.D.?

    33._____

(b) In what year did you obtain your M.D.?

    34._____

15(a) In what hospital did you intern? (*Please give name and city where hospital is located.*)

    35._____

(b) In what hospital(s) have you been a resident or fellow? (*Please give name and city where hospital is located.*)

    36. 1st year _____
           2nd year _____
           3rd year_____

(c) What is your status now?

    37. _____ 1. Resident.
           _____ 2. Full-time physician on hospital staff.
           _____ 3. Private practice.

(d) If private practice, do you admit patients to more than one hospital?

    _____ Yes   _____ No

(e) What proportion of your patients do you admit to the hospital named in the covering letter?

    _____

(f) Are you board certified in internal medicine?

    38. _____ 1. Yes.
           _____ 2. No.

16. What is your citizenship?

    39. _____

17. What is your marital status?

    40. _____ 1. Single.
           _____ 2. Married.
           _____ 3. Divorced or separated.
           _____ 4. Widowed.

18. What is your sex?

    41. _____ 1. Male.
           _____ 2. Female.

19. What is your race?

    42. _____ 1. Black.
           _____ 2. White.
           _____ 3. Other.

20.(a) In what religious denomination were you raised? (*Check one of the following.*)

    43. _____ 1. Catholic.
           _____ 2. Jewish.
           _____ 3. Protestant. (*Please specify denomination, e.g. Congregationalist.*)

    _____
           _____ 4. Other. (*Please specify religion, e.g. Buddhist.*) _____
           _____ 5. None.

(b) If you have *changed* your religion, please indicate your new faith.

    _____

(c) In general, how important would you say your religion is to you? (*Check one of the following.*)

    44. _____ 1. Extremely important.
           _____ 2. Fairly important.

_____ 3. Fairly unimportant.
_____ 4. Not at all important.

---

21. What is your father's occupation? *(If he is retired or deceased, please indicate his occupation before his retirement or decease.)*

    45. _____

PLEASE MAIL THE POSTCARD WHICH IS ENCLOSED WITH THE QUESTIONNAIRE. THIS WILL INDICATE THAT YOU HAVE RETURNED IT WITHOUT REVEALING YOUR IDENTITY ON THE QUESTIONNAIRE IN ANY WAY. THESE POSTCARDS WILL BE USED TO COMPILE A MAILING LIST OF PHYSICIANS TO WHOM COPIES OF THE FINDINGS FROM THIS STUDY WILL BE SENT.

IF YOU HAVE ANY COMMENTS ON THESE QUESTIONS OR A PERSONAL PHILOSOPHY CONCERNING THESE ISSUES, PLEASE WRITE THEM BELOW. THANK YOU VERY MUCH FOR YOUR COOPERATION.

Critical Decisions in Medical Practice: B

Instructions-- Either pen or pencil may be used to complete the questionnaire. Please disregard the numbers which appear in the text of the questions. They are for the use of IBM tabulating machine operators.

The following cases are designed to simulate the decision-making process which the physician faces in dealing with patients suffering from chronic diseases. In responding to these questions, please keep in mind similar cases which you have treated in the hospital named in the covering letter.

B (1) A 45 year old lawyer with a history of mild hypertension and biopsy-proven carcinoma of the upper esophagus develops a severe esophageal obstruction. He is not able to swallow liquids and has considerable local discomfort requiring morphine on admission to the hospital. Chest x-rays reveal an enlarged cardiac silhouette and it is suspected that he may have pericardial effusion. His wife and three teenage sons are deeply concerned. You are aware that his illness is exhausting the family's resources. Which of the following would you be likely to perform? *(Check yes, maybe or no for each item).*

Yes	Maybe	No		
☐	☐	☐	*10.*	Intravenous fluids for dehydration.
☐	☐	☐	*11.*	Heart scan for diagnosis.
☐	☐	☐	*12.*	Pericardiocentesis for cardiac tamponade.
☐	☐	☐	*13.*	Thoracotomy and pericardial window for recurrent tamponade due to spread of cancer.
☐	☐	☐	*14.*	Colon bypass for palliation if liver biopsy contains tumor and life expectancy is 9 months.
☐	☐	☐	*15.*	Feeding gastrostomy if liver biopsy contains tumor and the life expectancy is one month.
☐	☐	☐	*16.*	If life expectancy is one month, and respiratory insufficiency due to pneumonia became severe, would you use endotrachial tube and respirator?
☐	☐	☐	*17.*	If respiratory distress lasted 2 days, would you perform tracheostomy?
☐	☐	☐	*18.*	If cardiac arrest occurred, would you begin resuscitation?
☐	☐	☐	*19.*	If resuscitation was unsuccessful after 15 minutes, would you continue?

B (2) A 65 year old woman with severe cerebral atrophy cannot walk, feed herself or communicate meaningfully with others. She is admitted to the ward service dehydrated and septic. Her family is unwilling to care for her at home if discharged from the hospital following treatment. Which of the following would you be likely to perform? *(Check yes, maybe, or no for each item).*

Yes	Maybe	No		
☐	☐	☐	*20.*	Intravenous feeding for dehydration.
☐	☐	☐	*21.*	Lumbar puncture for stiff neck and fever.
☐	☐	☐	*22.*	Urine culture for pyuria.
☐	☐	☐	*23.*	Six blood cultures for fever and murmur.

235

☐ ☐ ☐ 24. Appendectomy for incidental suspected appendicitis.

☐ ☐ ☐ 25. Small bowel resection for suspected infarcted bowel.

☐ ☐ ☐ 26. If respiratory insufficiency due to pneumonia became severe, would you use endotrachial tube and respirator?

☐ ☐ ☐ 27. If respiratory distress lasted 2 days, would you perform tracheostomy?

☐ ☐ ☐ 28. If cardiac arrest occurred, would you begin resuscitation?

☐ ☐ ☐ 29. If resuscitation was unsuccessful after 15 minutes, would you continue?

B (3) A 67 year retired social worker is admitted to your service. She has previously been in excellent health except for shortness of breath. You treat the patient for pulmonary edema and during rigorous accepted therapy, the patient's heart suddenly stops. After three minutes, you insert endotracheal tube and restore respirations and a normal sinus rhythm. Which of the following would you be likely to perform? *(Check yes, maybe, or no for each item).*

Yes   Maybe   No

☐ ☐ ☐ 30. Monitor EKG constantly.

☐ ☐ ☐ 31. Order special nurses on 24-hour duty or place in an intensive care unit.

☐ ☐ ☐ 32. Measure arterial blood gases.

☐ ☐ ☐ 33. Respirations become labored, would you begin artificial ventilation?

☐ ☐ ☐ 34. Two days later respirations remain depressed, would you perform a tracheostomy?

☐ ☐ ☐ 35. Acute renal shutdown with uremia develops; her heart functions but she is in coma; would you perform peritoneal dialysis when urea nitrogen reached indicated level?

☐ ☐ ☐ 36. One month later she opens eyes, follows objects, cannot speak or use extremities. Pneumonia recurs; would you give antibiotics?

☐ ☐ ☐ 37. Breathing is labored again, would you use respirator?

☐ ☐ ☐ 38. Two EEG's are flat in 24-hour period, heart is still beating; brother *reluctantly* agrees to consider donation if she *"dies"*; kidneys are needed by young patient with excellent match. Would you pronounce dead or call the death committee?

☐ ☐ ☐ 39. Two EEG's are flat in a 24-hour period; heart is still beating; brother agrees *willingly* to donation. Would you pronounce dead or call the death committee?

B (4) A 47 year old unemployed laborer with recent pneumonectomy for lung cancer is admitted to the hospital because he has become jaundiced. On the night of admission he has a myocardial infarction and a few PVC's. Which of the following would you be likely to perform? *(Check yes, maybe or no for each of the following).*

Yes   Maybe   No

☐ ☐ ☐ 40. Would you order 24-hour special nurses or place in intensive care unit?

☐ ☐ ☐ 41. Respirations become labored; would you use endotrachial tube and respirator?

☐ ☐ ☐ 42. Two days later, respirations are still poor; would you perform tracheostomy?

☐ ☐ ☐ 43. Ventricular tachycardia occurs. Would you use constant IV xylocaine if you had to sit by bed all night?

☐ ☐ ☐ 44. Would you use constant IV xylocaine if nurses monitored all night?

☐ ☐ ☐ 45. He survives MI but has acute tubular necrosis. Would you do peritoneal dialysis when urea nitrogen reached indicated level?

☐ ☐ ☐ 46. Would you use antibiotics for pneumonia?

☐ ☐ ☐ 47. He suddenly arrests; would you begin resuscitation?

☐ ☐ ☐ 48. After 20 minutes, no stable rhythm is obtained; would you continue resuscitation?

☐ ☐ ☐ 49. If chest cardiac massage did not produce an effective pulse, would you open the chest?

B (5) A 30 year old bachelor has multiple sclerosis and has become paraplegic. You have been treating him for several months on a out-patient basis. He then develops a severe urinary tract infection. He is admitted to the hospital, alert but septic and in severe distress. There is a small chance that he can be given additional weeks of life through vigorous therapy but he will be paraplegic. He requests that he not be treated vigorously. Which of the following would you be likely to perform? *(Check yes, maybe, or no for each item).*

Yes   Maybe   No

☐ ☐ ☐ 50. Intravenous fluids for dehydration.

☐ ☐ ☐ 51. Antibiotics.

☐ ☐ ☐ 52. Lumbar puncture because he has stiff neck and fever.

☐ ☐ ☐ 53. Urethral catheter for urinary retention.

☐ ☐ ☐ 54. Suprapubic tube if catheter can't be inserted.

☐ ☐ ☐ 55. Appendectomy for incidental appendicitis.

☐ ☐ ☐ 56. Upper G.I. series for acute upper G.I. bleeding.

☐ ☐ ☐ 57. Esophagoscopy and gastroscopy for acute upper G.I. bleeding.

☐ ☐ ☐ 58. If cardiac arrest occurred, would you begin resuscitation?

☐ ☐ ☐ 59. If resuscitation was unsuccessful after 15 minutes, would you continue?

B (6) A 35 year old drug addict is brought to the hospital by the police. He has a history of severe chronic pulmonary fibrosis and for three years has been unable to climb stairs or walk more than 10 feet due to shortness of breath. He is found to have pneumococcal pneumonia, but during his first hospital day he becomes cyanotic and semicomatose. If a tracheostomy is performed, he will probably survive without further impairment of lung function. His only relative, a brother, is reluctant to authorize this procedure. Which of the following would you be likely to perform? *(Check yes, maybe, or no for each item).*

Yes   Maybe   No

☐ ☐ ☐ 60. Would you attempt to persuade his brother to authorize tracheostomy?

☐ ☐ ☐ 61. Intravenous feeding for dehydration.

☐	☐	☐	62.	Antibiotics.
☐	☐	☐	63.	Arterial puncture for blood gas analysis.
☐	☐	☐	64.	Urine culture for pyuria.
☐	☐	☐	65.	Urethral catheter for urinary obstruction.
☐	☐	☐	66.	Appendectomy for incidental suspected appendicitis.
☐	☐	☐	67.	Small bowel resection for suspected infarcted bowel.
☐	☐	☐	68.	If cardiac arrest occurred, would you begin resuscitation?
☐	☐	☐	69.	If resuscitation was unsuccessful after 15 minutes, would you continue?

B (7) A 75 year old man is brought to the hospital by his concerned family. Chest x-ray reveals a mass in the right hilum which is thought by the radiologist to represent lung cancer. He admits to smoking and hemoptysis. His family expresses concern for his welfare and asks you to do all you can for him. While you are talking to the family, the nurse tells you that he has become dyspneic while getting into bed and has developed hypotension. Which of the following would you be likely to perform? *(Check yes, maybe or no for each item).*

Yes   Maybe   No

☐	☐	☐	70.	Do EKG.
☐	☐	☐	71.	Lung scan for suspected pulmonary emboli.
☐	☐	☐	72.	Pulmonary arteriogram for suspected emboli.
☐	☐	☐	73.	Heparin therapy for proven pulmonary emboli.
☐	☐	☐	74.	A proven massive embolus occurs and he has approximately a 20% chance of living only if he has embolectomy. Would you ask surgeon to operate?
☐	☐	☐	75.	He survives embolus only to have a myocardial infarction and develops shock requiring your constant monitoring of an intravenous infusion of Levophed. Would you stay by bed all night?
☐	☐	☐	76.	After he recovers from MI and if respiratory insufficiency due to pneumonia became severe, would you use endotrachial tube and respirator?
☐	☐	☐	77.	If respiratory distress lasted 2 days, would you perform tracheostomy?
☐	☐	☐	78.	If cardiac arrest occurred, would you begin resuscitation?

☐ ☐ ☐ 79. If resuscitation was unsuccessful after 15 minutes, would you continue?

8 (a) In the hospital named in the covering letter, what is the average number of patients which you treat per month?

10. _____

(b) On the average, how many of these patients require decisions of the type described above?

11. _____

(c) Do you generally refer these patients or do you treat them yourself?

_____ I generally refer these patients.

_____ I generally treat them myself.

9 (a) A 25 year old man with head trauma is in deep coma on a respirator. There is no evidence of intracranial hematoma. He has had two flat EEG's over a 2-day period and is unresponsive to painful stimuli. Brain stem reflexes are absent. Cardiac activity is present but there is no spontaneous respiratory activity. Which of the following would you be likely to perform? *(Check one of the following).*

12. _____ 1. Leave respirator running until spontaneous cardiac activity ceases.

_____ 2. Turn off respirator without consulting colleagues or family.

_____ 3. Turn off respirator after consulting colleagues and finding a consensus of their opinion in favor of doing so.

_____ 4. Turn off respirator after consulting family and finding that they will accept this decision.

_____ 5. Turn off respirator after consulting both colleagues and family and finding both groups in favor of it.

(b) In the past year, how many patients have you treated on the respirator in whom there was a question of brain death?

13. _____

10. A 45 year old, 140 pound man in the last stages of terminal cancer has been receiving 40 mg. of morphine p.r.n. Later 40 mg. of morphine no longer gives him relief from pain. Which of the following would you be likely to prescribe? *(Check one of the following).*

14. _____ 1. No increase in dosage.

_____ 2. Increased dosage but not to the extent that there is danger of producing respiratory arrest.

_____ 3. Increased dosage to the point where pain is relieved even if it might risk respiratory arrest.

_____ 4. If dosage described in (3) was not effective, increased dosage to the point where pain is relieved even if it will probably lead to respiratory arrest.

11. (a) Assuming that the patient is a 45 year old man with a concerned family, please rank the following illnesses in terms of how actively you would treat them. Place a 1 next to the illness which you would treat *most* actively, an 8 next to the illness you would treat *least* actively, and 2, 3, 4, 5, 6, and 7 next to the illnesses to which you would give intermediate degrees of attention.

15. _____ a. Chronic pulmonary disease.

_____ b.   Chronic uremia.

_____ c.   Meningitis.

_____ d.   Metastatic carcinoma to the brain.

_____ e.   Metastatic carcinoma to the spine.

_____ f.   Multiple strokes.

_____ g.   Myocardial infarction.

_____ h.   Pneumonia.

(b) *Approximately* how many cases of these illnesses do you treat in an average year in the hospital named in the covering letter?

16. _____ a.   Chronic pulmonary disease.

17. _____ b.   Chronic uremia.

18. _____ c.   Meningitis.

_____ d.   Metastatic carcinoma to the brain.

_____ e.   Metastatic carcinoma to the spine.

_____ f.   Multiple strokes.

_____ g.   Myocardial infarction.

_____ h.   Pneumonia.

12.(a) When you are uncertain about how actively to treat a patient with debilitating chronic disease, how much do the following *professional considerations* influence your decision? Please place a 1 next to the factor which influences you most, a 6 next to the factor which influences you least, and a 2,3,4, and 5 next to the factors which have intermediate degrees of influence upon your decision.

19. _____ a. Your previous success in treating a similar and equally difficult case.

20. _____ b. The advice of residents and interns.

21. _____ c. The advice of senior physicians.

22. _____ d. Legal consequences which might ensue if medically indicated therapy were omitted.

23. _____ e. Scientific studies showing the success rate of a particular type of treatment.

24. _____ f. Opportunity to learn, practice or teach new techniques.

(b) When you are uncertain about how actively to treat such a patient, how much do the following *characteristics of the patient* influence your decision? Please place a 1 next to the factor which influences you most, a 7 next to the factor which influences you least, and a 2,3,4,5, and 6 next to the factors which have intermediate degrees of influence upon your decision.

25. _____ a. The patient's chronological age.

26. _____ b. The patient's physiological age.

27. _____ c. The patient's desire to die.

28. _____ d. The family's concern for the patient.

29. _____ e. The financial burden of his illness to his family.

30. _____ f. The financial burden to society (i.e. insurance and welfare).

31. _____ g. The patient's potential usefulness to society or family if he recovers.

13. How would you rate the quality of intensive nursing care on the medical service of the hospital named in the covering letter? (*Check one of the following.*)

32. _____ 1. Very good.
    _____ 2. Good.
    _____ 3. Fair.
    _____ 4. Poor.
    _____ 5. Very poor.

14.(a) What is the name of the medical school from which you obtained your M.D.?

33. _____

(b) In what year did you obtain your M.D.?

34. _____

15(a) In what hospital did you intern? *(Please give name and city where hospital is located.)*

35. _____

(b) In what hospital(s) have you been a resident or fellow? *(Please give name and city where hospital is located.)*

36. 1st year _____
    2nd year _____
    3rd year_____

(c) What is your status now?

37. _____ 1. Resident.
    _____ 2. Full-time physician on hospital staff.
    _____ 3. Private practice.

(d) If private practice, do you admit patients to more than one hospital?

_____ Yes   _____ No

(e) What proportion of your patients do you admit to the hospital named in the covering letter?

_____

(f) Are you board certified in internal medicine?

38. _____ 1. Yes.
    _____ 2. No.

16. What is your citizenship?

39. _____

17. What is your marital status?

40. _____ 1. Single.
    _____ 2. Married.
    _____ 3. Divorced or separated.
    _____ 4. Widowed.

18. What is your sex?

41. _____ 1. Male.
    _____ 2. Female.

19. What is your race?

42. _____ 1. Black.
    _____ 2. White.
    _____ 3. Other.

20.(a) In what religious denomination were you raised? *(Check one of the following.)*

43. _____ 1. Catholic.
    _____ 2. Jewish.
    _____ 3. Protestant. *(Please specify denomination, e.g. Congregationalist.)*

    _____
    _____ 4. Other. *(Please specify religion, e.g. Buddhist.)* _____
    _____ 5. None.

(b) If you have *changed* your religion, please indicate your new faith.

_____

(c) In general, how important would you say your religion is to you? *(Check one of the following.)*

44. _____ 1. Extremely important.
    _____ 2. Fairly important.

_____ 3. Fairly unimportant.
_____ 4. Not at all important.

21. What is your father's occupation? *(If he is retired or deceased, please indicate his occupation before his retirement or decease.)*

45. _____

PLEASE MAIL THE POSTCARD WHICH IS ENCLOSED WITH THE QUESTIONNAIRE. THIS WILL INDICATE THAT YOU HAVE RETURNED IT WITHOUT REVEALING YOUR IDENTITY ON THE QUESTIONNAIRE IN ANY WAY. THESE POSTCARDS WILL BE USED TO COMPILE A MAILING LIST OF PHYSICIANS TO WHOM COPIES OF THE FINDINGS FROM THIS STUDY WILL BE SENT.

IF YOU HAVE ANY COMMENTS ON THESE QUESTIONS OR A PERSONAL PHILOSOPHY CONCERNING THESE ISSUES, PLEASE WRITE THEM BELOW. THANK YOU VERY MUCH FOR YOUR COOPERATION.

Instructions-- Either pen or pencil may be used to complete the questionnaire. Please disregard the numbers which appear in the text of the questions. They are for the use of IBM tabulating machine operators.

The following cases are designed to simulate the decision-making process which the physician faces in dealing with patients suffering from chronic diseases. In responding to these questions, please keep in mind similar cases which you have treated *in the hospital named in the covering letter.*

C (1) A 45 year old truck driver with a history of mild hypertension and biopsy-proven carcinoma of the upper esophagus develops a severe esophageal obstruction. He is not able to swallow liquids and has considerable local discomfort requiring morphine on admission to the hospital. Chest x-rays reveal an enlarged cardiac silhouette and it is suspected that he may have pericardial effusion. His wife and three teenage sons are deeply concerned. You are aware that his illness is exhausting the family's financial resources. Which of the following would you be likely to perform? *(Check yes, maybe, or no for each item).*

Yes	Maybe	No		
☐	☐	☐	*10.*	Intravenous fluids for dehydration.
☐	☐	☐	*11.*	Heart scan for diagnosis.
☐	☐	☐	*12.*	Pericardiocentesis for cardiac tamponade.
☐	☐	☐	*13.*	Thoracotomy and pericardial window for recurrent tamponade due to spread of cancer.
☐	☐	☐	*14.*	Colon bypass for palliation if liver biopsy contains tumor and life expectancy is 9 months.
☐	☐	☐	*15.*	Feeding gastrostomy if liver biopsy contains tumor and life expectancy is one month.
☐	☐	☐	*16.*	If life expectancy is one month and respiratory insufficiency due to pneumonia became severe, would you use endotrachial tube and respirator?
☐	☐	☐	*17.*	If respiratory distress lasted 2 days, would you perform tracheostomy?
☐	☐	☐	*18.*	If cardiac arrest occurred, would you begin resuscitation?
☐	☐	☐	*19.*	If resuscitation was unsuccessful after 15 minutes, would you continue?

C (2) A 65 year old woman had a severe stroke one year ago. As a result, she cannot walk, eats with difficulty and has mild difficulty expressing herself. She is admitted to the ward service dehydrated and septic. Her family is willing to care for her at home if discharged from the hospital following treatment. Which of the following would you be likely to perform? *(Check yes, maybe, or no for each item).*

Yes	Maybe	No		
☐	☐	☐	*20.*	Intravenous feeding for dehydration.
☐	☐	☐	*21.*	Lumbar puncture for stiff neck and fever.

☐ ☐ ☐   22. Urine culture for pyuria.

☐ ☐ ☐   23. Six blood cultures for fever and murmur.

☐ ☐ ☐   24. Appendectomy for incidental suspected appendicitis.

☐ ☐ ☐   25. Small bowel resection for suspected infarcted bowel.

☐ ☐ ☐   26. If respiratory insufficiency due to pneumonia became severe, would you use endotrachial tube and respirator?

☐ ☐ ☐   27. If respiratory distress lasted 2 days, would you perform tracheostomy?

☐ ☐ ☐   28. If cardiac arrest occurred, would you begin resuscitation?

☐ ☐ ☐   29. If resuscitation was unsuccessful after 15 minutes, would you continue?

C (3)   A 47 year old social worker is admitted to your service. She has previously been in excellent health except for shortness of breath. You obtain blood gases and treat the patient for pulmonary edema. After giving a second large dose of morphine, the patient's heart suddenly stops. Blood gas report is then called to the ward, indicating that PCO_2 before repeated morphine was 87 mm Hg. After three minutes, you insert endotracheal tube and restore respirations and a normal sinus rhythm. Which of the following would you be likely to perform? *(Check yes, maybe, or no for each item).*

Yes.   Maybe   No

☐ ☐ ☐   30. Monitor EKG constantly.

☐ ☐ ☐   31. Order special nurses on 24-hour duty or place in an intensive care unit.

☐ ☐ ☐   32. Measure arterial blood gases.

☐ ☐ ☐   33. Respirations become labored, would you begin artificial ventilation?

☐ ☐ ☐   34. Two days later respirations remain depressed, would you perform a tracheostomy?

☐ ☐ ☐   35. Acute renal shutdown with uremia develops; her heart functions but she is in coma; would you perform peritoneal dialysis when urea nitrogen reached indicated level?

☐ ☐ ☐   36. One month later she opens eyes, follows objects, cannot speak or use extremities. Pneumonia recurs, would you give antibiotics?

☐ ☐ ☐   37. Breathing is labored again, would you use respirator?

☐ ☐ ☐   38. Two EEG's are flat in a 24 hour period, heart is still beating; brother *reluctantly* agrees to consider donation if she *"dies"*; kidneys are needed by young patient with excellent match. Would you pronounce dead or call the death committee?

☐ ☐ ☐   39. Two EEG's are flat in a 24-hour period; heart is still beating; brother agrees *willingly* to donation. Would you pronounce dead or call the death committee?

C (4) A 47 year old married banker with recent pneumonectomy for lung cancer is brought to the hospital by his wife and daughter because he has become jaundiced. On the night of admission to the hospital he talks fatalistically about dying. Later that evening he has a myocardial infarction and a few PVC's. Which of the following would you be likely to perform? *(Check yes, maybe, or no for each item).*

Yes	Maybe	No		
☐	☐	☐	40.	Would you order 24-hour special nurses or place in intensive care unit?
☐	☐	☐	41.	Respirations become labored; would you use endotrachial tube and respirator?
☐	☐	☐	42.	Two days later, respirations are still poor; would you perform tracheostomy?
☐	☐	☐	43.	Ventricular tachycardia occurs. Would you use IV xylocaine if you had to sit by bed all night?
☐	☐	☐	44.	Would you use constant IV xylocaine if nurses monitored all night?
☐	☐	☐	45.	He survives MI but has acute tubular necrosis. Would you perform peritoneal dialysis when urea nitrogen reached indicated level?
☐	☐	☐	46.	Antibiotics for pneumonia.
☐	☐	☐	47.	He suddenly arrests; would you begin resuscitation?
☐	☐	☐	48.	After 20 minutes, no stable rhythm is obtained; would you continue to resuscitate?
☐	☐	☐	49.	If chest cardiac massage did not produce an effective pulse would you open the chest?

C (5) A 30 year old bachelor has been suffering from melanoma of the leg that has metastasized to the spinal cord and he becomes paraplegic. You have been treating him for several months on an out-patient basis. He then develops a severe urinary tract infection. He is admitted to the hospital, alert but septic and in severe distress. He requests that he be treated vigorously. Which of the following would you be likely to perform? *(Check yes, maybe or no for each item).*

Yes	Maybe	No		
☐	☐	☐	50.	Intravenous fluids for dehydration.
☐	☐	☐	51.	Antibiotics.
☐	☐	☐	52.	Lumbar puncture because he has stiff neck and fever.
☐	☐	☐	53.	Urethral catheter for urinary retention.
☐	☐	☐	54.	Suprapubic tube if catheter can't be inserted.
☐	☐	☐	55.	Appendectomy for incidental appendicitis.
☐	☐	☐	56.	Upper G.I. series for acute upper G.I. bleeding.
☐	☐	☐	57.	Esophagoscopy and gastroscopy for acute upper G.I. bleeding.
☐	☐	☐	58.	If cardiac arrest occurred, would you begin resuscitation?
☐	☐	☐	59.	If resuscitation was unsuccessful after 15 minutes, would you continue?

C (6) A 65 year old man is brought to the hospital by his wife. He has a history of severe chronic pulmonary fibrosis and for three years has been unable to climb stairs or walk more than 10 feet due to shortness of breath. He is found to have pneumococcal pneumonia but during his first hospital day he becomes cyanotic and semicomatose. If a tracheostomy is performed, he will probably survive without further impairment of lung function. His wife is reluctant to authorize this procedure. Which of the following would you be likely to perform? *(Check yes, maybe, or no for each of the following).*

Yes	Maybe	No	
☐	☐	☐	60. Would you attempt to persuade his wife to authorize tracheostomy?
☐	☐	☐	61. Intravenous feeding for dehydration.
☐	☐	☐	62. Antibiotics.
☐	☐	☐	63. Arterial puncture for blood gas analysis.
☐	☐	☐	64. Urine culture for pyuria.
☐	☐	☐	65. Urethral catheter for urinary obstruction.
☐	☐	☐	66. Appendectomy for incidental suspected appendicitis.
☐	☐	☐	67. Small bowel resection for suspected infarcted bowel.
☐	☐	☐	68. If cardiac arrest occurred, would you begin resuscitation?
☐	☐	☐	69. If resuscitation was unsuccessful after 15 minutes, would you continue?

C (7) A 75 year old man is brought to the hospital by his concerned family. Chest x-ray reveals a mass in the right hilum which is thought by the radiologist to represent lung cancer. He admits to smoking and hemoptysis. His family cannot be located. While you are examining another patient, the nurse tells you that he has become dyspneic while getting into bed and has developed hypotension. Which of the following would you be likely to perform? *(Check yes, maybe, or no for each item).*

Yes	Maybe	No	
☐	☐	☐	70. Do EKG.
☐	☐	☐	71. Lung scan for suspected pulmonary emboli.
☐	☐	☐	72. Pulmonary arteriogram for suspected emboli.
☐	☐	☐	73. Heparin therapy for proven pulmonary emboli.
☐	☐	☐	74. A proven massive embolus occurs and he has approximately a 20% chance of living only if he has embolectomy. Would you ask surgeon to operate?
☐	☐	☐	75. He survives embolus only to have a myocardial infarction and develops shock requiring your constant monitoring of an intravenous infusion of Levophed. Would you stay by bed all night?
☐	☐	☐	76. After he has recovered from MI and if respiratory insufficiency due to pneumonia became severe, would you use endotrachial tube and respirator?
☐	☐	☐	77. If respiratory distress lasted 2 days, would you perform tracheostomy?
☐	☐	☐	78. If cardiac arrest occurred, would you begin resuscitation?

☐ ☐ ☐ 79. If resuscitation was unsuccessful after 15 minutes, would you continue?

8 (a) In the hospital named in the covering letter, what is the average number of patients which you treat per month?

10. _____

(b) On the average, how many of these patients require decisions of the type described above?

11. _____

(c) Do you generally refer these patients or do you treat them yourself?

_____ I generally refer these patients.

_____ I generally treat them myself.

9 (a) A 25 year old man with head trauma is in deep coma on a respirator. There is no evidence of intracranial hematoma. He has had two flat EEG's over a 2-day period and is unresponsive to painful stimuli. Brain stem reflexes are absent. Cardiac activity is present but there is no spontaneous respiratory activity. Which of the following would you be likely to perform? *(Check one of the following).*

12. _____ 1. Leave respirator running until spontaneous cardiac activity ceases.

_____ 2. Turn off respirator without consulting colleagues or family.

_____ 3. Turn off respirator after consulting colleagues and finding a consensus of their opinion in favor of doing so.

_____ 4. Turn off respirator after consulting family and finding that they will accept this decision.

_____ 5. Turn off respirator after consulting both colleagues and family and finding both groups in favor of it.

(b) In the past year, how many patients have you treated on the respirator in whom there was a question of brain death?

13. _____

10. A 45 year old, 140 pound man in the last stages of terminal cancer has been receiving 40 mg. of morphine p.r.n. Later 40 mg. of morphine no longer gives him relief from pain. Which of the following would you be likely to prescribe? *(Check one of the following).*

14. _____ 1. No increase in dosage.

_____ 2. Increased dosage but not to the extent that there is danger of producing respiratory arrest.

_____ 3. Increased dosage to the point where pain is relieved even if it might risk respiratory arrest.

_____ 4. If dosage described in (3) was not effective, increased dosage to the point where pain is relieved even if it will probably lead to respiratory arrest.

11. (a) Assuming that the patient is a 45 year old man with a concerned family, please rank the following illnesses in terms of how actively you would treat them. Place a 1 next to the illness which you would treat *most* actively, an 8 next to the illness you would treat *least* actively, and 2, 3, 4, 5, 6, and 7 next to the illnesses to which you would give intermediate degrees of attention.

15. _____ a. Chronic pulmonary disease.

_____ b. Chronic uremia.

_____ c. Meningitis.

_____ d. Metastatic carcinoma to the brain.

_____ e. Metastatic carcinoma to the spine.

_____ f. Multiple strokes.

_____ g. Myocardial infarction.

_____ h. Pneumonia.

(b) *Approximately* how many cases of these illnesses do you treat in an average year in the hospital named in the covering letter?

16. _____ a. Chronic pulmonary disease.

17. _____ b. Chronic uremia.

18. _____ c. Meningitis.

_____ d. Metastatic carcinoma to the brain.

_____ e. Metastatic carcinoma to the spine.

_____ f. Multiple strokes.

_____ g. Myocardial infarction.

_____ h. Pneumonia.

12.(a) When you are uncertain about how actively to treat a patient with debilitating chronic disease, how much do the following *professional considerations* influence your decision? Please place a 1 next to the factor which influences you most, a 6 next to the factor which influences you least, and a 2,3,4, and 5 next to the factors which have intermediate degrees of influence upon your decision.

19. _____ a. Your previous success in treating a similar and equally difficult case.

20._____ b. The advice of residents and interns.

21. _____ c. The advice of senior physicians.

22._____ d. Legal consequences which might ensue if medically indicated therapy were omitted.

23._____ e. Scientific studies showing the success rate of a particular type of treatment.

24._____ f. Opportunity to learn, practice or teach new techniques.

(b) When you are uncertain about how actively to treat such a patient, how much do the following *characteristics of the patient* influence your decision? Please place a 1 next to the factor which influences you most, a 7 next to the factor which influences you least, and a 2,3,4,5, and 6 next to the factors which have intermediate degrees of influence upon your decision.

25._____ a. The patient's chronological age.

26._____ b. The patient's physiological age.

27._____ c. The patient's desire to die.

28._____ d. The family's concern for the patient.

29._____ e. The financial burden of his illness to his family.

30._____ f. The financial burden to society (i.e. insurance and welfare).

31. _____ g. The patient's potential usefulness to society or family if he recovers.

13. How would you rate the quality of intensive nursing care on the medical service of the hospital named in the covering letter? *(Check one of the following.)*

    *32.*_____ 1. Very good.
        _____ 2. Good.
        _____ 3. Fair.
        _____ 4. Poor.
        _____ 5. Very poor.

14.(a) What is the name of the medical school from which you obtained your M.D.?

    *33.*_____

(b) In what year did you obtain your M.D.?

    *34.*_____

15(a) In what hospital did you intern? *(Please give name and city where hospital is located.)*

    *35.*_____

(b) In what hospital(s) have you been a resident or fellow? *(Please give name and city where hospital is located.)*

    36. 1st year _____
        2nd year _____
        3rd year_____

(c) What is your status now?

    *37.*_____ 1. Resident.
        _____ 2. Full-time physician on hospital staff.
        _____ 3. Private practice.

(d) If private practice, do you admit patients to more than one hospital?

    _____ Yes   _____ No

(e) What proportion of your patients do you admit to the hospital named in the covering letter?

    _____

(f) Are you board certified in internal medicine?

    *38.*_____ 1. Yes.
        _____ 2. No.

16. What is your citizenship?

    *39.*_____

17. What is your marital status?

    *40.*_____ 1. Single.
        _____ 2. Married.
        _____ 3. Divorced or separated.
        _____ 4. Widowed.

18. What is your sex?

    *41.*_____ 1. Male.
        _____ 2. Female.

19. What is your race?

    *42.*_____ 1. Black.
        _____ 2. White.
        _____ 3. Other.

20.(a) In what religious denomination were you raised? *(Check one of the following.)*

    *43.*_____ 1. Catholic.
        _____ 2. Jewish.
        _____ 3. Protestant. *(Please specify denomination, e.g. Congregationalist.)*

        _____ 4. Other. *(Please specify religion, e.g. Buddhist.)* _____
        _____ 5. None.

(b) If you have *changed* your religion, please indicate your new faith.

    _____

(c) In general, how important would you say your religion is to you? *(Check one of the following.)*

    *44.*_____ 1. Extremely important.
        _____ 2. Fairly important.

———— 3. Fairly unimportant.
———— 4. Not at all important.

---

21. What is your father's occupation? *(If he is retired or deceased, please indicate his occupation before his retirement or decease.)*

    45. ————————————————————————————————

PLEASE MAIL THE POSTCARD WHICH IS ENCLOSED WITH THE QUESTIONNAIRE. THIS WILL INDICATE THAT YOU HAVE RETURNED IT WITHOUT REVEALING YOUR IDENTITY ON THE QUESTIONNAIRE IN ANY WAY. THESE POSTCARDS WILL BE USED TO COMPILE A MAILING LIST OF PHYSICIANS TO WHOM COPIES OF THE FINDINGS FROM THIS STUDY WILL BE SENT.

IF YOU HAVE ANY COMMENTS ON THESE QUESTIONS OR A PERSONAL PHILOSOPHY CONCERNING THESE ISSUES, PLEASE WRITE THEM BELOW. THANK YOU VERY MUCH FOR YOUR COOPERATION.

3: Treatment of Congenital Anomalies and Severe Birth Defects in Newborns: A

Instructions-- Either pen or pencil may be used to complete the questionnaire. Please disregard the numbers which appear in the text of the questions. They are for the use of IBM tabulating machine operators.

The following cases are designed to simulate the decision-making process which the pediatrician faces in dealing with *newborn* infants who have congenital anomalies or severe birth defects. In responding to these questions, please keep in mind cases which you have treated in the hospital named in the covering letter.

A (1) An infant has been born with anencephalia and has lived for three days. The mother is beginning to express a desire to see the child. Which of the following would you be likely to perform? *(Check yes, maybe, or no for each item).*

(a) If no research studies are planned:

Yes   Maybe   No

☐ ☐ ☐   *10.* Intravenous fluids for maintenance.

☐ ☐ ☐   *11.* Gavage feedings.

☐ ☐ ☐   *12.* Antibiotics for infection.

☐ ☐ ☐   *13.* Blood transfusion for anemia.

☐ ☐ ☐   *14.* Correct blood sugar for hypoglycemia and hypocalcemia.

☐ ☐ ☐   *15.* Intravenous injection of a lethal dose of potassium chloride or a sedative drug.

☐ ☐ ☐   *16.* Resuscitation for cardio-respiratory arrest.

(b) If diagnostic tests performed on the infant can contribute to ongoing research and the parents give their consent:

Yes   Maybe   No

☐ ☐ ☐   *17.* Intravenous fluids for maintenance.

☐ ☐ ☐   *18.* Gavage feedings.

☐ ☐ ☐   *19.* Antibiotics for infection.

☐ ☐ ☐   *20.* Blood transfusion for anemia.

☐ ☐ ☐   *21.* Correct blood sugar for hypoglycemia and hypocalcemia.

☐ ☐ ☐   *22.* Resuscitation for cardio-respiratory arrest.

☐ ☐ ☐   *23.* Diagnostic tests for research purposes.

A (2) An infant is born with high lumbar myelomeningocele. He has no nerve function in his legs and no bladder or rectal sphincter control. The parents of the child are well educated and financially comfortable. Which of the following would you be likely to perform? *(Check yes, maybe, or no for each item).*

Yes   Maybe   No

☐ ☐ ☐   *24.* Treat myelomeningocele locally by painting the area with an antibiotic preparation.

☐ ☐ ☐   *25.* Arrange for operation for early closure of defect.

☐ ☐ ☐   *26.* Manage urinary tract infection.

251

Yes	Maybe	No	
☐	☐	☐	27. Perform credé massage on the bladder.
☐	☐	☐	28. Arrange shunt operation if hydrocephalus developed.
☐	☐	☐	29. If the infant developed meningitis, would you treat him?
☐	☐	☐	30. If the infant had a cardiac arrest, would you resuscitate him?

A (3) A 1500 gram infant is born with all the clinical characteristics of a mongoloid (Downs' syndrome). Six hours later, he develops severe respiratory distress. Chest film is read as compatible with hyaline membrane disease or pneumonia. The mother of the child, whose husband is a physician, has 4 healthy children of normal intelligence and does not appear to be anxious to save the child. Which of the following would you be likely to perform? *(Check yes, maybe, or no for each item).*

Yes	Maybe	No	
☐	☐	☐	31. Perform appropriate cultures (blood, CSF, etc.).
☐	☐	☐	32. Treat with antibiotics.
☐	☐	☐	33. Correct acidosis.
☐	☐	☐	34. If he develops pneumothorax, would you aspirate the chest?
☐	☐	☐	35. If he stops breathing for two minutes, would you bag-breathe him for two to three hours?
☐	☐	☐	36. Would you place him on a respirator if he continued to have apneic spells?
☐	☐	☐	37. If he then has a cardiac arrest, would you resuscitate him?

A (4) As a result of premature separation of the placenta, an infant was without oxygen in the uterus for an indeterminate period. He weighs 1500 grams. Seizures develop within two or three hours of birth and persist in spite of therapy. Marked spasticity and hypertonia develop. An electroencephalogram is highly abnormal. This is the first birth for a professional woman who has had several miscarriages. She wants the child very much. Which of the following would you be likely to perform? *(Check yes, maybe, or no for each item).*

Yes	Maybe	No	
☐	☐	☐	38. Intravenous fluids for maintenance.
☐	☐	☐	39. Monitor blood pH and correct as needed.
☐	☐	☐	40. Antibiotics for infection.
☐	☐	☐	41. If he develops pneumothorax, would you aspirate the chest?
☐	☐	☐	42. If he stops breathing for more than two minutes, would you bag-breathe him for two to three hours?
☐	☐	☐	43. Would you place him on a respirator if he continues to have apneic spells?
☐	☐	☐	44. If he then has a cardiac arrest, would you resuscitate him?

A (5) During the process of delivery, a 1400 gram infant's umbilical cord is torn. A short stump remains which is not carefully clamped. He goes to the nursery in good condition but soon after begins to bleed from the retracted vessel into the peritoneal cavity. Because of involvement in other emergencies in the nursery, the seriousness of the problem is not recognized until the infant goes into shock and is bleeding everywhere. Which of the following would you be likely to perform? *(Check yes, maybe, or no for each item).*

Yes	Maybe	No	
☐	☐	☐	45. Blood transfusion.

Yes   Maybe   No

46. Surgery to tie off the vessel.

47. Evacuation of blood from the peritoneal cavity.

48. Antibiotics for infection.

49. Oxygen.

50. The infant has a cardiac arrest. Would you resuscitate?

51. Assuming he has already been resuscitated once, would you resuscitate him if he had a second cardiac arrest?

6. (a) In the hospital named in the covering letter, what is the average number of newborns which you treat per month?

   10. _____

6. (b) On the average, how many of these require decisions of the type described here?

   11. _____

6. (c) Do you generally refer these patients or do you treat them yourself?

   _____ I generally refer these patients.

   _____ I generally treat them myself.

7. (a) An infant weighing 1500 grams has not breathed upon delivery. He has been placed on a respirator. He has had two flat EEG's over a 2-day period and is unresponsive to painful stimuli. Brain stem reflexes are absent. Cardiac activity is present but there is no spontaneous respiratory activity. Which of the following would you be likely to do? *(Check one of the following)*.

   12. _____ 1. Leave respirator running until spontaneous cardiac activity ceases.

   _____ 2. Turn off respirator without consulting colleagues or family.

   _____ 3. Turn off respirator after consulting colleagues and finding a consensus of their opinion in favor of doing so.

   _____ 4. Turn off respirator after consulting family and finding that they will accept this decision.

   _____ 5. Turn off respirator after consulting both colleagues and family and finding both groups in favor of it.

7. (b) In the past year, how many infants have you treated on respirators in whom there was a question of brain death?

   13. _____

8. (a) Assuming that the infant's family wants you to do everything possible for him, please indicate how actively you would treat an acute illness if it developed in conjunction with each of the following conditions. Place a 1 next to the condition in which you would treat an acute illness *most actively* and a 7 next to the condition in which you would treat an acute illness *least actively*. Place a 2,3,4,5, or 6 next to conditions in which you would treat acute illnesses with intermediate degrees of activism.

   14. _____ a. Anencephalia.

   15. _____ b. Hypoplastic left ventricle.

   16. _____ c. myelomeningocele.

   17. _____ d. Mongolism (Downs' syndrome).

18. _____   e.   Primary apnea.

19. _____   f.   Rubella syndrome.

20. _____   g.   Seizures combined with spasticity and hypertonia.

(b) *Approximately* how many newborns with these conditions do you see in the average year in the hospital named in the covering letter?

21. _____   a.   Anencephalia.

22. _____   b.   Hypoplastic left ventricle.

23. _____   c.   myelomeningocele.

24. _____   d.   Mongolism (Downs' syndrome).

25. _____   e.   Primary apnea.

26. _____   f.   Rubella syndrome.

27. _____   g.   Seizures combined with spasticity and hypertonia.

9. (a) When you are uncertain about how actively to treat an infant with congenital anomalies, how much do the following *professional considerations* influence your decision? Please place a 1 next to the factor which influences you most, a 6 next to the factor which influences you least, and a 2,3,4, and 5 next to the factors which have intermediate degrees of influence upon your decision.

28. _____   a.   Your previous success in treating a similar and equally difficult case.

29. _____   b.   The advice of residents and interns.

30. _____   c.   The advice of senior physicians.

31. _____   d.   Legal consequences which might ensue if medically indicated therapy were omitted.

32. _____   e.   Scientific studies showing the success rate of a particular type of treatment.

33. _____   f.   Opportunity to learn, practice or teach new techniques.

(b) When you are uncertain about how actively to treat such an infant, how much do the following *characteristics of the infant* influence your decision? Please place a 1 next to the factor which influences you most, a 7 next to the factor which influences you least, and a 2,3,4,5 and 6 next to the factors which have intermediate degrees of influence upon your decision.

34. _____   a.   The anticipated impact of the severely deformed or brain damaged infant upon the family with whom he will live.

35. _____   b.   The infant's potential usefulness to society or family.

36. _____   c.   The mother's attitude toward a mongoloid infant.

37. _____   d.   The mother's attitude toward a severely deformed infant.

38. _____   e.   The mother's desire to have a baby combined with the fact that she has been unable to complete previous pregnancies successfully.

39. _____   f.   The financial burden of the infant's condition to his family.

40. _____   g.   The financial burden of the infant's condition to the state (i.e. insurance and welfare).

10. How would you rate the quality of intensive nursing care in the nursery of the hospital named in the covering letter?

   41. _____ 1. Very good.
   _____ 2. Good.
   _____ 3. Fair.
   _____ 4. Poor.
   _____ 5. Very poor.

11. (a) What is the name and location of the medical school from which you obtained your M.D.?

   42. _____

   (b) In what year did you obtain your M.D.?

   43. _____

12. (a) In what hospital did you intern? *(Please give name and city where hospital is located).*

   44. _____

   (b) In what hospital (s) have you been a resident or fellow? *(Please give name and city where hospital is located).*

   45. _____

   (c) What is your status now?

   46. _____ 1. Resident.
   _____ 2. Full-time physician on hospital staff.
   _____ 3. Private practice.

   (d) If private practice, do you admit patients to more than one hospital?

   _____ Yes _____ No

   (e) What proportion of your patients do you admit to the hospital named in the covering letter?

   47. _____

   (f) Are you board-certified in pediatrics?
   48. _____ 1. Yes.
   _____ 2. No.

13. What is your citizenship?
   49. _____

14. What is your marital status? *(Check one of the following).*

   50. _____ 1. Single.
   _____ 2. Married.
   _____ 3. Divorced or separated.
   _____ 4. Widowed.

15. How many children do you have?
   51. _____

16. What is your sex?
   52. 1. Male _____ 2. Female _____

17. What is your race?
   53. _____ 1. Black.
   _____ 2. White.
   _____ 3. Other.

18. (a) In what religious denomination were you raised? *(Check one of the following).*

   54. _____ 1. Catholic.
   _____ 2. Jewish.
   _____ 3. Protestant. *(Please specify denomination, e.g. Congregationalist).*

   _____

   _____ 4. Other. *(Please specify denomination, e.g. Buddhist).*

   _____

   _____ 5. None.

   (b) If you have *changed* your religion, please indicate your new faith.

   _____

   (c) In general, how important would you say your religion is to you? *(Check one of the following).*

   55. _____ 1. Extremely important.
   _____ 2. Fairly important.
   _____ 3. Fairly unimportant.
   _____ 4. Not at all important.

19. What is your father's occupation? *(If he is retired or deceased, please indicate his occupation before his retirement or decease).*

   56. _____

PLEASE MAIL THE POSTCARD WHICH IS ENCLOSED WITH THE QUESTIONNAIRE. THIS WILL INDICATE THAT YOU HAVE RETURNED IT WITHOUT REVEALING YOUR IDENTITY ON THE QUESTIONNAIRE IN ANY WAY. THESE POSTCARDS WILL BE USED TO COMPILE A MAILING LIST OF PHYSICIANS TO WHOM COPIES OF A REPORT OF THE FINDINGS FROM THIS STUDY WILL BE SENT.

IF YOU HAVE ANY COMMENTS ON THESE QUESTIONS OR A PERSONAL PHILOSOPHY CONCERNING THESE ISSUES, PLEASE WRITE THEM ON THE FOLLOWING PAGE. THANK YOU VERY MUCH FOR YOUR COOPERATION.

Treatment of Congenital Anomalies and Severe Birth Defects in Newborns: B

Instructions-- Either pen or pencil may be used to complete the questionnaire. Please disregard the numbers which appear in the text of the questions. They are for the use of IBM tabulating machine operators.

The following cases are designed to simulate the decision-making process which the pediatrician faces in dealing with *newborn* infants who have congenital anomalies or severe birth defects. In responding to these questions, please keep in mind similar cases which you have treated in the hospital named in the covering letter.

B (1) Within the first day of life, an infant develops congestive heart failure and has a course which is thought to be compatible with hypoplastic left ventricle. The parents indicate that they understand the medical problem and request that you make no vigorous effort to maintain the child's life. Which of the following would you be likely to perform? *(Check yes, maybe, or no for each item).*

   a. The infant's kidneys are a good match for a transplant to which the parents give their consent:

Yes	Maybe	No		
☐	☐	☐	*10.*	Intravenous fluids for maintenance.
☐	☐	☐	*11.*	Oxygen for congestive heart failure.
☐	☐	☐	*12.*	Catheterization for diagnosis.
☐	☐	☐	*13.*	Antibiotics for infection.
☐	☐	☐	*14.*	Bag-breathing for respiratory distress.
☐	☐	☐	*15.*	Respirator for respiratory distress.
☐	☐	☐	*16.*	Resuscitation for cardio-respiratory arrest.

   b. No kidney transplant is planned:

Yes	Maybe	No		
☐	☐	☐	*17.*	Intravenous fluids for maintenance.
☐	☐	☐	*18.*	Medical management of congestive heart failure (i.e. digitalis, diuretics, oxygen).
☐	☐	☐	*19.*	Catheterization for diagnosis.
☐	☐	☐	*20.*	Antibiotics for infection.
☐	☐	☐	*21.*	Bag-breathing for respiratory distress.
☐	☐	☐	*22.*	Respirator for respiratory distress.
☐	☐	☐	*23.*	Resuscitation for cardio-respiratory arrest.

257

B (2) An infant is born with high lumbar myelomeningocele. He has no nerve function in his legs and no bladder or rectal sphincter control. This is the first child of twenty year old parents, neither of whom have completed high school. Which of the following would you be likely to perform? *(Check yes, maybe, or no for each item).*

Yes	Maybe	No		
☐	☐	☐	24.	Treat myelomeningocele locally by painting the area with an antibiotic preparation.
☐	☐	☐	25.	Arrange for operation for early closure of defect.
☐	☐	☐	26.	Manage urinary tract infection.
☐	☐	☐	27.	Perform credé massage on the bladder.
☐	☐	☐	28.	Arrange shunt operation if hydrocephalus developed.
☐	☐	☐	29.	If the infant developed meningitis, would you treat him?
☐	☐	☐	30.	If the infant had a cardiac arrest, would you resuscitate him?

B (3) A 1500 gram infant is born with all the clinical characteristics of a mongoloid (Downs' syndrome). Six hours later, he develops severe respiratory distress. Chest film is read as compatible with hyaline membrane disease or pneumonia. This is the first child of a 35 year old woman who has been trying for a number of years to become pregnant. She wants the child very much. She and her husband have limited financial resources. Which of the following would you be likely to perform? *(Check yes, maybe, or no for each item).*

Yes	Maybe	No		
☐	☐	☐	31.	Perform appropriate cultures (blood, CSF, etc.).
☐	☐	☐	32.	Treat with antibiotics.
☐	☐	☐	33.	Correct acidosis.
☐	☐	☐	34.	If he develops pneumothorax, would you aspirate the chest?
☐	☐	☐	35.	If he stops breathing for two minutes, would you bag-breathe him for two to three hours?
☐	☐	☐	36.	Would you place him on a respirator if he continued to have apneic spells?
☐	☐	☐	37.	If he then has a cardiac arrest, would you resuscitate him?

B (4) As a result of premature separation of the placenta, an infant was without oxygen in the uterus for an indeterminate period. He weighs 1500 grams. Seizures develop within two or three hours of birth and persist in spite of therapy. Marked spasticity and hypertonia develop. An electroencephalogram is highly abnormal. The mother is unmarried and does not want the child. Which of the following would you be likely to perform? *(Check yes, maybe, or no for each item).*

Yes	Maybe	No		
☐	☐	☐	38.	Intravenous fluids for maintenance.
☐	☐	☐	39.	Monitor blood pH and correct as needed.
☐	☐	☐	40.	Antibiotics for infection.

Yes	Maybe	No	
☐	☐	☐	41. If he develops pneumothorax, would you aspirate the chest?
☐	☐	☐	42. If he stops breathing for two minutes, would you bag-breathe him for two to three hours?
☐	☐	☐	43. Would you place him on a respirator if he continued to have apneic spells.
☐	☐	☐	44. If he has a cardiac arrest, would you resuscitate him?

B (5) As a result of a mechanical failure in an incubator, a 1400 gram infant is exposed to a temperature of 107 degrees Fahrenheit for an indeterminate period of at least 30 minutes. After this insult, he is febrile, markedly lethargic, lacks reflexes, is dehydrated, and acidotic. Which of the following would you be likely to perform? *(Check yes, maybe, or no for each item).*

Yes	Maybe	No	
☐	☐	☐	45. Intravenous fluids to counteract shock.
☐	☐	☐	46. Sponging to reduce temperature.
☐	☐	☐	47. Sodium bicarbonate to correct acidosis.
☐	☐	☐	48. Oxygen.
☐	☐	☐	49. Blood transfusion to counteract shock.
☐	☐	☐	50. If he has a cardiac arrest, would you resuscitate him?
☐	☐	☐	51. Would you resuscitate him again if he had a second cardiac arrest?

6. (a) In the hospital named in the covering letter, what is the average number of newborns which you treat per month?

10. _____

6. (b) On the average, how many of these require decisions of the type described here?

11. _____

6. (c) Do you generally refer these patients or do you treat them yourself?

_____ I generally refer these patients.

_____ I generally treat them myself.

7. (a) An infant weighing 1500 grams has not breathed upon delivery. He has been placed on a respirator. He has had two flat EEG's over a 2-day period and is unresponsive to painful stimuli. Brain stem reflexes are absent. Cardiac activity is present but there is no spontaneous respiratory activity. Which of the following would you be likely to do? *(Check one of the following).*

12. _____ 1. Leave respirator running until spontaneous cardiac activity ceases.

_____ 2. Turn off respirator without consulting colleagues or family.

_____ 3. Turn off respirator after consulting colleagues and finding a consensus of their opinion in favor of doing so.

_____ 4. Turn off respirator after consulting family and finding that they will accept this decision.

_____ 5. Turn off respirator after consulting both colleagues and family and finding both groups in favor of it.

7. (b) In the past year, how many infants have you treated on respirators in whom there was a question of brain death?

13. _____

---

8. (a) Assuming that the infant's family wants you to do everything possible for him, please indicate how actively you would treat an acute illness if it developed in conjunction with each of the following conditions. Place a 1 next to the condition in which you would treat an acute illness *most actively* and a 7 next to the condition in which you would treat an acute illness *least actively*. Place a 2,3,4,5, or 6 next to conditions in which you would treat acute illnesses with intermediate degrees of activism.

14. _____ a. Anencephalia.

15. _____ b. Hypoplastic left ventricle.

16. _____ c. Myelomeningocele.

17. _____ d. Mongolism (Downs' syndrome).

18. _____ e. Primary apnea.

19. _____ f. Rubella syndrome.

20. _____ g. Seizures combined with spasticity and hypertonia.

(b) *Approximately* how many newborns with these conditions do you see in the average year in the hospital named in the covering letter?

21. _____ a. Anencephalia.

22. _____ b. Hypoplastic left ventricle.

23. _____ c. Myelomeningocele.

24. _____ d. Mongolism (Downs' syndrome).

25. _____ e. Primary apnea.

26. _____ f. Rubella syndrome.

27. _____ g. Seizures combined with spasticity and hypertonia.

---

9. (a) When you are uncertain about how actively to treat an infant with congenital anomalies, how much do the following *professional considerations* influence your decision? Place a 1 next to the factor which influences you most, a 6 next to the factor which influences you least, and a 2,3,4, and 5 next to the factors which have intermediate degrees of influence upon your decision.

28. _____ a. Your previous success in treating a similar and equally difficult case.

29. _____ b. The advice of residents and interns.

30. _____ c. The advice of senior physicians.

31. _____ d. Legal consequences which might ensue if medically indicated therapy were omitted.

32. _____ e. Scientific studies showing the success rate of a particular type of treatment.

33. _____ f. Opportunity to learn, practice or teach new techniques.

(b) When you are uncertain about how actively to treat such an infant, how much do the following *characteristics of the infant* influence your decision? Place a 1 next to the factor which influences you most, a 7 next to the factor which influences you least, and a 2,3,4,5 and 6 next to the factors which have intermediate degrees of influence upon your decision.

34. _____ a. The anticipated impact of the severely deformed or brain damaged infant upon the family with whom he will live.

35. _____ b. The infant's potential usefulness to society or family.

36. _____ c. The mother's attitude toward a mongoloid infant.

37. _____ d. The mother's attitude toward a severely deformed infant.

38. _____ e. The mother's desire to have a baby combined with the fact that she has been unable to complete previous pregnancies successfully.

39. _____ f. The financial burden of the infant's condition to his family.

40. _____ g. The financial burden of the infant's condition to the state (i.e. insurance and welfare).

10. How would you rate the quality of intensive nursing care in the nursery of the hospital named in the covering letter?

41. _____ 1. Very good.
    _____ 2. Good.
    _____ 3. Fair.
    _____ 4. Poor.
    _____ 5. Very poor.

11. (a) What is the name and location of the medical school from which you obtained your M.D.?

42. _____

(b) In what year did you obtain your M.D.?

43. _____

12. (a) In what hospital did you intern? *(Please give name and city where hospital is located).*

44. _____

(b) In what hospital (s) have you been a resident or fellow? *(Please give name and city where hospital is located).*

45. _____

(c) What is your status now?

46. _____ 1. Resident.
    _____ 2. Full-time physician on hospital staff.
    _____ 3. Private practice.

(d) If private practice, do you admit patients to more than one hospital?

_____ Yes _____ No

(e) What proportion of your patients do you admit to the hospital named in the covering letter?

47. _____

(f) Are you board-certified in pediatrics?

48. _____ 1. Yes.
    _____ 2. No.

13. What is your citizenship?

49. _____

14. What is your marital status? *(Check one of the following).*

50. _____ 1. Single
    _____ 2. Married.
    _____ 3. Divorced or separated.
    _____ 4. Widowed.

15. How many children do you have?

51. _____

16. What is your sex?

52. _____ 1. Male
    _____ 2. Female

17. What is your race?

53. _____ 1. Black,
    _____ 2. White.
    _____ 3. Other.

18. (a) In what religious denomination were you raised? *(Check one of the following).*

54. _____ 1. Catholic.
    _____ 2. Jewish.

_____ 3. Protestant. *(Please specify denomination, e.g., Congregationalist).*

_____

_____ 4. Other. *(Please specify denomination,e.g., Buddhist).*

_____

_____ 5. None.

(b) If you have *changed* your religion, please indicate your new faith.

_____

(c) In general, how important would you say your religion is to you? *(Check one of the following).*

55. _____ 1. Extremely important.

_____ 2. Fairly important.

_____ 3. Fairly unimportant.

_____ 4. Not at all important.

19. What is your father's occupation? *(If he is retired or deceased, please indicate his occupation before his retirement of decease).*

56. _____

PLEASE MAIL THE POSTCARD WHICH IS ENCLOSED WITH THE QUESTIONNAIRE. THIS WILL INDICATE THAT YOU HAVE RETURNED IT WITHOUT REVEALING YOUR IDENTITY ON THE QUESTIONNAIRE IN ANY WAY. THESE POSTCARDS WILL BE USED TO COMPILE A MAILING LIST OF PHYSICIANS TO WHOM COPIES OF A REPORT OF THE FINDINGS FROM THIS STUDY WILL BE SENT.

IF YOU HAVE ANY COMMENTS ON THESE QUESTIONS OR A PERSONAL PHILOSOPHY CONCERNING THESE ISSUES, PLEASE WRITE THEM BELOW. THANK YOU VERY MUCH FOR YOUR COOPERATION.

4: Critical Decisions in Pediatric Cardiac Surgery

Instructions-- Either pen or pencil may be used to complete the questionnaire. Please disregard the numbers which appear in the text of the questions. They are for the use of IBM tabulating machine operators.

The object of this survey is to determine your attitudes toward performing operations upon children born with congenital anomalies. In responding to these questions, please keep in mind similar cases which you have treated in the hospital where you perform most of your operations.

Operation 1: To correct tetralogy of Fallot in an 8 year old child with mongolism (Downs' syndrome). Would you perform the operation under either of the following circumstances?

    (a) The child is living with his parents who are anxious to have the operation performed. *(Check one of the following).*

        5. ☐ 1. Would *usually* perform.

           ☐ 2. Would *sometimes* perform.

           ☐ 3. Would *rarely* perform.

    (b) The child is living in an institution for mentally retarded children. *(Check one of the following).*

        6. ☐ 1. Would *usually* perform.

           ☐ 2. Would *sometimes* perform.

           ☐ 3. Would *rarely* perform.

Operation 2: To correct the atrio-ventricular canal in an 8 year old child with mongolism (Downs' syndrome). Would you perform the operation under either of the following circumstances?

    (a) The child is living with his parents who are anxious to have the operation performed. *(Check one of the following).*

        7. ☐ 1. Would *usually* perform.

           ☐ 2. Would *sometimes* perform.

           ☐ 3. Would *rarely* perform.

    (b) The child is living in an institution for mentally retarded children. *(Check one of the following).*

        8. ☐ 1. Would *usually* perform.

           ☐ 2. Would *sometimes* perform.

           ☐ 3. Would *rarely* perform.

Operation 3: To correct the atrio-ventricular canal in an 8 year old child with IQ less than 50. The child is living in an institution for mentally retarded children. *(Check one of the following).*

        9. ☐ 1. Would *usually* perform.

           ☐ 2. Would *sometimes* perform.

           ☐ 3. Would *rarely* perform.

263

Operation 4: To correct tetralogy of Fallot in a child with a severe but treatable urogenital anomaly. Would you perform the operation under either of the following circumstances?

(a) The parents are financially comfortable and ask you to spare no expense in the treatment of their child. *(Check one of the following).*

    10. ☐ 1. Would *usually* perform.
        ☐ 2. Would *sometimes* perform.
        ☐ 3. Would *rarely* perform.

(b) The parents have three other healthy children and have limited financial resources. *(Check one of the following).*

    11. ☐ 1. Would *usually* perform.
        ☐ 2. Would *sometimes* perform.
        ☐ 3. Would *rarely* perform.

Operation 5: To correct the atrio-ventricular canal in a child with a severe but treatable urogenital anomaly. Would you perform the operation under either of the following circumstances?

(a) The parents of the child are financially comfortable and ask you to spare no expense in the treatment of their child. *(Check one of the following).*

    12. ☐ 1. Would *usually* perform.
        ☐ 2. Would *sometimes* perform.
        ☐ 3. Would *rarely* perform.

(b) The parents have three other healthy children and have limited financial resources. *(Check one of the following).*

    13. ☐ 1. Would *usually* perform.
        ☐ 2. Would *sometimes* perform.
        ☐ 3. Would *rarely* perform.

Operation 6: To correct patent ductus arteriosus in a 2 year old child with defective hearing cataracts, and retarded growth (e.g. rubella syndrome). Would you perform the operation under either of the following circumstances?

(a) He does not have developmental retardation. *(Check one of the following).*

    14. ☐ 1. Would *usually* perform.
        ☐ 2. Would *sometimes* perform.
        ☐ 3. Would *rarely* perform.

(b) He does have developmental retardation. *(Check one of the following).*

    15. ☐ 1. Would *usually* perform.
        ☐ 2. Would *sometimes* perform.
        ☐ 3. Would *rarely* perform.

Question 1: Which of the following best describes the attitude of the majority of pediatric heart surgeons in the department of surgery in the hospital where you perform most of your operations?

(a) Toward operations to correct the atrio-ventricular canal in a child with mongolism (Downs' syndrome). *(Check one of the following).*

16. ☐ 1. They are in favor of performing such operations in most cases.
   ☐ 2. They are *not* in favor of performing such operations in most cases.
   ☐ 3. There is no consensus among them about such operations.

(b) Toward operations to correct the atrio-ventricular canal in a child with a severe but treatable urogenital anomaly. *(Check one of the following).*

17. ☐ 1. They are in favor of performing such operations in most cases.
   ☐ 2. They are *not* in favor of performing such operations in most cases.
   ☐ 3. There is no consensus among them about such operations.

Question 2:   *Approximately* how many cases of the following conditions do you see in an average year?

18. _____ a. Tetralogy of Fallot combined with mongolism.
19. _____ b. Defect in the atrio-ventricular canal combined with mongolism.
20. _____ c. Tetralogy of Fallot combined with severe but treatable urogenital anomaly.
21. _____ d. Defect in the atrio-ventricular canal combined with a severe but treatable urogenital anomaly.
22. _____ e. Patent ductus arteriosus combined with rubella syndrome.

Question 3: (a) A 10 year old boy in deep coma is on a respirator. There is no evidence of intra-cranial hematoma. He has had two flat EEG's over a 2-day period and is unresponsive to painful stimuli. Brain stem reflexes are absent. Cardiac activity is present but there is no spontaneous respiratory activity. Which of the following would you be likely to do? *(Check one of the following).*

23.
   ☐ 1. Leave respirator running until spontaneous cardiac activity ceases.
   ☐ 2. Turn off respirator without consulting colleagues or family.
   ☐ 3. Turn off respirator after consulting colleagues and finding a consensus of their opinion in favor of doing so.
   ☐ 4. Turn off respirator after consulting family and finding that they will accept this decision.
   ☐ 5. Turn off respirator after consulting both colleagues and family and finding both groups in favor of it.

(b) In the past year, how many children have you treated on the respirator in whom there was a question of brain death?
   24. _____

Question 4: (a) When you are uncertain about whether to operate upon a child born with congenital anomalies, how much do the following *professional considerations* influence your decision? Please place a 1 next to the factor which influences you most, a 6 next to the factor which influences you least, and a 2, 3, 4, and 5 next to the factors which have intermediate degrees of influence upon your decision.

25._____ a. Your previous success in treating a similar case against all odds.

26._____ b. The advice of residents and interns.

27._____ c. The advice of senior physicians.

28._____ d. Legal consequences which might ensue if medically indicated therapy were omitted.

29._____ e. Scientific studies showing the success rate of a particular type of treatment.

30._____ f. Opportunity to learn, practice or teach new techniques.

(b) When you are uncertain about whether to operate upon such a child, how much do the following *characteristics of the child or his family* influence your decision? Please place a 1 next to the factor which influences you most, a 7 next to the factor which influences you least, and a 2, 3, 4, 5, and 6 next to the factors which have intermediate degrees of influence upon your decision.

31._____ a. The impact of the severely deformed child upon his family.

32._____ b. The impact of the severely brain damaged child upon his family.

33._____ c. The mother's attitude toward a mongoloid child.

34._____ d. The mother's attitude toward a severely deformed child.

35._____ e. The financial burden of the child's condition to the family.

36._____ f. The financial burden of the child's condition to the state (i.e. insurance and welfare).

37._____ g. The child's potential usefulness to society or family.

Question 5: (a) *Approximately* how many cardiac operations of all types (excluding diagnostic procedures) do you perform on children per year?

38._____

(b) In what type of hospital do you perform the *majority* of these operations? *(Check one of the following).*

39. ☐ 1. A teaching hospital which is the major unit in a medical school's teaching program.

☐ 2. A teaching hospital which is used to a limited extent in a medical school's teaching program.

☐ 3. A teaching hospital which is used for graduate training only in a medical school's teaching program.

☐ 4. A teaching hospital with no medical school affiliation.

☐ 5. A hospital with no teaching program.

Question 6: (a) In what year did you receive your M.D.?

40._____

(b) In what hospital(s) did you do your surgical residency? *(Please give name and city where hospital is located for each hospital).*

41._____

(c) What is your status now?

42. ☐ 1. Full-time surgeon on hospital staff.

☐ 2. Part-time surgeon on hospital staff (private practice).

Question 7: Are you board certified in thoracic surgery?

43 ☐ 1. Yes.

☐ 2. No.

Question 8: (a) What is your marital status? *(Check one of the following).*

    44. ☐ I. Single.
        ☐ 2. Married.
        ☐ 3. Divorced or separated.
        ☐ 4. Widowed.

    (b) How many children do you have?

    45. _____

Question 9: (a) In what religious faith were you raised? *(Check one of the following).*

    46. ☐ I. Catholic.
        ☐ 2. Jewish.
        ☐ 3. Protestant *(Please specify denomination, e.g. Congregationalist).*

        _____

        ☐ 4. Other *(Please specify religion, e.g. Buddhist).*

        _____

        ☐ 5. None.

    (b) If you have changed your religion, please indicate your new faith.

    _____

    (c) How important is your religion to you now? *(Check one of the following).*

    47. ☐ I. Extremely important.
        ☐ 2. Fairly important.
        ☐ 3. Fairly unimportant.
        ☐ 4. Not at all important.

Question 10: What is your father's occupation? (If he is retired or deceased, please indicate his occupation before his retirement or decease).

    48. _____

PLEASE MAIL THE POSTCARD WHICH IS ENCLOSED WITH THE QUESTIONNAIRE. THIS WILL INDICATE THAT YOU HAVE RETURNED IT WITHOUT REVEALING YOUR IDENTITY ON THE QUESTIONNAIRE IN ANY WAY. THESE POSTCARDS WILL BE USED TO COMPILE A MAILING LIST OF PHYSICIANS TO WHOM COPIES OF A REPORT OF THE FINDINGS FROM THE STUDY WILL BE SENT.

IF YOU HAVE ANY COMMENTS ON THESE QUESTIONS OR A PERSONAL PHILOSOPHY CONCERNING THESE ISSUES, PLEASE WRITE THEM BELOW. THANK YOU VERY MUCH FOR YOUR COOPERATION.

Glossary of Medical Terms[1]

Anencephaly.   A child born without the portions of the brain that control conscious and voluntary processes and coordinate muscular movements. The condition is invariably fatal.

Catheterization, Cardiac.   A diagnostic procedure for heart ailments in which tubes are inserted in veins and arteries to measure pressures in the heart or to inject dyes in order to be able to x-ray the heart chambers.

Dialysis, Chronic.   A form of treatment for chronic renal failure in which the patient's blood is circulated through an artificial kidney machine in order to remove poisons from the bloodstream.

Dyspnea.   Increased effort in breathing that causes discomfort. Often a part of heart or lung disease.

Embolectomy.   An embolus is a clot or some other solid debris that travels in the blood stream and wedges in an artery thereby stopping blood flow. An embolectomy is an operation to remove an embolus.

Gastrostomy.   An operation that opens a hole in the stomach often for the purpose of feeding a patient who cannot swallow.

Hematoma.   A swelling filled with blood, e.g. a bruise.

Hemoptysis.   Coughing up blood.

---

[1] Based on definitions contained in American Medical Association, *Current Medical Terminology,* 3rd Edition, Chicago, 1966, and *The Random House Dictionary of the English Language,* New York: Random House, 1966.

Hyaline Membrane Disease. A frequently fatal disease of the lungs of new-born babies, especially premature infants, that is characterized by a fibrinous membrane lining the air sacs in association with rapid, difficult, ineffective ventilation.

Hydrocephalus. A condition in which an excess amount of fluid accumulates in the head of a child so that the head increases in size and the brain is squeezed.

Hypertonia. Abnormally high tone of the muscles.

Hypocalcemia. Low calcium levels in the blood.

Hypoglycemia. Abnormally low level of glucose in the blood.

Hypotension. Low blood pressure.

Melanoma. A type of cancer, usually of the skin.

Metastasis. The transfer of a cancer from one part of the body to another, with development of a similar lesion in the new location.

Myelomeningocele. (also called meningomyelocele) An abnormality seen at birth resulting in a protrusion of the spinal cord through a defect in the vertebral canal. In severe cases of this congenital condition, the infant's legs are paralyzed, he lacks the capacity to develop bladder and bowel control, and, if untreated, he frequently develops hydrocephalus.

Nephrotomy. Surgical incision into the kidney, usually when urine drainage has been stopped as by a stone.

Pericardial Effusion. A collection of fluid in the sac that surrounds the heart.

Pericardiocentesis. Draining a pericardial effusion with a needle.

Peritoneal Dialysis. A form of treatment used for acute and chronic kidney failure which involves washing toxins out of the blood by passing fluids through the peritoneal cavity (the lining of the abdominal cavity and viscera).

Primary Apnea. At birth the infant does not breathe.

Pulmonary Edema. Fluid in the lungs.

Pulmonary Fibrosis. A form of respiratory disease leading to the formation of excess fibrous connective tissue in the lung, usually making the patient short of breath during exercise.

PVC. Premature (abnormal) ventricular contraction in the heart.

Spasticity. Increased muscle tension.

Thoracotomy. Cutting into the chest wall (for example, to operate on the lungs).

Tracheostomy. Opening a hole into the windpipe so that the patient can breathe.

Bibliography

Abram, H. S., *et al.* Suicidal behavior in chronic dialysis patients. *American Journal of Psychiatry*, 127 (1971), 1199–1204.

Ad Hoc Committee of the Harvard Medical School to Examine Brain Death. A definition of irreversible coma. *Journal of the American Medical Association*, 205 (1968), 85–88.

Adams, S. Trends in occupational origins of physicians. *American Sociological Review*, 18 (August, 1953), 404–409.

Ariès, P. La mort inversée: le changement des attitudes devant la mort dans les sociétés occidentales. *European Journal of Sociology*, 8 (1967), 169–195.

Babbie, E. R. *Science and Morality in Medicine: A Survey of Medical Educators.* Berkeley: University of California Press, 1970.

Barber, B. Experimenting with humans. *The Public Interest*, 6 (Winter, 1967), 91–102.

Barber, B., *et al. Research on Human Subjects: Problems of Social Control in Medical Experimentation.* New York: Russell Sage Foundation, 1973.

Beecher, H. K. The new definition of death: some opposing views. Paper presented at the meetings of the American Association for the Advancement of Science, 1970.

Bell, D. *The Reforming of General Education.* New York: Columbia University Press, 1966.

Blake, J. Abortion and public opinion: the 1960–70 decade. *Science*, 171 (12 February 1971), 540–549.

Blalock, H. M. *Social Statistics.* New York: McGraw-Hill, 1960.

Bluestone, S. S., and Deaver, G. G. Habilitation of the child with spina bifida and myelomeningocele. *Journal of the American Medical Association,* 161 (1956), 1248–51.

Bowers, M., *et al. Counseling the Dying.* New York: Thomas Nelson, 1964.

Brown, N. K., *et al.* The preservation of life. *Journal of the American Medical Association,* 211 (January 5, 1970), 76–81.

Bucy, P. C. A philosophy of neurosurgery. *Clinical Neurosurgery,* 8 (1960), 64–77.

Cantor, N. L. A patient's decision to decline life-saving medical treatment: bodily integrity versus the preservation of life. *Rutgers Law Review,* 26 (Winter, 1973), 228–264.

Caplow, T. *Principles of Organization.* New York: Harcourt, Brace and World, 1964.

Cappon, D. Attitudes of and toward the dying. *Canadian Medical Association Journal,* 87 (September, 1962), 693–700.

Capron, A. M., and Kass, L. R. A statutory definition of the standards for determining human death: an appraisal and proposals. *University of Pennsylvania Law Review,* 121 (November, 1972), 87–117.

Carlin, J. E. *Lawyers' Ethics: A Survey of the New York City Bar.* New York: Russell Sage Foundation, 1966.

Cassell, E. Being and becoming dead. *Social Research,* 39 (Autumn, 1972), 528–542.

Charlebois, P. A. Emergency resuscitation in a community hospital. *Canadian Anesthetics Society Journal,* 15 (July, 1968), 383–393.

Congress of Neurological Surgeons, *World Directory of Neurological Surgeons,* Part I. Bakersfield, California, 1969.

Coser, R. L. *Life in the Ward.* East Lansing, Michigan: Michigan State University Press, 1962.

Crafton, J. Doc: ethics made me save heart man. *Daily News,* January 29, 1972.

Crane, D. The academic marketplace revisited: a study of faculty mobility in six disciplines, *American Journal of Sociology,* 75 (May, 1970), 953–964.

Crane, D., and Matthews, D. Heart transplant operations: diffusion of a medical innovation. Paper presented at the 64th Annual Meeting of the American Sociological Association. San Francisco, California, September 4, 1969.

Department of Health Affairs, United States Catholic Conference. Ethical and religious directives for Catholic health facilities. Washington, D. C., 1971 (booklet).

Dilemma in Dying. *Time* Magazine, July 19, 1971, 44.

Dorpat, T. L., and Ripley, H. S. A study of suicide in the Seattle area. *Comprehensive Psychiatry,* 1 (1960), 349–359.

Duff, R. S., and Campbell, A. G. M. Moral and ethical dilemmas in the special-care nursery. *New England Journal of Medicine,* 289 (Oct. 25, 1973), 890–894.

Duff, R. S., and Hollingshead, A. B. *Sickness and Society.* New York: Harper and Row, 1968.

Durkheim, E. *Suicide.* Glencoe: Free Press, 1951.

Farber, B. *Mental Retardation: Its Social Context and Social Consequences.* Boston: Houghton Mifflin, 1968.

Feifel, H. (ed.) *The Meaning of Death.* New York: McGraw-Hill, 1959.

Feifel, H., et al. Physicians consider death. *Proceedings of the 75th Annual Convention of the American Psychological Association,* 2 (1967), 201–202.

Fletcher, G. P. Legal aspects of the decision not to prolong life. *Journal of the American Medical Association,* 203 (January 1, 1968), 119–122.

Ford, A. B. Casualties of our time. *Science,* 167 (January 16, 1970), 256–263.

Fox, R. C. *Experiment Perilous.* Glencoe: Free Press, 1959.

Fox, R. C. Ethical and existential developments in contemporaneous American medicine: their implications for culture and society. Paper prepared for presentation at the Conference on Medical Sociology, sponsored by the Polish Academy of Sciences and endorsed by the Research Committee on the Sociology of Medicine of the International Sociological Association. Warsaw (Jablonna), Poland, August 20-25, 1973.

Fox, R. C., and Crane, D. The death and dying movement. Forthcoming.

Fox, R. C., and Swazey, J. P. *The Courage to Fail: A Social View of Organ Transplants and Dialysis.* Chicago: University of Chicago Press, 1974.

Freeman, H., Levine, S., and Reeder, L. (eds.). *Handbook of Medical Sociology.* Englewood Cliffs, New Jersey: Prentice-Hall, 1972.

Freeman, J. M. Is there a right to die — quickly? *Journal of Pediatrics,* 80 (May, 1972), 904–5.

Freeman, L. C. *Elementary Applied Statistics for Students in Behavioral Science.* New York: Wiley, 1965.

Freidson, E. *Profession of Medicine.* New York: Dodd Mead and Company, 1970.

Fulton, R., and Geis, G. *Death and Identity.* New York: Wiley, 1965.

Giertz, G. B. Ethical problems in medical procedures in Sweden. In G. E. W. Wolstenholme and M. O'Connor (eds.), *Ethics in Medical Progress.* Boston: Little Brown, 1966, 139–148.

Glaser, B. G., and Strauss, A. L. *Awareness of Dying.* Chicago: Aldine, 1965.

Glaser, B. G., and Strauss, A. L. *Time for Dying.* Chicago: Aldine, 1968.

Glaser, W. A. *Social Settings and Medical Organization: A Cross-National Study of the Hospital.* Chicago: Aldine, 1970.

Glock, C. Y., and Stark, R. *Religion and Society in Tension.* Chicago: Rand McNally, 1965.

Goss, M. E. W. Organizational goals and the quality of medical care. *Journal of Health and Social Behavior,* 11 (December, 1970), 255–268.

Hendin, D. *Death as a Fact of Life.* New York: W. W. Norton, 1973.

Herberg, W. Religion in a secularized society: some aspects of America's three-religion pluralism. In Knudten, R. D. (ed.), *The Sociology of Religion — An Anthology*. New York: Appleton-Century Crofts, 1967.

Hinton, J. *Dying*. Baltimore: Penguin Books, 1967.

Holman, E. J. Adult Jehovah's Witnesses and blood transfusions. *Journal of the American Medical Association*, 219 (January 10, 1972), 273–274.

Isaacs, B., *et al*. The concept of pre-death. *The Lancet*, May 29, 1971, 1115–18.

Jakobovits, I. *Jewish Medical Ethics*. New York: Bloch, 1962.

Jung, M. A., *et al*. Value of a cardiac arrest team in a university hospital. *Canadian Medical Association Journal*, 98 (January 13, 1968), 74–78.

Kalish, R. A. Social distance and the dying. *Community Mental Health Journal*, 2 (Summer, 1966), 152–155.

Kalish, R. A. Life and death: dividing the indivisible. *Social Science and Medicine*, 2 (1968), 249–259.

Kamisar, Y. Euthanasia legislation: some non-religious objections. In A. B. Downing (ed.), *Euthanasia and the Right to Death*. London: Peter Owen, 1969.

Karnofsky, D. A. Why prolong the life of a patient with advanced cancer? *CA Bulletin of Cancer Progress*, 10 (January-February, 1960), 9–11.

Kasl, S., and Cobb, S. Health behavior, illness behavior, and sick role behavior. *Archives of Environmental Health*, 12 (1966), 246–266.

Kass, L. R. Death as an event: a commentary on Robert Morison. *Science*, 173 (August 20, 1971), 698–702.

Kendall, P. L. The learning environments of hospitals. In E. Freidson (ed.), *The Hospital in Modern Society*. London: The Free Press, 1963, 195–230.

Kendall, P. L. *The Relationship between Medical Educators and Medical Practitioners*. Evanston, Ill.: Association of American Medical Colleges, 1965.

Kirkpatrick, C. Religion and humanitarianism: a study of institutional implications. *Psychological Monographs*, 63 (no. 304, 1949).

Knutson, A. L. Body transplants and ethical values. *Social Science and Medicine*, 2 (1968–69), 393–414.

Kübler-Ross, E. *On Death and Dying*. New York: Macmillan, 1969.

Kuty, O. *Le Pouvoir du Malade: Analyse sociologique des Unités de Rein artificiel*. Thèse de doctorat présentée à la Faculté des Lettres et des Sciences humaines de Paris-V (René Descartes), 1973.

Lasagna, L. Physicians' behavior toward the dying patient. In O. B. Brim *et al*. (eds.), *The Dying Patient*. New York: Russell Sage Foundation, 1970, 83–101.

Lerner, M. When, why, and where people die. In O. B. Brim *et al*. (eds.), *The Dying Patient*. New York: Russell Sage Foundation, 1970, 5–29.

Lester, D. Experimental and correlational studies of the fear of death. *Psychological Bulletin*, 67 (1967), 27–36.

Lewis, A. British doctor urges end of obligation to keep aged patients alive.

New York Times, Wednesday, April 30, 1969, p. 16.

Lilienfeld, A. M. *Epidemiology of Mongolism.* Baltimore: The Johns Hopkins Press, 1969.

Lorber, J., Results of treatment of myelomeningocele. *Developmental Medicine and Child Neurology,* 13 (1971), 279–303.

Luckmann, T. *The Invisible Religion.* New York: Macmillan, 1967.

Mann, K. W. *Deadline for Survival: A Survey of Moral Issues in Science and Medicine.* New York: The Seabury Press, 1970.

McNemar, Q. *Psychological Statistics.* New York: Wiley, 1962 (3rd edition).

Meister, D. Survey of clergymen regarding ethical problems in medical advance. Unpublished paper, School of Hygiene and Public Health, Johns Hopkins University, 1971.

Meyers, D. W. The legal aspects of medical euthanasia. *Bioscience,* 23 (1973), 467–470.

Miller, S. *Prescription for Leadership.* Chicago: Aldine, 1970.

More, D. A note on occupational origins of health service professions. *American Sociological Review,* 25 (June, 1960), 403–404.

Morison, R. Death: process or event? *Science,* 173 (August 20, 1971), 694–698.

Mumford, E. *Interns: From Students to Physicians.* Cambridge, Mass.: Harvard University Press, 1970.

Pappworth, M. H. *Human Guinea Pigs: Experimentation on Man.* Boston: Beacon Press, 1968.

Parsons, T. *The Social System.* New York: The Free Press of Glencoe, 1951, Chapter 10.

Parsons, T. Definitions of health and illness in the light of American values and social structure. In E. Jaco (ed.), *Patients, Physicians and Illness.* New York: The Free Press of Glencoe, 1958.

Parsons, T. and Lidz, V. Death in American society. In E. Shneidman (ed.), *Essays in Self-Destruction.* New York: Science House, 1967.

Parsons, T., Fox, R. C., and Lidz, V. M. The "gift of life" and its reciprocation. *Social Research,* 39 (Autumn, 1972), 367–415.

Petersen, O. L., *et al.* Analytic study of North Carolina general practice. *Journal of Medical Education,* 31 (1956), 1–165, Part 2.

Quint, J. C. Mastectomy — symbol of cure or warning sign? *General Practice* (March, 1964), 119–124.

Ramsey, P. *The Patient as Person.* New Haven: Yale University Press, 1970.

Reeder, L. G. The patient-client as a consumer: some observations on the changing professional-client relationship. *Journal of Health and Social Behavior,* 13 (1972), 406–412.

Riley, J. W., Jr. What people think about death. In O. B. Brim *et al.* (eds.), *The Dying Patient.* New York: Russell Sage Foundation, 1970, 30–41.

Roemer, M. I., and Friedman, J. W. *Doctors in Hospitals.* Baltimore: The

Johns Hopkins Press, 1971.

Rokeach, M. *Beliefs, Attitudes and Values: A Theory of Organization and Change.* San Francisco: Jossey-Bass, Inc., 1970.

Rosner, F., Euthanasia. Position paper on Euthanasia for the Symposium on Psychosocial Aspects of Terminal Care, November 6 and 7, 1970.

Roth, J. A. Some contingencies in the moral evaluation and control of clientele: the case of the hospital emergency service. *American Journal of Sociology,* 77 (March, 1972), 839–856.

Sackett, W. W. Death with dignity. *Medical Opinion and Review* (June, 1969), 25–31.

Sanders, J. Euthanasia: None dare call it murder. *Journal of Criminal Law, Criminology, and Police Science,* 60 (1969), 351–359.

Scheff, T. J. Decision rules, types of error, and their consequences in medical diagnosis. *Behavioral Science,* 8 (1963), 97–107.

Schumacher, C. F. The 1960 medical school graduate: his biographical history. *Journal of Medical Education,* 36 (May, 1961), 398–406.

Shaw, A. On mongoloid babies: Do parents have a chance? *International Herald Tribune.* February 1, 1972, 6.

Shils, E. The sanctity of life. In D. H. Labby (ed.), *Life or Death: Ethics and Options.* Seattle: University of Washington Press, 1968, 2–38.

Shneidman, E. S. Suicide. In N. L. Farberow (ed.), *Taboo Topics.* New York: Atherton, 1963, 33–43.

Silverman, D., *et al.* Cerebral death and the electroencephalogram. *Journal of the American Medical Association,* 209 (September 8, 1969), 1505–1510.

Simmons, R. G., and Simmons, R. L. Sociological and psychological aspects of transplantation and dialysis as a special case. In J. Nazarian and R. G. Simmons (eds.), *Transplantation.* Philadelphia: Lea and Febiger, 1970.

Simmons, R. G., and Simmons, R. L. Organ transplantation: a societal problem. *Social Problems,* 19 (1971), 36–57.

Simmons, R. G., *et al.* Family decision-making and the selection of a kidney transplant donor. Paper presented at the Meetings of the American Sociological Association. New Orleans, La., August 26, 1972.

Smelser, N. J. *Theory of Collective Behavior.* New York: Free Press, 1962.

Spray, S. L., and Marx, J. H. The origins and correlates of religious adherence and apostasy among mental health professionals. Paper presented at the Meeting of the American Sociological Association, August, 1968.

Stewart, I. Suicide: the influence of organic disease. *The Lancet,* 2 (October, 1960), 919–920.

Sudnow, D. *Passing On.* Englewood Cliffs, N.J.: Prentice-Hall, 1967.

Swazey, J. P., and Fox, R. C. The clinical moratorium: a case study of mitral valve surgery. In P. A. Freund (ed.), *Experimentation with Human Subjects.* New York: George Braziller, Inc., 1970, 315–357.

Tooley, M. Abortion and infanticide. *Philosophy and Public Affairs,* 2 (Fall, 1972), 37–65.

Trussell, R. E., *et al. The Quantity, Quality and Costs of Medical and Hospital Care Secured by a Sample of Teamster Families in the New York Area.* New York: Columbia University School of Public Health and Administrative Medicine, 1962.

Veatch, R. M. Allowing the dying patient to die: an ethical analysis of new policy proposals. Hastings-on-Hudson: Institute of Society, Ethics and the Life Sciences, 1972 (mimeo).

Veatch, R. M., and Sollitto, S. The refusal of treatment: summary of American cases. Institute of Society, Ethics, and the Life Sciences, Hastings-on-Hudson, New York, 1973, unpublished memorandum.

Walker, H. M., and Lev, J. *Statistical Inference.* New York: Henry Holt, 1953.

Warner, W. L. *Social Class in America.* New York: Harper Torchbooks, 1960.

Weisman, A., and Kastenbaum, R. *The Psychological Autopsy: A Study of the Terminal Phase of Life.* Community Mental Health Journal Monograph, No. 4, 1968.

Williams, R. H. Our role in the generation, modification and termination of life. *Archives of Internal Medicine,* 124 (August, 1969), 215–237.

Index

Abortion, 4, 13, 204, 207
Abram, H. S., 10, 197
Activism, 137, 143, 173–178; and
    physician age, 170–172; and
    religious variables, 175, 176, 178,
    179, 200, 203; scales of, 173–178
Adams, S., 172
Age, patient, and activism scales, 176;
    as determinant of treatment, 12,
    52, 58–61, 96, 99, 112; and
    religious variables, 146, 149, 164,
    165, 166–167, 168, 170
Age, physician, and activism, 170–172;
    and acute vs. chronic illness, 63;
    and administration of narcotics,
    72–73; and ethical guidelines, 206
Anencephalic infant, 39, 44, 71–72,
    76–77, 158, 162–163, 200, 202,
    205
Anencephaly, 23, 39, 205
Asians. See Religions, Asian

Babbie, E. R., 140, 163

Barber, B., 182, 183n, 190, 195, 196,
    197
Beecher, H. K., 7
Bell, D., 211
Blake, J., 207
Blalock, H. M., 32
Bluestone, S. S., 4
Brain damage, 3–4, 11, 13, 14, 23,
    36–40, 107, 208; attitudes toward,
    13, 41–46, 57, 68–71, 79, 89, 158,
    164, 167, 172, 199, 201–202; in
    children, 49–51; and resuscitation,
    91, 92. See also Damage, physical
Brain death, 7, 73–77, 84, 200, 205;
    attitudes toward, 74, 76
Brain Death, Ad Hoc Committee of the
    Harvard Medical School to
    Examine the Definition of, 73
Brown, N. K., 40
Bucy, P. C., 4, 6
Buddhism, 139

Campbell, A. G. M., 100

Cancer, 14, 23, 38, 46, 92, 93, 131; and resuscitation, 90. *See also* Patients, unsalvageable
Cancer chemotherapy, 181–194
Cantor, N. L. A., 207
Caplow, T., 107
Capron, A. M., 10, 210n
Carlin, J. E., 173
Case histories, 14–15, 22–25, 36–40
Cassell, E., 13
Catheterization, cardiac, 44n, 97n
Catholics, 138–140, 141, 143, 146, 152, 154, 155–157, 158, 160, 162, 164–165, 167–168, 170, 178–179, 203; and activism, 175–179; and euthanasia, 138
Charlebois, P. A., 78
Christianity, 138
Citizenship, of residents, 154, 155, 160–162, 163, 170, 176, 177, 178, 203
Clinical mentality, 18, 19–21
Cobb, S., 11
Comfort, as criterion for treatment, 5
Communication, problems of, 47–48
Consensus, colleague, 123–127; on treatment of critically ill patients, 201–202
Consent, voluntary, 182, 184, 190–194
Controversy, 2–6, 21–22; in the hospital setting, 117–136. *See also* Consensus
Coser, R. L., 125–127
Crafton, J., 208
Crane, D., 5n, 10, 107

Damage, physical, 14, 23, 36–46, 51, 68–71, 78, 89, 107, 158, 197, 201–202, 208. *See also* Brain damage
Death, definitions of, 2–6, 7, 67, 71–77, 210n; hastening, 71–77, 83–84, 155, 162, 200 (*see also* Euthanasia; Narcotics; Respirator); interest in, 1, 8–10; reversing, 78–83 (*see also* Resuscitation)

Deaver, G. G., 4
Decision-making, and clinical mentality, 19–22; and hospital records, 88–95, 96–100; and hospital setting, 107–114; influence of colleagues on, 123–134, 135; normative criteria for, 6–8; religious influences on, 143–170; social criteria for, 13–14, 40–61, 68–71, 78–83. *See also* Internists; Neurosurgeons; Pediatric heart surgeons; Pediatricians
Deviance, as determinant of treatment, 12, 52, 57–58, 96
Diagnosis, certainty of, 52, 64–65, 146, 170
Disability, levels of, 9
Diseases, acute vs. chronic, 1; types of, 61–65, 90, 95n
Doctor-patient relationship in medical research, 181, 182, 187, 190, 194, 195
Dorpat, T. L., 9
Drugs, effects of, 67, 183. *See also* Narcotics
Duff, R. S., 100
Durkheim, E., 164–166
Dying, the, treatment of, 67–71. *See also* Life; Death; Patients

Episcopal Church, 154; and euthanasia, 138
Ethics, 17; 84, 101; codes of, 183–184, 195, 205; and social organization, 190–194; and the unsalvageable, 194–197
Euthanasia, current practice of, 206–212; definition of, 8; and definitions of death, 71–77; and infants, 4–5; legal practice concerning, 8; legislation, 209–210; negative vs. positive, 67, 200; and religions, 138–140, 162–163, 203; and religious variables, 162–163; studies of, 40

Euthanasia movement, 3
Euthanasia Society, 10
Experimentation, medical, 181–197

Family attitude, as determinant of
    treatment, 49–51, 56–57, 71n, 83,
    113, 159, 167, 192–193, 199–200
Farber, B., 51, 57n
Fletcher, G. P., 8
Fletcher, J., 138
Ford, A. B., 9
Foundation of Thanatology, 10
Fox, R. C., 10, 181, 182, 194, 196
Freeman, H., 138n
Freeman, J. M., 171, 205
Freeman, L. C., 32
Freidson, E., 11, 18, 135, 211
Friedman, J. W., 106

Giertz, G. B., 3
Glaser, B. G., 12, 47
Glaser, W. A., 139–140
Glock, C. Y., 143n, 178
Goss, M. E. W., 27, 105, 106

Heart transplants, 5n, 196n
Hendin, D., 207
Herberg, W., 178
Hinduism, 139
Holman, E. J., 207, 210n
Hospital records, 25; vs.
    questionnaires, 88–90; study of
    resuscitations in, 58, 85–95, 201;
    study of mongoloids with heart
    defects in, 85–86, 96–100
Hospital setting, and activism, 175,
    203; prestige of, 88n, 107–108,
    110–116, 122, 134, 135, 162, 173,
    202; and quality of care, 105–107;
    and religious variables, 141–142,
    155–156, 162; and sampling,
    27–29; and social class level of
    patient population, 122–123n;
    and treatment of critically ill
    patients, 107–116, 134, 202–203
Hospitals, samples of, 27–30

Humanitarianism, 7, 8

Ideology, and experimentation, 185,
    188–189, 195
Illness, acute vs. chronic, 1, 8, 9,
    61–65, 211. *See also* Diseases
Individuality, sanctity of, 6, 209
Infants. *See* Newborns; Pediatricians
Institute of Society, Ethics and the
    Life Sciences, 10
Internal medicine, case histories in,
    37–38; controversy in, 22;
    interviews in, 18; questionnaire
    for, 23–24; response rates in
    samples for, 30; samples for,
    27–29; scales for, 25–26. *See
    also* Internists, Medical
    residents
Internists, activism of, 174–175; and
    brain death, 75–77; and certainty
    of diagnosis, 64–65; and colleague
    consensus, 123–127; and
    consensus on treatment of
    critically ill patients, 201–202;
    and decisions to treat critically ill
    patients, 41–43, 47, 49, 52, 119,
    122, 134; and departmental
    policy, 127–129, 131; and
    euthanasia, 72; and family
    attitude, 49; and hospital setting,
    108–110, 116–122, 134, 135; and
    narcotics, 200; and patient
    attitude, 172; and professional
    age, 171–172; ranking of illnesses
    by, 63; and religiosity, 141, 151,
    152; and religious affiliation,
    140–151, 152, 155–157, 163–170;
    and resuscitation, 78–84, 119,
    201; samples of, 27, 28–31; social
    class origin of, 172–173; and
    treatment withdrawal, 68–70
Interviews, 17–22, 182
Isaacs, B., 9
Islam, 139

Jakobovits, I., 139

Jews, 138–140, 141, 143, 146, 152, 154, 155, 156, 157, 158, 160, 162–163, 164–168, 178–179, 203; and activism, 175–179, 203
Judaism, 138–139
Jung, M. A., 88

Kamisar, Y., 3
Karnofsky, D. A., 2
Kasl, S., 11
Kass, L. R., 7, 10, 210n
Kastenbaum, R., 5
Kendall, P. L., 26, 106, 118n, 122
Kirkpatrick, C., 152
Knutson, A. L., 139
Kübler-Ross, E., 10, 47
Kuty, O., 195

Lasagna, L., 61
Law, the, and social interpretation of life, 8; and treatment refusal, 9, 206–210. *See also* Euthanasia
Lerner, M., 1, 23
Lester, D., 1
Lidz, V., 58
Life, defining, 3, 6, 199, 206–208; preservation of, 164–168, 170, 178–179 (*see also* Patient attitude; Respirator; Resuscitation); prolongation of, 5–6, 7, 178, 191–192, 197 (*see also* Experimentation); quality of, 5n, 14, 69; sanctity of, 6–7
Lorber, J., 205
Luckmann, T., 178

Mann, K. W., 138
Matthews, D., 5n
McNemar, Q., 31
Medical residents, and departmental policy, 127–129, 135; and experimentation, 186–187; and hospital setting, 108–112, 113, 116–122, 135, 202–203. *See also* Internal medicine, Internists
Meister, D., 162–163

Miller, S., 106, 113n, 129
Mongoloids, 5, 43, 45n, 50, 51, 71, 112, 158, 201–202; hospital records of, 96–100
Mongolism, 39, 98–99, 131; and cardiac anomalies, 45–46
Morality, and euthanasia, 140. *See also* Religions
More, D., 172
Morison, R., 2–3, 3n, 7
Mumford, E., 106, 110, 118
Myelomeningocele, 4, 9, 38–39, 43, 53, 71, 158, 171, 202, 205

Narcotics, administration of, 67, 72–73, 83, 152–154, 155, 156, 157, 164, 168, 175, 193, 200
Neurosurgeons, and age, 54, 59–60; and brain death, 75–77; and colleague consensus, 124–126, 135; and consensus on treatment of critically ill patients, 201; and decisions to operate upon critically ill patients, 40–41, 43, 49, 53; and departmental policy, 125; and family attitude, 49, 50–51, 54; and hospital setting, 108, 108n, 109, 134; and professional age, 171–172; and religiosity, 141, 151; and religious affiliation, 143–151, 155–157, 158, 165–167; sample of, 26, 30–31; social backgrounds of, 172; and socioeconomic status of patient's family, 56; and withdrawal of treatment, 71
Neurosurgery, case histories in, 36; interviews in, 18; questionnaire for, 23–24; response rate in sample of, 30; sample for, 26; values of profession of, 156–157
Newborns, 4, 13, 78, 157, 199. *See also* Pediatricians
Norm-oriented social movements, definition of, 10n
Nuremberg Code, 183n, 190, 191, 193

Nurses, in premature nursery, 133; and resuscitation, 80–81, 82; in wards for medical experimentation, 185, 189

Ombudsmen, 210–211
Organizational setting, and experimentation, 181–197

Pappworth, M. H., 197
Parental attitudes. *See* Family attitude
Parsons, Talcott, 11–12, 58
Patient attitude, 14, 46–48, 82–83, 200, 209; and activism scales, 176; and age of internist, 172; and experimentation, 192; and hospital setting, 110; and religious affiliation of internist, 146, 150, 170
Patient care, and psychiatrists, 187, 193; quality of, 105–107; residents and, 108–114
Patients, "Bill of Rights" for, 9, 210; critically ill, 17, 35–65; geriatric, 4, 5, 9; non-private service, 48, 95–96; private service, 48; and refusal of treatment, 9, 47, 94–95, 206–207, 209; and refusal of resuscitation, 81–82; salvage-ability of, 13–14; salvageable, 13, 14, 36–46, 49, 68, 69, 78, 89, 151, 199, 201–202, 208; social value of, 12, 14, 51–61, 200; social value of, in experimentation, 196; treatable vs. untreatable, 11, 61, 199; types of, 2–5; unsalvageable, 14, 36–46, 49, 52, 68, 69, 78, 89, 108, 110, 181, 194, 197, 199, 201–202, 208. *See also* Brain Damage, Damage, physical, Salvageability
Pediatric cardiologists, 22, 46, 97, 123, 124
Pediatric heart surgeons, and brain death, 75–77; and colleague consensus, 123–126, 135; and consensus concerning treatment of critically ill patients, 201; and

departmental policy, 123–125; and decisions to operate upon critically ill patients, 45–46, 49–51; and family attitude, 49, 50–51; and hospital records, 96–100; and hospital setting, 108n, 113n; and mongoloids, 45, 49–51, 96–100, 201; and religiosity, 141, 158; and religious affiliation, 141, 158, 165–167; sample of, 26–27, 30; social class origin of, 172; and withdrawal of treatment, 71
Pediatric heart surgery, case histories in, 39–40; controversy in, 22; interviews in, 18; questionnaire for, 23–24; response rate in, 30; sample for, 26; values of profession of, 165
Pediatric residents, and departmental policy, 129–134, 135; and hospital setting, 108, 112–113, 116, 135, 203. *See also* Pediatricians; Pediatrics
Pediatricians, and activism, 175–178; and brain death, 74–77; and colleague consensus, 123–127; and consensus concerning treatment of patients, 202; and decisions to treat critically ill patients, 43–45, 49, 119, 120–121, 134; and departmental policy, 129–134; and euthanasia, 71–72, 200; and family attitude toward patient, 49–50; and hospital setting, 108–110, 116–122, 134, 135; and professional age, 171; ranking of illnesses by, 63; and religiosity, 141, 158; and religious affiliation, 141, 158–170; and resuscitation, 78–84, 119, 129; samples of, 26–31; social background of, 173; and socioeconomic status of patient's family, 56, 57; and with-drawal of treatment, 71

Pediatrics, case histories in, 38–39; controversy in, 22; interviews in, 18; questionnaire for, 23; response rates in, 30; samples for, 26–30; scales for, 25–26

Peer review, 123–127, 197, 206

Physicians, and clinical mentality, 18, 19–21; vs. residents, 116–122, 203; role of, 11–12, 211. *See specifically* Internists; Neurosurgeons; Pediatric Heart Surgeons; Pediatricians

Policy, of department, 125–134; recommendations, 203–206

Potential, social, of patient, vs. social value, 51–61, 200

Professional values, 81

Prognoses, 13–14, 40–46. *See also* Salvageability

Protestants, 138–140, 141, 143, 146, 152, 154, 155–157, 158, 160, 162, 164–165, 166, 167, 178–179, 203; and activism, 175–179, 203

Psychiatrists, and research patients, 186–187, 193

Questionnaires, development of, 22–26; vs. hospital records, 88–90

Quint, J. C., 47

Ramsey, P., 5

Records, hospital. *See* Hospital records

Reeder, L. G., 211

Religions, and activism, 175–176, 203; Asian, 139, 146, 152, 154, 158, 160–162, 163, 170, 176, 177, 178; and attitudes toward critically ill patients, 138–170, 178–179, 203; and hospital setting, 141–142, 156, 162. *See also* Catholics; Jews; Protestants

Religiosity, 140, 141, 151, 152, 155, 157, 158, 178

Research, codes of ethics for medical, 183–184, 190–194; treatment of patients in medical, 184–197

Residents. *See* Medical residents; Pediatric residents

Respirator, and brain death, 73–76, 84, 154, 155, 160–162, 164, 172, 174–175, 200, 210n

Resuscitation, 23, 68, 85n, 101, 200–203; and activism, 173–176; and age of patient, 52, 58–61; and brain damage, 91, 92; decisions concerning, 78–84, 128; as experiment, 192; and hospital records, 86–95; and religious affiliation, 146–150, 158–163, 164, 169, 170; and the terminally ill, 78–79, 84

Ripley, H. S., 9

Roemer, M. I., 106

Rosner, F., 8

Rounds, system of, 128–129; ward, 113–114

Sackett, W. W., 4

Salvageability, 5, 13–14, 36, 70, 79, 90, 92, 107, 199. *See also* Patients

Samples, 14; design of, 26–31

Sanders, J., 8, 208

Scales, construction of, 25–26, 68n, 173–176

Scheff, T. J., 204

Schumacher, C. F., 172

Senility, 5

Sex, of physician, 173

Shaw, A., 5

Shils, E., 4, 6

Sibling characteristics, and treatment of mongoloids, 99–100

Sick role, 11–12, 13

Silverman, D., 73

Simmons, R. G., 20n, 182, 197

Simmons, R. L., 182, 197

Smelser, N., 10

Social class, of physicians, 172–173

Social characteristics of patients, physicians' rankings of, 53–57, 155, 172, 176–178

Social roles, performance of, 13–14, 35; resumption of, 10–14

Socialization, of physicians, 106, 123, 134–135, 178, 182

Socioeconomic status of patient, as determinant of treatment, 52–57, 112; and religious affiliation of physician, 146, 164–165, 168, 170

Socioeconomic status of patient's family, as determinant of treatment, 53, 56–57, 112; and religious affiliation of physician, 158–160, 164–165, 170

Stark, R., 143n, 178

Stewart, I., 9

Strauss, A. L., 12, 47

Sudnow, D., 12, 52, 57, 61

Suicide, 8–9, 165–167, 197

Surgeons. *See* Neurosurgeons; Pediatric heart surgeons

Surgery, decision-making in, 123–127, 135–136; experimental, 196. *See* Neurosurgeons; Pediatric heart surgeons

Swazey, J. P., 181, 196

Technology, 1, 67, 170, 171; development of medical, 181–197; and disability levels, 9–10

Terminal patients, attitude of, 47; treatment of, 2–3, 67–84, 96

Thalidomide babies, 9, 163

Tooley, M., 4

Transplantation, 194

Treatment, heroic, 1–2, 5, 15, 21, 173–175; guidelines for withdrawal of, 204–206; observations of, 95–96; refusal of, 9, 10, 94–95, 206–210; withdrawal of, 68–71

Trussell, R. E., 106

Utilitarianism, 7–8

Value, social, vs. social potential, 14, 51–61; of patient in experimental treatment, 182, 196

Values, social. *See* Social characteristics of patients

Veatch, R. M., 10, 209, 210n

Warner, W. L., 172n

Weisman, A., 5

Williams, R. H., 40

"Wills, living," 10, 210n

Printed in the United States
by Baker & Taylor Publisher Services.

Printed in the United States
by Baker & Taylor Publisher Services